# PHYSICAL REHABILITATION: MEDICINE AND THERAPY

## SOURCEBOOK

**FIRST EDITION**

Health Reference Series

# PHYSICAL REHABILITATION: MEDICINE AND THERAPY SOURCEBOOK

**FIRST EDITION**

Basic Consumer Health Information about Physical Rehabilitation, Different Types of Disabilities, Focus Areas of Physical Rehabilitation, Treatment Plans and Physical Modalities, Exercise Regimens, Coping with Physical Limitations, Populations with Physical Rehabilitation Concerns, Rehabilitation for Major Diseases and Conditions, Disability Inclusion, Employment, Transport Facilities, and Financial Support

Along with Facts about Peer Support and Assistive Technology, a Glossary, and Directory of Organizations That Provide Services for Physical Rehabilitation

OMNIGRAPHICS

*615 Griswold St., Ste. 520, Detroit, MI 48226*

Bibliographic Note

Because this page cannot legibly accommodate all the copyright notices, the Bibliographic Note portion of the Preface constitutes an extension of the copyright notice.

* * *

OMNIGRAPHICS
Angela L. Williams, Managing Editor

* * *



ISBN 978-0-7808-1774-6
E-ISBN 978-0-7808-1775-3

Library of Congress Cataloging-in-Publication Data

Names: Williams, Angela, 1963- editor.

Title: Physical rehabilitation, medicine, and therapy sourcebook / edited by Angela L. Williams.

Description: First edition. | Detroit, MI: Omnigraphics, [2020] | Series: Health reference series | Includes index. | Summary: "Offers basic consumer health information about barriers physical rehabilitation, disabilities and types, treatment plans, modalities, physical limitations, co-occurring conditions, employment, and transportation, as well as insurance benefits. A directory of organizations that provide services for physical rehabilitation and therapy"-- Provided by publisher.

Identifiers: LCCN 2019044339 (print) | LCCN 2019044340 (ebook) | ISBN 9780780817746 (library binding) | ISBN 9780780817753 (ebook)

Subjects: LCSH: Medical rehabilitation. | Medicine, Physical. | Physical therapy. | People with disabilities--Rehabilitation.

Classification: LCC RM700 .P49 2020 (print) | LCC RM700 (ebook) | DDC 615.8/2--dc23

LC record available at https://lccn.loc.gov/2019044339

LC ebook record available at https://lccn.loc.gov/2019044340

This book is printed on acid-free paper meeting the ANSI Z39.48 Standard. The infinity symbol that appears above indicates that the paper in this book meets that standard.

Printed in the United States

# Table of Contents

**Part 3. Treatment Plans, Exercise Regimens, and Physical Modalities**

**Part 4. Physical Limitations: Impact and Coping**



**Part 5. Populations with Distinctive Physical Rehabilitation Concerns**

**Part 6. Rehabilitation for Major Diseases or Conditions**



**Part 7. Disability Inclusion and Support Services**

**Part 8. Additional Help and Information**

# Preface

## ABOUT THIS BOOK

Physical rehabilitation is the process of regaining physical strength and restoring the functional ability and quality of life in those who have an impairment or long-term loss in body functions. The Centers for Disease Control and Prevention (CDC) reports that 1 in 4 adults in the United States have some type of disability. The CDC also reports that 13.7 percent of adults have serious difficulties in walking or climbing stairs. Rehabilitation provides the tools needed to attain independence and self-determination.

*Physical Rehabilitation: Medicine and Therapy Sourcebook, First Edition* provides information about physical rehabilitation along with its components. This book also describes focus areas of physical rehabilitation, medicine, and therapy. Information on treatment plans and modalities used in physical therapy is also provided. It gives facts about populations with distinctive physical rehabilitation concerns. This book elaborates on disability inclusion and living with a disability with the help of assistive technologies.

## HOW TO USE THIS BOOK

This book is divided into parts and chapters. Parts focus on broad areas of interest. Chapters are devoted to single topics within a part.

*Part 1: Physical Rehabilitation: An Overview* explains physical rehabilitation and its components. It mentions disabilities along with disability types. It also discusses diagnostic procedures such as radiodiagnostics, electromyography (EMG), and nerve conduction studies (NCS). It also covers rehabilitation facilities and the development of physical wellness.

*Part 2: Focus Areas of Physical Rehabilitation* outlines physical therapy, occupational therapy, and creative arts therapy. It discusses orthopedic and musculoskeletal rehabilitation. It covers neurorehabilitation, pediatric rehabilitation, geriatric rehabilitation, and sports injury rehabilitation.

*Part 3: Treatment Plans, Exercise Regimens, and Physical Modalities* focuses on physical-therapy assessments and evaluation. It explains the modalities used in physical therapy. It outlines therapeutic exercises for improving motor function and community-based rehabilitation.

*Part 4: Physical Limitations: Impact and Coping* gives information about physical limitations and coping. It gives facts about the impact of disability on society.

*Part 5: Populations with Distinctive Physical Rehabilitation Concerns* describes physical health in sports and recreation and physical activity for people with disabilities. It talks about early mobilization and rehabilitation.

*Part 6: Rehabilitation for Major Diseases or Conditions* focuses on depression associated with physical therapy and obesity and disability. It also gives insight on vestibular disorders.

*Part 7: Disability Inclusion and Support Services* discusses rehabilitative and assistive technology and the role of caregivers. It highlights disability inclusion along with strategies. It talks about insurance benefits, community support, financial support, and housing support. It provides information about employment and transport facilities for people with disabilities.

*Part 8: Additional Help and Information* includes a glossary of terms related to physical rehabilitation and directory of resources for additional help and support.

## BIBLIOGRAPHIC NOTE

This volume contains documents and excerpts from publications issued by the following U.S. government agencies: Administration for Community Living (ACL); Agency for Healthcare Research and Quality (AHRQ); Centers for Disease Control and Prevention (CDC); Centers for Medicare & Medicaid Services (CMS); Division of Occupational Health and Safety (DOHS); *Eunice Kennedy Shriver* National Institute of Child Health and Human Development (NICHD); Federal Communications Commission (FCC); Federal Trade Commission (FTC); *Go4Life*; Lawrence Berkley National Laboratory; National Cancer Institute (NCI); National Center for Complementary and Integrative Health (NCCIH); National Council on Disability (NCD); National Highway Traffic Safety Administration (NHTSA); National Institute of Arthritis and Musculoskeletal and Skin Diseases (NIAMS); National Institute of Biomedical Imaging and Bioengineering (NIBIB); National Institute of Diabetes and Digestive and Kidney Diseases (NIDDK); National Institute of Mental Health (NIMH); National Institute of Neurological Disorders and Stroke (NINDS); National Institute of Standards and Technology (NIST); National Institute on Aging (NIA); National Institute on Deafness and Other Communication Disorders (NIDCD); National Institutes of Health (NIH); National Science Foundation (NSF); *NIH News in Health*; NIH Osteoporosis and Related Bone Diseases—National Resource Center (NIH ORBD—NRC); Office of Disease

Prevention and Health Promotion (ODPHP); Office of the Assistant Secretary for Planning and Evaluation (ASPE); Office on Women's Health (OWH); USA.gov; U.S. Bureau of Labor Statistics (BLS); U.S. Department of Health and Human Services (HHS); U.S. Department of Justice (DOJ); U.S. Department of Transportation (DOT); U.S. Department of Veterans Affairs (VA); and U.S. Social Security Administration (SSA).

It may also contain original material produced by Omnigraphics and reviewed by medical consultants.

## ABOUT THE HEALTH REFERENCE SERIES

The *Health Reference Series* is designed to provide basic medical information for patients, families, caregivers, and the general public. Each volume takes a particular topic and provides comprehensive coverage. This is especially important for people who may be dealing with a newly diagnosed disease or a chronic disorder in themselves or in a family member. People looking for preventive guidance, information about disease warning signs, medical statistics, and risk factors for health problems will also find answers to their questions in the *Health Reference Series*. The *Series*, however, is not intended to serve as a tool for diagnosing illness, in prescribing treatments, or as a substitute for the physician–patient relationship. All people concerned about medical symptoms or the possibility of disease are encouraged to seek professional care from an appropriate healthcare provider.

## A NOTE ABOUT SPELLING AND STYLE

*Health Reference Series* editors use *Stedman's Medical Dictionary* as an authority for questions related to the spelling of medical terms and *The Chicago Manual of Style* for questions related to grammatical structures, punctuation, and other editorial concerns. Consistent adherence is not always possible, however, because the individual volumes within the *Series* include many documents from a wide variety of different producers, and the editor's primary goal is to present material from each source as accurately as is possible. This sometimes means that information in different chapters or sections may follow other guidelines and alternate spelling authorities. For example, occasionally a copyright holder may require that eponymous terms be shown in possessive forms (Crohn's disease vs. Crohn disease) or that British spelling norms be retained (leukaemia vs. leukemia).

## MEDICAL REVIEW

Omnigraphics contracts with a team of qualified, senior medical professionals who serve as medical consultants for the *Health Reference Series*. As necessary, medical consultants review reprinted and originally written material for currency and accuracy. Citations including the phrase "Reviewed (month, year)" indicate material reviewed by this team. Medical consultation services are provided to the *Health Reference Series* editors by:

Dr. Vijayalakshmi, MBBS, DGO, MD
Dr. Senthil Selvan, MBBS, DCH, MD
Dr. K. Sivanandham, MBBS, DCH, MS (Research), PhD

## OUR ADVISORY BOARD

We would like to thank the following board members for providing initial guidance on the development of this series:

- Dr. Lynda Baker, Associate Professor of Library and Information Science, Wayne State University, Detroit, MI
- Nancy Bulgarelli, William Beaumont Hospital Library, Royal Oak, MI
- Karen Imarisio, Bloomfield Township Public Library, Bloomfield Township, MI
- Karen Morgan, Mardigian Library, University of Michigan-Dearborn, Dearborn, MI
- Rosemary Orlando, St. Clair Shores Public Library, St. Clair Shores, MI

## HEALTH REFERENCE SERIES UPDATE POLICY

The inaugural book in the *Health Reference Series* was the first edition of *Cancer Sourcebook* published in 1989. Since then, the *Series* has been enthusiastically received by librarians and in the medical community. In order to maintain the standard of providing high-quality health information for the layperson the editorial staff at Omnigraphics felt it was necessary to implement a policy of updating volumes when warranted.

Medical researchers have been making tremendous strides, and it is the purpose of the *Health Reference Series* to stay current with the most recent advances. Each decision to update a volume is made on an individual basis. Some of the considerations include how much new information is available and the feedback we receive from people who use the books. If there is a topic you would like to see added to the update list, or an area of medical concern you feel has not been adequately addressed, please write to:

Managing Editor
*Health Reference Series*
Omnigraphics
615 Griswold St., Ste. 520
Detroit, MI 48226

# Part 1 | **Physical Rehabilitation: An Overview**

# Chapter 1 | Understanding Rehabilitation Medicine

## WHAT IS REHABILITATION MEDICINE?

Rehabilitation medicine describes efforts to improve function and minimize impairment related to activities that have been hampered by disease, injuries, or developmental disorders.

Injuries, illnesses, or conditions that may cause or contribute to disability can include stroke, traumatic brain injury (TBI), spinal cord injury (SCI), musculoskeletal injuries, pain, a number of intellectual and developmental disorders such as cerebral palsy (CP), fragile X syndrome (FXS), and autism spectrum disorders (ASDs), and other conditions and injuries.

The primary effects of many such conditions are physical—perhaps mobility or sensory limitations. But, individuals facing them can also experience intellectual, behavioral, and communication difficulties. They might have challenges involving making decisions, paying attention, or speaking. These may also require rehabilitation medical care.

Rehabilitation medicine differs from drug and alcohol rehabilitation, which aims to help a person control or eliminate her or his substance use, and from the rehabilitation that is commonly referred to within the context of the criminal justice system.

This chapter contains text excerpted from the following sources: Text under the heading "What Is Rehabilitation Medicine?" is excerpted from "Rehabilitation Medicine: Topic Information," *Eunice Kennedy Shriver* National Institute of Child Health and Human Development (NICHD), December 1, 2016. Reviewed November 2019; Text under the heading "Why Do We Need Rehabilitation Medicine?" is excerpted from "Why Might Someone Need Rehabilitation Medicine?" *Eunice Kennedy Shriver* National Institute of Child Health and Human Development (NICHD), December 1, 2016. Reviewed November 2019; Text under the heading "What Types of Activities Are Involved with Rehabilitation Medicine?" is excerpted from "What Types of Activities Are Involved with Rehabilitation Medicine?" *Eunice Kennedy Shriver* National Institute of Child Health and Human Development (NICHD), December 1, 2016. Reviewed November 2019; Text beginning with the heading "How Do I Find an Accredited Rehabilitation Medicine Facility?" is excerpted from "Rehabilitation Medicine: Other FAQs" *Eunice Kennedy Shriver* National Institute of Child Health and Human Development (NICHD), December 1, 2016. Reviewed November 2019.

## WHY DO WE NEED REHABILITATION MEDICINE?

There are many reasons why a person may need care related to rehabilitation medicine. For example:

- Injuries and trauma, such as:
    - Burns
    - Limb loss or amputation
    - Fractures, including multiple fractures to the long bones in the limbs and fractures of the hip, spine, or skull
    - Traumatic brain injury (TBI) or concussion (mild TBI)
    - Spinal cord injury
    - Loss of sight or hearing
- Diseases and conditions that can cause loss of mobility function, such as:
    - Muscular dystrophy
    - Spina bifida
    - Cerebral palsy
    - Arthritis
    - Scoliosis or curvature of the spine
    - Damage to muscles, ligaments, tendons, or cartilage
    - Knee arthroplasty/replacement
    - Hip replacement
    - Stroke
    - Multiple sclerosis
    - Parkinson disease and related degenerative disorders
- Surgery or prolonged treatment for other diseases or illnesses that can cause loss of function, such as:
    - Chronic pain/neuropathy
    - Severe infection
    - Diabetes
    - Cancers (including chemo and radiation therapies)
    - Peripheral artery disease
    - Cardiac arrest

Likewise, certain intellectual and developmental disabilities, such as autism spectrum disorders, may benefit from rehabilitation medicine in the form of occupational or physical therapy or other rehabilitation services.

In general, though, any person might need care related to rehabilitation medicine at some point in her or his life, for a variety of reasons.

### Secondary Conditions

Many people who experience the disorders listed above also face their secondary effects—limitations that are not necessarily part of the main diagnosis, but that can also have an impact on patients' health, independence, and quality of life.

Rehabilitation medicine may include treatments for these and other secondary symptoms:

- Muscle atrophy (wasting), blood clots or circulation issues, obesity, or other symptoms resulting from disuse
- Problems caused by overuse of prosthetics or medical devices
- Ulcers, bedsores, or other challenges involving skin integrity
- Local or widespread infections or sepsis
- Injuries resulting from falls
- Challenges involving balance or vision
- High blood pressure, diabetes, and other conditions
- Bladder and bowel problems
- Breathing problems, including those related to mechanical ventilation
- Emotional or cognitive difficulties, such as anger, depression, or difficulty controlling emotions or behavior

If not addressed in a timely manner, many of these secondary conditions can become serious, some of them fatal.

## WHAT TYPES OF ACTIVITIES ARE INVOLVED WITH REHABILITATION MEDICINE?

Rehabilitation medicine uses many kinds of assistance, therapies, and devices to improve function. The type of rehabilitation a person receives depends on the condition causing impairment, the bodily function that is affected, and the severity of the impairment.

The following are some common types of rehabilitation:

- Cognitive rehabilitation therapy involves relearning or improving skills, such as thinking, learning, memory, planning, and decision making that may have been lost or affected by brain injury.
- Occupational therapy helps a person carry out daily life tasks and activities in the home, workplace, and community.
- Pharmacorehabilitation involves the use of drugs to improve or restore physical or mental function.
- Physical therapy involves activities and exercises to improve the body's movements, sensations, strength, and balance.
- Rehabilitative/assistive technology refers to tools, equipment, and products that help people with disabilities move and function. This technology includes (but is not limited to):
    - Orthotics, which are devices that aim to improve movement and prevent contracture in the upper and lower limbs. For instance, pads inserted into a shoe, specially fitted shoes, or ankle or leg braces can

improve a person's ability to walk. Hand splints and arm braces can help the upper limbs remain supple and unclenched after a spinal cord injury.
    - Prosthetics, which are devices designed to replace a missing body part, such as an artificial limb.
    - Wheelchairs, walkers, crutches, and other mobility aids
    - Augmentative/Alternative Communication (AAC) devices, which aim to either make a person's communication more understandable or take the place of a communication method. They can include electronic devices, speech-generating devices, and picture boards.
    - Hearing aids and cochlear implants
    - Retinal prostheses, which can restore useful vision in cases in which it has been lost due to certain degenerative eye conditions
    - Telemedicine and telerehab technologies, which are devices or software to deliver care or monitor conditions in the home or community
    - Rehabilitation robotics
    - Mobile apps to assist with speech/communication, anxiety/stress, memory, and other functions or symptoms
- Recreational therapy helps improve symptoms and social and emotional well-being through arts and crafts, games, relaxation training, and animal-assisted therapy.
- Speech and language therapy aims to improve impaired swallowing and movement of the mouth and tongue, as well as difficulties with the voice, language, and talking.
- Surgery includes procedures to correct a misaligned limb or to release a constricted muscle, skin grafts for burns, insertion of chips into the brain to assist with limb or prosthetic movement, and placement of skull plates or bone pins.
- Vocational rehabilitation aids in building skills for going to school or working at a job.
- Music or art therapy can specifically aid in helping people express emotion, in cognitive development, or in helping to develop social connectedness.

These services are provided by a number of different healthcare providers and specialists, including (but not limited to):

- Physiatrists (also called "rehabilitation physicians")
- Occupational therapists
- Physical therapists
- Cognitive rehabilitation therapists

- Gait and clinical movement specialist
- Rehabilitation technologists
- Speech therapists
- Audiologists
- Orthopedists/surgeons
- Neurologists
- Psychiatrists/psychologists
- Biomedical engineers
- Rehabilitation engineers

## HOW DO I FIND AN ACCREDITED REHABILITATION MEDICINE FACILITY?

The Joint Commission, which evaluates and accredits over 20,000 healthcare organizations in the United States, offers a search engine to locate accredited and certified facilities by city and state, by name, by zip code, or type of care. The Commission on Accreditation of Rehabilitation Facilities (CARF) search engine finds facilities within and outside the United States by location, program type, company name, or keyword.

## WHAT IS "PLASTICITY"? HOW IS PLASTICITY RELATED TO REHABILITATION MEDICINE?

In biology, plasticity is a healing process in which the body reorganizes in response to changes in the environment. For example, the cells in our brains constantly form new connections.

Scientists used to believe that people with brain injury were not able to recover or relearn lost functions and that the brain was not capable of plasticity. Scientists have found that training—such as physical therapy—can help harness the brain's natural plasticity and help people with brain injuries regain lost function by stimulating new connections between brain cells. Researchers now believe the brain has a significant amount of plasticity and that certain rehabilitation methods can harness this ability.

Using techniques that harness or enhance the body's natural plasticity is an important aspect of rehabilitation medicine. The *Eunice Kennedy Shriver* National Institute of Child Health and Human Development (NICHD) supports research on the biology of plasticity and research to develop new rehabilitation approaches that engage and enhance human plasticity and aid in restoring function.

# Chapter 2 | The Components of Physical Rehabilitation

The components of physical medicine and rehabilitation services (PM&RS) consist of a direct service provider and a consultative service that provides medical and rehabilitative preventative strategies and acute and chronic management of disorders that alter functional status. This treating specialty emphasizes restoration and optimization of function through physical modalities, therapeutic exercise and interventions, adaptive equipment, modification of the environment, education, and assistive devices.

## ORGANIZATIONAL STRUCTURE

The organizational structure of PM&R varies system-wide. Physiatry physicians typically lead core rehabilitation services. Physiatrists specialize in diagnosing, treating, and directing an interdisciplinary rehabilitation plan for individuals with acute and chronic disability and pain to maximize the patient's functional status.

Other core components of PM&RS disciplines include physical therapy (PT), occupational therapy (OT), and kinesiotherapy (KT).

Physical therapists diagnose and manage movement dysfunction and enhance physical and functional abilities. Movement disorders physical therapists treat impairments of the musculoskeletal, cardiovascular/pulmonary, neuromuscular and integumentary (skin) systems.

Occupational therapists provide evaluation and treatment in areas of self-care, work, and productive activities, and play/leisure activities to achieve outcomes that support patients' participation in their everyday life occupations.

Kinesiotherapists provide service to patients through the application of scientifically-based exercise principles adapted to enhance the strength, endurance, and mobility of individuals with functional limitations.

This chapter includes text excerpted from "Physical Medicine and Rehabilitation Fact Sheet," U.S. Department of Veterans Affairs (VA), March 2018.

## POPULATION SERVED

The population served by the components of PM&RS consists of children, young adults to geriatric, with a wide spectrum of neurological, orthopedic, medical, psychological, and surgical conditions.

Special populations include age-related disability, stroke, spinal cord injury (SCI), brain dysfunction or traumatic brain injury (TBI), orthopedic injury and dysfunction, and amputation.

Services are provided in physical rehabilitation-based clinics and inpatient units, including specialized programs for drivers training, polytrauma, brain injury, assistive technology, pain management, telerehabilitation, and amputation care.

## OUTPATIENT AND RESIDENTIAL REHABILITATION PROGRAMS

Patients throughout the continuum of care settings often need rehabilitation services, including outpatient and residential services, to improve their functional status.

Referrals to rehabilitation services may originate from a range of sources, but regardless of the origin of the rehabilitation referral, the patient will be evaluated for the most appropriate rehabilitation treatment plan of care based on their specific needs.

## INPATIENT REHABILITATION PROGRAM

Patients who require the intensity of medical and rehabilitation services that can only be provided at an inpatient facility are admitted to a Comprehensive Integrated Inpatient Rehabilitation Program (CIIRP).

The CIIRP services are goal-oriented, comprehensive, patient-centric inpatient care designed to optimize functional recovery after an acute illness, injury, or exacerbation of a disease process.

While the delivery of expert and compassionate care by the rehabilitation team working in concert with the patient and their family is the mainstay of rehabilitation, inpatient care offered also includes high technology monitoring, complex diagnostic procedures, and state-of-the-art evidence-based treatment protocols. The second level of inpatient services, subacute rehabilitation is also available at multiple sites, specifically designed to provide rehabilitation therapies for individuals who have a lower level of tolerance for exercise and activity, but still require the holistic, interdisciplinary approach in an inpatient setting.

Subacute rehabilitation care is generally more intensive than traditional nursing facility care and less intensive than acute inpatient rehabilitation care.

# Chapter 3 | What Is a Disability?

A disability is any condition of the body or mind (impairment) that makes it more difficult for the person with the condition to do certain activities (activity limitation) and interact with the world around them (participation restrictions).

There are many types of disabilities, such as those that affect a person's:

- Vision
- Movement
- Thinking
- Remembering
- Learning
- Communicating
- Hearing
- Mental health
- Social relationships

Although "people with disabilities" sometimes refers to a single population, this is actually a diverse group of people with a wide range of needs. Two people with the same type of disability can be affected in very different ways. Some disabilities may be hidden or not easy to see.

According to the World Health Organization (WHO), disability has three dimensions:

1. **Impairment** in a person's body structure or function, or mental functioning; examples of impairments include loss of a limb, loss of vision, or memory loss.
2. **Activity limitation**, such as difficulty seeing, hearing, walking, or problem-solving.

This chapter includes text excerpted from "Disability and Health Overview," Centers for Disease Control and Prevention (CDC), September 4, 2019.

3. **Participation restrictions** in normal daily activities, such as working, engaging in social and recreational activities, and obtaining healthcare and preventive services.

Disability can be:

- Related to conditions that are present at birth and may affect functions later in life, including cognition (memory, learning, and understanding), mobility (moving around in the environment), vision, hearing, behavior, and other areas. These conditions may be:
    - Disorders in single *genes* (for example, Duchenne muscular dystrophy)
    - Disorders of *chromosomes* (for example, Down syndrome), and
    - The result of the mother's exposure during pregnancy to infections (for example, rubella) or substances, such as alcohol or cigarettes
- Associated with developmental conditions that become apparent during childhood (for example, autism spectrum disorder and attention deficit hyperactivity disorder (ADHD))
- Related to an injury (for example, traumatic brain injury or spinal cord injury)
- Associated with a long-standing condition (for example, diabetes), which can cause a disability such as vision loss, nerve damage, or limb loss
- Progressive (for example, muscular dystrophy), static (for example, limb loss), or intermittent (for example, some forms of multiple sclerosis)

## WHAT IS IMPAIRMENT?

Impairment is an absence of or significant difference in a person's body structure or function or mental functioning. For example, irregularities in the structure of the brain can result in difficulty with mental functions, or challenges involving the structure of the eyes or ears can result in difficulty with the functions of vision or hearing.

- **Structural impairments** are significant problems with an internal or external component of the body. Examples of these include a type of nerve damage that can result in multiple sclerosis, or a complete loss of a body component, as when a limb has been amputated.
- **Functional impairments** include the complete or partial loss of function of a body part. Examples of these include pain that does not go away or joints that no longer move easily.

## WHAT IS THE DIFFERENCE BETWEEN ACTIVITY LIMITATION AND PARTICIPATION RESTRICTION?

The World Health Organization (WHO) published the International Classification of Functioning, Disability and Health (ICF) in 2001. The ICF provides a standard language for classifying body function and structure, activity, participation levels, and conditions in the world around us that influence health. This description helps to assess the health, functioning, activities, and factors in the environment that either help or create barriers for people to fully participate in society.

According to the ICF:

- **Activity** is the execution of a task or action by an individual
- **Participation** is a person's involvement in a life situation

The ICF acknowledges that the distinction between these two categories is somewhat unclear and combines them, although basically, activities take place at a personal level and participation involves engagement in life roles, such as employment, education, or relationships. Activity limitations and participation restrictions have to do with difficulties an individual experiences in performing tasks and engaging in social roles. Activities and participation can be made easier or more difficult as a result of environmental factors, such as technology, support, and relationships, services, policies, or the beliefs of others.

The ICF includes the following in the categories of activities and participation:

- Learning and applying knowledge
- Managing tasks and demands
- Mobility (moving and maintaining body positions, handling and moving objects, moving around in the environment, moving around using transportation)
- Managing self-care tasks
- Managing domestic life
- Establishing and managing interpersonal relationships and interactions
- Engaging in major life areas (education, employment, managing money or finances)
- Engaging in community, social, and civic life

It is very important to improve the conditions in communities by providing accommodations that decrease or eliminate activity limitations and participation restrictions for people with disabilities, so they can participate in the roles and activities of everyday life.

# Chapter 4 | Types of Disabilities

Disability is a restriction or limitation in the function of an individual's ability in performing one's everyday activities. This does not mean that a differently abled person cannot participate equally in activities of daily living. Many differently abled persons can prevail over their restrictions with the use of suitable aids and support services.

Disability can be categorized into various types based on the parts and organs of the body that are disabled.

The various types of disabilities are:

- Physical disability
- Intellectual disability
- Learning disability
- Visual disability
- Hearing disability
- Speech disability

## PHYSICAL DISABILITY

Physical disability is a condition in which a person lives with physiological, functional, or mobility impairments. Physical disabilities fall under two broad categories:

- **Congenital or hereditary.** A person either has had the disability since birth or acquired it later as the result of a genetic disorder, injury during birth, or because of a muscular problem.
- **Acquired.** A person acquires the disability as a result of an accident, polio infection, or diseases such as cancer or stroke.

Two major classifications of physical disabilities are discussed below.

### Musculoskeletal Disability

A musculoskeletal disability is defined as the inability to carry out different activities related to the movement of the body due to muscle or bone deformities, disease, or degeneration. A few musculoskeletal disabilities are:

- Loss or deformity of limbs
- Osteogenesis imperfecta
- Muscular dystrophy

### Neuromuscular Disability

Neuromuscular disability is defined as the lack of ability to perform controlled movements of body parts due to degeneration or disorder of the nervous system. Neuromuscular disabilities include:

- Cerebral palsy
- Spina bifida
- Poliomyelitis
- Stroke
- Head injury
- Paraplegia
- Tetraplegia
- Multiple sclerosis

Physical disabilities can also be classified as temporary and permanent disabilities based on the length of time the condition is expected to last.

- Temporary disability is a disabling condition that affects a person for a short period of time (usually days, weeks, months, or a couple of years). Eventually, the person recovers completely from the disabling condition. Temporary disabilities include illnesses or injuries that hinder a person from temporarily participating in daily or routine activities, such as walking, showering without help, taking care of the kids, or working.
- Permanent disability is also known as "long-term disability." It can be due to an injury or illness that results in permanent impairment of routine activities, such as competing in the job market or sports activities, for the duration of one's life. It is an injury or illness from which the person is not expected to recover and will live with that disability for the rest of her or his life.

## INTELLECTUAL DISABILITY

An intelligence quotient (IQ) testing is a series of exams used to determine one's general intelligence in relation to other people of the same age. A person who has an IQ level of less than 70 is considered to have an intellectual disability, which is determined by the fact that the median IQ level is 100. Such a person will have a notable difficulty in performing the tasks of daily living, such as taking care of oneself, communicating effectively, and conforming to social norms. People with intellectual disabilities may face challenges in abstract concepts such as money and time as well. The most common causes of intellectual disability are genetic conditions, problems during birth, complications during pregnancy or from diseases, and toxic exposure.

A few types of intellectual disability can happen during birth, while others can happen before birth or soon after birth, and they are:

- Fragile X syndrome
- Down syndrome
- Fetal alcohol syndrome
- Apert syndrome
- Prader-Willi syndrome
- Autism
- Cerebral palsy

## LEARNING DISABILITY

This is a neurological disorder, and a person with a learning disability may find activities such as reading, writing, reasoning, recalling, or organizing difficult.

A learning disorder could be passed down from generation to generation or could be due to certain medical conditions such as neurological illness or chronic childhood ear infections, which can alter brain functioning or neurological development and cause a learning disability.

Some examples of learning disabilities are:

- Dyslexia
- Dyscalculia
- Dysgraphia
- Auditory processing disorder
- Language processing disorder

## VISUAL DISABILITY

Visual impairment can range from mild vision loss in one or both eyes to a complete loss of eyesight. A lack of sensitivity to certain colors that makes it difficult to distinguish colors is another example. The most common causes of visual disabilities are an inherited condition, eye injury, or eye infection.

Visual impairments include:

- Color blindness
- Low vision
- Blindness

## HEARING DISABILITY

Hearing loss is a partial to moderate hearing impairment in one or both ears. The major causes of hearing loss are heredity, aging, and chronic exposure to loud noises.

Hearing loss falls into three categories:

- Conductive, which involves the outer and middle ear
- Sensorineural, which involves the inner ear, and
- Mixed, which involves the combination of the two

Hearing impairment leads to:

- Hard of hearing
- Deafness

## SPEECH DISABILITY

Speech disability is a communication disorder characterized by the inability to speak or articulate words in a manner that allows other people to understand you.

Speech disability can be categorized into two types:

- **Speech impairment:** Difficulty in articulation, fluency, and voice are called "speech impairment."
- **Language impairment:** Morphological disorders, semantic disorders, syntactical deficits, and pragmatic difficulties are the basic areas of language impairment.

The inability to speak due to mental illness, cognitive impairments, or the inability to learn to speak is called "muteness."

## References

1. "General Information on Physical Disabilities," Handicaps Welfare Association (HWA), February 1, 2001.
2. "The Difference between Temporary Disability and Permanent Disability," Young, Marr & Associates Law Firm, September 5, 2015.
3. "Types of Learning Disabilities," Learning Disabilities Association of America (LDA), November 10, 2013.
4. "Types of Disabilities," Yale University, August 26, 2017.

# Chapter 5 | Disability and Health Information for Women with Disabilities

About 36 million women in the United States have disabilities—and the number is growing. About 44 percent of those aged 65 years or older are living with a disability. The most common cause of disability for women is arthritis or rheumatism.

Women with disabilities may need specialty care to address their individual needs. In addition, they need the same general healthcare as women without disabilities, and they may also need additional care to address their specific needs. However, research has shown that many women with disabilities may not receive regular health screenings within recommended guidelines.

## VIOLENCE AGAINST WOMEN WITH DISABILITIES

Women with disabilities are more likely to experience domestic violence, emotional abuse, and sexual assault than women without disabilities. Women with disabilities may also feel more isolated and feel they are unable to report the abuse, or they may be dependent on the abuser for their care. Like many women who are abused, women with disabilities are usually abused by someone they know, such as a partner or family member.

### How Can I Recognize Signs of Abuse in a Loved One with a Disability?

Relatives must be strong advocates for their loved ones with disabilities. If you have a relative with a disability, learn the signs of abuse, especially if your relative has trouble communicating.

This chapter contains text excerpted from the following sources: Text in this chapter begins with excerpts from "Disability and Health Information for Women with Disabilities," Centers for Disease Control and Prevention (CDC), October 28, 2019; Text under the heading "Violence against Women with Disabilities" is excerpted from " Violence against Women with Disabilities," Office on Women's Health (OWH), U.S. Department of Health and Human Services (HHS), September 13, 2018.

Report abuse to adult protective services if you notice any of the following with a loved one who has a disability:

- Suddenly being unable to meet essential day-to-day living needs that affect health, safety, or well-being
- Lack of contact with friends or family
- Visible handprints or bruising on the face, neck, arms, or wrists
- Burns, cuts, or puncture wounds
- Unexplained sprains, fractures, or dislocations
- Signs of injuries to internal organs, such as vomiting
- Wearing torn, stained, soiled, or bloody clothing
- Appearing hungry, malnourished, disoriented, or confused

### How Common Is Violence or Abuse against Women with Disabilities?

Women with a disability are more likely to experience violence or abuse compared to women without a disability. Some studies show that women with a disability may be more likely to experience violence or abuse by a current or former partner compared to women without disabilities.

### Who Commits Violence or Abuse against Women with Disabilities?

Most often, violence or abuse against women with disabilities is by their spouses or partners. But women with disabilities can also face abuse from caregivers or personal assistants. Women with disabilities who need help with daily activities like bathing, dressing, or eating may be more at risk of abuse because they are physically or mentally more vulnerable and can have many different caregivers in their life.

### What Should I Do If I Suspect Abuse against a Woman with a Disability?

Report any suspected abuse to adult protective services. Each state has an adult protective services agency.

# Chapter 6 | Disability and Health Information for People with Disabilities

The Americans with Disabilities Act (ADA) was enacted in 1990, many social barriers have been removed or reduced for people with disabilities. But, there is more work that needs to be done for people with disabilities to become more independent and involved in their world. Good health is important to be able to work, learn, and be engaged within a community.

## HEALTHY LIVING

People with disabilities need healthcare and health programs for the same reasons anyone else does—to stay well, active, and a part of the community.

Having a disability does not mean a person is not healthy or that she or he cannot be healthy. Being healthy means the same thing for all of us—getting and staying well so we can lead full, active lives. That means having the tools and information to make healthy choices and knowing how to prevent illness.

## SAFETY

People with disabilities can be at higher risk for injuries and abuse. It is important for parents and other family members to teach their loved one how to stay safe and what to do if they feel threatened or have been hurt in any way.

## ASSISTIVE TECHNOLOGY

Assistive technologies (AT) are devices or equipment that can be used to help a person with a disability fully engage in life activities. AT's can help enhance functional indcpendence and make daily living tasks easier through the use of aids that help a person travel, communicate with others, learn, work, and participate in social and recreational activities. An example of assistive technology can

This chapter includes text excerpted from "Disability and Health Information for People with Disabilities," Centers for Disease Control and Prevention (CDC), October 28, 2019.

be anything from a low-tech device, such as a magnifying glass, to a high tech device, such as a special computer that talks and helps someone communicate. Other examples are wheelchairs, walkers, and scooters, which are mobility aids that can be used by persons with physical disabilities.

## SCHOOL

In order to help a child fully participate in school, plans can be developed around the child's specific needs. These plans, known as "504 plans," are used by general education students not eligible for special education services. By law, children may be eligible to have a 504 plan which lists accommodations related to a child's disability. The 504 plan accommodations may be needed to give the child an opportunity to perform at the same level as their peers. For example, a 504 plan may include your child's assistive technology needs, such as a tape recorder or keyboard for taking notes and a wheelchair-accessible environment.

A different plan is needed for children taking special education classes. An Individual Education Plan (IEP) is a legal document that tells the school its duties to your child.

## TRANSITIONS

For some people with disabilities and their parents, change can be difficult. Planning ahead of time may make transitions easier for everyone. Transitions occur at many stages of life. For example, the transition from teen years to adulthood can be especially challenging. There are many important decisions to make, such as deciding whether to go to college, a vocational school, or enter the workforce. It is important to begin thinking about this transition in childhood, so that educational transition plans are put in place. Ideally, transition plans from teen years to adulthood are in place by age 14, but no later than age 16. This makes sure the person has the skills she or he needs to begin the next phase of life. This stage in life also involves transitioning one's healthcare services from pediatricians to physicians who primarily treat adults.

## INDEPENDENT LIVING

Independent living means that a person lives in her or his own apartment or house and needs limited or no help from outside agencies. The person may not need any assistance or might need help with only complex issues such as managing money, rather than day-to-day living skills. Whether an adult with disabilities continues to live at home or moves out into the community depends in large part on her or his ability to manage everyday tasks with little or no help. For example, can the person clean the house, cook, shop, and pay bills? Is she or he able to use public transportation? Many families prefer to start with some supported living arrangements and move towards increased independence.

## FINDING SUPPORT

For many people with disabilities and those who care for them, daily life may not be easy. Disabilities affect the entire family. Meeting the complex needs of a person with a disability can put families under a great deal of stress—emotional, financial, and sometimes even physical.

However, finding resources, knowing what to expect, and planning for the future can greatly improve the overall quality of life (QOL). If you have a disability or care for someone who does, it might be helpful to talk with other people who can relate to your experience.

### Find a Support Network

By finding support within your community, the needs of families and people with disabilities. This can help increase confidence, enhance QOL, and assist in meeting the needs of family members.

A national organization that focuses on the disability, such as Spina Bifida Association (SBA), that has a state or local branch, such as Spina Bifida Association in your state, might exist. State or local area Centers for Independent Living (CIL) icon could also be helpful. United Way offices may be able to point out resources. Look in the phone book or on the web for phone numbers and addresses.

Other ways to connect with other people include camps, organized activities, and sports for people with disabilities. In addition, there are online support groups and networks for people with many different types of disabilities.

### Talk with a Mental-Health Professional

Psychologists, social workers, and counselors can help you deal with the challenges of living with or caring for someone with a disability. Talk to your primary care physician for a referral.

# Chapter 7 | Disability and Health Information for Family Caregivers

If you are a family member who cares for someone with a disability, whether a child or an adult, combining personal, caregiving, and everyday needs can be challenging. This site has information for family caregivers such as yourself to help you and those you care for stay safe and healthy.

## CAREGIVING TIPS FOR FAMILIES OF PEOPLE WITH DISABILITIES

These general caregiving tips provide families with information on how to stay healthy and positive. Keep in mind that these tips can be used to address many family issues. Information, support, advocacy, empowerment, care, and balance can be the foundation for a healthy family and are appropriate no matter what the challenge.

### Be Informed

- Gather information about your family member's condition, and discuss issues with others involved in the care of your family member. Being informed will help you make more knowledgeable health decisions and improve your understanding about any challenges your family might face.
- Notice how others care for the person with special needs. Be aware of signs of mental or physical abuse.

### Get Support

- Family members and friends can provide support in a variety of ways and oftentimes want to help. Determine if there are big or small things they can do to assist you and your family.

This chapter includes text excerpted from "Disability and Health Information for Family Caregivers," Centers for Disease Control and Prevention (CDC), October 28, 2019.

- Join a local or online support group. A support group can give you the chance to share information and connect with people who are going through similar experiences. A support group may help combat the isolation and fear you may experience as a caregiver
- Do not limit your involvement to support groups and associations that focus on a particular need or disability. There are also local and national groups that provide services, recreation, and information for people with disabilities.
- Friends, family, healthcare providers, support groups, community services, and counselors are just a few of the people available to help you and your family.

## Be an Advocate

- Be an advocate for your family member with a disability. Caregivers who are effective advocates may be more successful at getting better service.
- Ask questions. For example, if your family member with a disability uses a wheelchair and you want to plan a beach vacation, find out if the beaches are accessible via a car, ramp, portable walkway mat, or other equipment.
- Inform other caregivers of any special conditions or circumstances. For example, if your family member with a disability has a latex allergy, remind dental or medical staff each time you visit them.
- Document the medical history of your family member with a disability, and keep this information current.
- Make sure your employer understands your circumstances and limitations. Discuss your ability to travel or to work weekends or evenings. Arrange for flexible scheduling when needed.
- Become familiar with the Americans with Disabilities Act, the Family Medical Leave Act, and other state and national provisions. Know how and when to apply them to your situation.

## Be Empowering

- Focus on what you and your family member with a disability can do.
- Find appropriate milestones and celebrate them.
- If someone asks you questions about the family member with a disability, let her or him answer when possible. Doing so may help empower the individual to engage with others.
- When appropriate, teach your family member with a disability to be as independent and self-assured as possible. Always keep health and safety issues in mind.

## Take Care of Yourself

- Take care of yourself as well. Caring for a family member with a disability can wear out even the strongest caregiver. Stay healthy for yourself and those you care for.
- Work hard to maintain your personal interests, hobbies, and friendships. Do not let caregiving consume your entire life. This is not healthy for you or those you care for. Balance is key.
- Allow yourself not to be the perfect caregiver. Set reasonable expectations to lower stress and make you a more effective caregiver.
- Delegate some caregiving tasks to other reliable people.
- Take a break. Short breaks, like an evening walk or relaxing bath, are essential. Long breaks are nurturing. Arrange a retreat with friends or get away with a significant other when appropriate.
- Do not ignore signs of illness: if you get sick, see a healthcare provider. Pay attention to your mental and emotional health as well. Remember, taking good care of yourself can help the person you care for as well. Exercising and eating healthy are also important.

## Keep Balance in the Family

- Family members with a disability may require extra care and attention. Take time for all family members, taking into account the needs of each individual. For example, it is important for parents of a child with a disability to also spend time with each other and with any other children they might have.
- Consider respite care. "Respite" refers to short-term, temporary care provided to people with disabilities so that their families can take a break from the daily routine of caregiving

# DISABILITY AND HEALTHY LIVING

People with disabilities need healthcare and health programs for the same reasons anyone else does—to stay well, active, and a part of the community.

Having a disability does not mean a person is not healthy or that she or he cannot be healthy. Being healthy means the same thing for all of us—getting and staying well so we can lead full, active lives. That means having the tools and information to make healthy choices and knowing how to prevent illness.

For people with disabilities, it also means knowing that health problems related to a disability can be treated. These problems, also called "secondary conditions," can include pain, depression, and a greater risk for certain illnesses.

To be healthy, people with disabilities require healthcare that meets their needs as a whole person, not just as a person with a disability. Most people with or without disabilities can stay healthy by learning about and living healthy lifestyles.

## EMERGENCY AND DISASTER PREPAREDNESS

It is important that people with disabilities and their caregivers make plans to protect themselves in the event of an emergency or disaster. Emergencies and disasters can strike quickly and without warning and can force people to leave their home or be confined in their home. For the millions of Americans who have disabilities, emergencies such as acts of terrorism and disasters such as fires and floods present a real challenge.

# Chapter 8 | Rehabilitation Facilities

**Chapter Contents**

## Section 8.1 | **Inpatient Facilities**

This section includes text excerpted from "Inpatient Rehabilitation Therapy Services: Complying with Documentation Requirements," Centers for Medicare & Medicaid Services (CMS), July 2012. Reviewed November 2019.

Inpatient rehabilitation facility (IRF) provide intensive rehabilitation services using an interdisciplinary team approach in a hospital environment. Admission to an IRF is appropriate for patients with complex nursing, medical management, and rehabilitative needs.

### MEDICAL NECESSITY AT THE TIME OF ADMISSION

Determinations of whether IRF stays are reasonable and necessary must be based on an assessment of each patient's individual care needs. For IRF care to be considered reasonable and necessary, the documentation in the patient's IRF medical record must demonstrate a reasonable expectation that the following criteria were met at the time of admission to the IRF. The patient must:

- Require active and ongoing intervention of multiple therapy disciplines (physical therapy (PT), occupational therapy (OT), speech-language pathology (SLP), or prosthetics/orthotics), at least one of which must be PT or OT;
- Require an intensive rehabilitation therapy program, generally consisting of:
    - 3 hours of therapy per day at least 5 days per week; or
    - In certain well-documented cases, at least 15 hours of intensive rehabilitation therapy within a 7-consecutive-day period, beginning with the date of admission;
- Reasonably be expected to actively participate in, and benefit significantly from, the intensive rehabilitation therapy program (the patient's condition and functional status are such that the patient can reasonably be expected to make measurable improvement, expected to be made within a prescribed period of time and as a result of the intensive rehabilitation therapy program, that will be of practical value to improve the patient's functional capacity or adaptation to impairments);
- Require physician supervision by a rehabilitation physician, with face-to-face visits at least three days per week to assess the patient both medically and functionally and to modify the course of treatment as needed; and
- Require an intensive and coordinated interdisciplinary team approach to the delivery of rehabilitative care.

## INTENSIVE LEVEL OF REHABILITATION SERVICES

The information in the patient's IRF medical record must document a reasonable expectation that, at the time of admission to the IRF, the patient generally required the intensive rehabilitation-therapy services that are uniquely provided in IRFs. Although the intensity of these services can be reflected in various ways, the generally accepted standard by which it is typically demonstrated in IRFs is by the provision of intensive therapies at least 3 hours a day for 5 days a week. However, this is not a "rule of thumb," and intensity may also be demonstrated by the provision of 15 hours in a 7-consecutive-day period starting from the date of admission, in certain well-documented cases.

Therapy evaluations done in the IRF constitute initiation of the required therapy services. The standard of care for IRF patients is one-on-one therapy. Group therapy is acceptable and may not constitute the majority of therapy provided to the patient.

While patients requiring an IRF stay are expected to need and receive an intensive rehabilitation-therapy program, this may not be true for a limited number of days during a patient's IRF stay because the patient's needs vary over time.

## INTERDISCIPLINARY TEAM APPROACH TO THE DELIVERY OF CARE

The complexity of the patient's condition must be such that the rehabilitation goals indicated in the preadmission screening, the postadmission physician evaluation, and the overall plan of care can only be achieved through periodic conferences of an interdisciplinary team of medical professionals. The purpose of the interdisciplinary team is to foster frequent, structured, and documented communication among disciplines to establish, prioritize, and achieve treatment goals.

Team conferences must be held once a week; a week is defined as a 7-consecutive-day period, beginning with the date of admission. A regularly scheduled weekly team conference meets this requirement. At a minimum, the interdisciplinary team must document participation by professionals from each of the following disciplines (each of whom must have current knowledge of the patient as documented in the IRF medical record):

- A rehabilitation physician with specialized training and experience in rehabilitation services
- A registered nurse with specialized training or experience in rehabilitation
- A social worker or a case manager (or both), and
- A licensed or certified therapist from each discipline involved in treating the patient

The weekly interdisciplinary team meeting must be led by a rehabilitation physician who is responsible for making the final decisions regarding the patient's treatment in the IRF. The physician must document concurrence with all decisions made by the interdisciplinary team. Documentation must include the name and professional designation of each interdisciplinary team member in attendance.

The periodic interdisciplinary team conferences must focus on:

- Assessing the patient's progress toward rehabilitation goals;
- Considering possible resolutions to any impediment that could impede the patient's progress toward the goals;
- Reassessing the validity of the rehabilitation goals previously established; and
- Monitoring and revising the treatment plan, as needed.

## MEASURABLE IMPROVEMENT

To justify a continued IRF stay, the documentation in the patient's medical record must demonstrate an ongoing requirement for an intensive level of rehabilitation services and an interdisciplinary team approach to care. The IRF medical record must demonstrate the patient is making functional improvements that are ongoing, sustainable, and of practical value, as measured against the patient's condition at the start of treatment.

# Section 8.2 | **Outpatient Facilities**

This section includes text excerpted from the following sources: Text beginning with the heading "Who Can Give Me Outpatient Therapy Services?" is excerpted from "Medicare Coverage of Therapy Services," Centers for Medicare & Medicaid Services (CMS), December 2018; Text under the heading "Outpatient Rehabilitation Providers" is excerpted from "Outpatient Rehabilitation Providers," Centers for Medicare & Medicaid Services (CMS), April 11, 2013. Reviewed November 2019.

## WHO CAN GIVE ME OUTPATIENT THERAPY SERVICES?

- Physical therapists
- Speech-language pathologists
- Occupational therapists

Doctors and other healthcare professionals (such as nurse practitioners, clinical nurse specialists, and physician assistants) may also offer physical therapy, speech-language pathology, and occupational therapy services.

## WHERE CAN I GET OUTPATIENT THERAPY SERVICES?

- Offices of privately practicing therapists
- Many medical offices
- Outpatient hospital departments

- Critical access hospital (CAH) outpatient departments
- Rehabilitation agencies (sometimes called "other rehabilitation facilities" (ORFs))
- Comprehensive outpatient rehabilitation facilities (CORFs)
- Skilled nursing facilities (SNFs)
- At home, from certain therapy providers, such as privately practicing therapists

## OUTPATIENT REHABILITATION PROVIDERS

There are three types of organizations that may qualify as Optional Practical Training (OPT) or Other Service Provider (OSP) providers:

- **Rehabilitation agency**—An agency that provides an integrated, multidisciplinary program designed to upgrade the physical functions of individuals with disabilities by bringing together, as a team, specialized rehabilitation personnel.
- **Clinic**—A facility established primarily for the provision of outpatient physicians' services.
  - The medical services of the clinic are provided by a group of three or more physicians practicing medicine together; and
  - A physician is present in the clinic at all times during hours of operation to perform medical services.
- **Public health agency**—An official agency established by a state or local government, the primary function of which is to maintain the health of the population served by providing environmental health services, preventive medical services, and in certain instances, therapeutic services.

# Chapter 9 | Healthy Living for People with Disability

People with disabilities need healthcare and health programs for the same reasons anyone else does—to stay well, active, and a part of the community.

Having a disability does not mean a person is not healthy or that she or he cannot be healthy. Being healthy means the same thing for all of us—getting and staying well so we can lead full, active lives. That means having the tools and information to make healthy choices and knowing how to prevent illness.

For people with disabilities, it also means knowing that health problems related to a disability can be treated. These problems, also called "secondary conditions," can include pain, depression, and a greater risk for certain illnesses.

To be healthy, people with disabilities require healthcare that meets their needs as a whole person, not just as a person with a disability. Most people with or without disabilities can stay healthy by learning about and living healthy lifestyles.

## LEADING A LONG AND HEALTHY LIFE

Although people with disabilities sometimes have a harder time getting and staying healthy than people without disabilities, there are things we can all do to get and stay healthy.

Tips for leading a long and healthy life:

- Be physically active every day.
- Eat healthy foods in healthy portions.
- Do not get too much sun.
- Get regular checkups.
- Do not smoke.

This chapter contains text excerpted from the following sources: Text in this chapter begins with excerpts from "Disability and Health Healthy Living," Centers for Disease Control and Prevention (CDC), September 4, 2019; Text under the heading "Disability and Health-Related Conditions" is excerpted from "Disability and Health-Related Conditions," Centers for Disease Control and Prevention (CDC), September 9, 2019.

- Use medicines wisely.
- If you drink alcoholic beverages, drink in moderation.
- Get help for substance abuse.
- Stay in touch with family and friends.
- If you need help, talk with your healthcare professional.

## GETTING THE BEST POSSIBLE HEALTHCARE

People with disabilities must get the care and services they need to help them be healthy.

If you have a disability, there are many things you can do to make sure you are getting the best possible healthcare:

- Know your body, how you feel when you are well and when you are not.
- Talk openly with your healthcare professional about your concerns.
- Find healthcare professionals that you are comfortable within your area.
- Check to be sure you can physically get into your healthcare professional's office, such as having access to ramps or elevators if you use an assistive device such as a wheelchair or scooter.
- Check to see if your healthcare professional's office has the equipment you need, such as an accessible scale or examining table.
- Ask for help from your healthcare professional's office staff if you need it.
- Think about your questions and health concerns before you visit your healthcare professional so that you are prepared.
- Bring your health records with you.
- Take a friend with you if you are concerned you might not remember all your questions or what is said by the healthcare professional.
- Get it in writing. Write down, or have someone write down for you, what is said by the healthcare professional.

## PHYSICAL ACTIVITY

Adults of all shapes, sizes, and abilities can benefit from being physically active, including those with disabilities. For important health benefits, all adults should do both aerobic and muscle-strengthening physical activities. Regular aerobic physical activity increases heart and lung functions; improves daily living activities and independence; decreases chances of developing chronic diseases; and improves mental health.

Adults with disabilities should try to get at least 2 hours and 30 minutes (150 minutes) a week of moderate-intensity aerobic physical activity (i.e., brisk walking; wheeling oneself in a wheelchair) or at least 1 hour and 15 minutes (75 minutes) a week of vigorous-intensity aerobic physical activity (i.e., jogging, wheelchair basketball) or a mix of both moderate- and vigorous-intensity aerobic physical activities each week. A rule of thumb is that 1 minute of vigorous-intensity activity is about the same as 2 minutes of moderate-intensity activity. They should avoid inactivity as some physical activity is better than none.

Muscle-strengthening activities should include moderate and high intensity, and involve all major muscle groups on two or more days a week (i.e., working with resistance-band, adapted yoga) as these activities provide additional health benefits. All children and adolescents should do 1 hour (60 minutes) or more of physical activity each day.

If a person with a disability is not able to meet the physical activity guidelines, they should engage in regular physical activity based on their abilities and should avoid inactivity. Adults with disabilities should talk to their healthcare provider about the amounts and types of physical activity that are appropriate for their abilities.

Tips for getting fit:

- Talk to your doctor about how much and what kind of physical activity is right for you.
- Find opportunities to increase physical activity regularly in ways that meet your needs and abilities.
- Start slowly, based on your abilities and fitness level (e.g., be active for at least 10 minutes at a time, slowly increase activity over several weeks, if necessary).
- Avoid inactivity. Some activity is better than none!

## SEXUAL HEALTH AND SEXUALITY

People with disabilities should feel comfortable talking to healthcare professionals and each other about sexual health and sexuality. People with disabilities can ask their doctor questions about sexuality, sexual functioning, contraceptives, and reproductive concerns.

## MENTAL HEALTH AND WELL-BEING

For everyone, overall mental health and well-being are very important. Mental health is how we think, feel and act as we cope with life. People need to feel good about their life and value themselves.

All people, including those with disabilities, might feel isolated from others, or have low self-esteem. They may be depressed. There are different ways to treat depression. Exercise may be effective for some people. Counseling, medication, or both might also be needed.

Everyone feels worried, anxious, sad or stressed sometimes. If these feelings do not go away and they interfere with your daily life, you should talk with other people about your feelings, such as a family member or healthcare professional.

## DISABILITY AND HEALTH-RELATED CONDITIONS

Studies have shown that individuals with disabilities are more likely than people without disabilities to report:

- Poorer overall health
- Less access to adequate healthcare
- Smoking and physical inactivity

People with disabilities need healthcare and health programs for the same reasons anyone else does—to stay well, active, and a part of the community.

Although a smaller percentage than people without disabilities, most people with disabilities report their health to be good, very good, or excellent. Being healthy means the same thing for all of us—getting and staying well so we can lead full, active lives. That means having the tools and information to make healthy choices and knowing how to prevent illness. For people with disabilities, it also means knowing that health problems related to a disability can be treated. These problems (also called "secondary conditions") can include pain, depression, and a greater risk for certain illnesses.

### Secondary Conditions

People with disabilities often are at greater risk for health problems that can be prevented. As a result of having a specific type of disability, such as a spinal cord injury, spina bifida, or multiple sclerosis, other physical or mental-health conditions can occur.

Some of these other health conditions are also called "secondary conditions" and might include:

- Bowel or bladder problems
- Fatigue
- Injury
- Overweight and obesity
- Pain
- Pressure sores or ulcers

#### Bowel and Bladder

Some disabilities, such as spinal cord injuries, can affect how well a person's bladder and bowel work.

#### Fatigue

Fatigue is a feeling of weariness, tiredness, or lack of energy. Fatigue can affect the way a person thinks and feels. It can also interfere with a person's activities of daily living.

### Injury

Injuries—including unintentional injury, homicide, and suicide—are the leading cause of death for people 1 through 44 years of age. The consequences of injuries can include physical, emotional, and financial consequences that can affect the lives of individuals, their families, and society.

### Overweight and Obesity

Children and adults with disabilities are less likely to be of a healthy weight and more likely to be obese than children and adults without disabilities. Overweight and obesity can have serious health consequences for all people.

### Pain

Pain is commonly reported by people with many types of disabilities. For some, pain can affect functioning and activities of daily living. The length of time a person experiences pain can be classified as either long-term (also called "chronic") or short-term.

### Pressure Sores or Ulcers

Pressure ulcers, also known as "bedsores," "pressure sores," or "decubitus ulcers," are wounds caused by constant pressure on the skin. They usually develop on body parts such as the elbow, heel, hip, shoulder, back, and back of the head.

People with disabilities who are bedridden or use a wheelchair are at risk of developing pressure sores.

## Other Concerns, Conditions, and Prevention

Many related health conditions and chronic diseases can be prevented. Chronic diseases are among the most common and costly of all health problems, even though many chronic diseases can be prevented. Some chronic diseases can be prevented by living a healthy lifestyle, visiting a healthcare provider for preventive care and routine screenings, and learning how to manage health issues.

### Arthritis

Arthritis—or joint inflammation—is the most common cause of disability among adults residing in the United States. It limits everyday activities for 24 million Americans. People with disabilities can be at greater risk of having arthritis.

### Asthma

Asthma is a disease that affects the lungs. It is one of the most common long-term diseases among children, but adults can have asthma, too. Asthma is the most common chronic disease of childhood and a leading cause of disability among children.

### Cancer

Getting screened for breast, cervical, and colorectal cancers as recommended helps find these diseases at an early, often highly treatable, stage. Research shows that women with disabilities are less likely to be screened for breast and cervical cancer within the recommended guidelines. Some reasons identified by women include encountering inaccessible facilities and equipment, and having to focus on other health issues.

### Chronic Fatigue Syndrome

Chronic fatigue syndrome (CFS) affects more than one million people in the United States. It is four times more common among females than males. People of both sexes and of every race and ethnicity and age (including adolescents) can develop CFS.

### Diabetes

Diabetes is a chronic disease for which care and treatment can help people to live normal and productive lives. However, some people might be limited in their everyday activities. People with diabetes, in general, report rates of disability that are significantly higher than those reported by the general U.S. population.

### Flu

People with certain types of disabilities have a higher risk of getting flu-related complications, such as pneumonia. Some physical disabilities can affect how well their body fights off infection. They should discuss their risk of illness with their healthcare provider.

### Substance Abuse

Alcohol, tobacco, illicit drugs, and prescription medications all can be substances of abuse. People with disabilities might have multiple risk factors that can increase their chances of substance abuse.

### Violence

Violence is a serious public-health problem in the United States. People with disabilities are 4 to 10 times more likely to become victims of violence, abuse, or neglect than people without disabilities. Children with disabilities are more than twice as likely to be physically or sexually abused as children without disabilities.

# Part 2 | **Focus Areas of Physical Rehabilitation**

# Chapter 10 | **Comprehensive Multidisciplinary Team Approach**

**Chapter Contents**

## Section 10.1 | **Physical Therapy**

This section includes text excerpted from "Fact Sheet for Physical Therapy," U.S. Department of Veterans Affairs (VA), March 2018.

### PHYSICAL THERAPY PRACTICE

Physical therapists diagnose and manage movement dysfunction, and enhance physical and functional abilities for movement disorders related to impairments of aging, and the musculoskeletal, cardiovascular/pulmonary, neuromuscular and integumentary (skin) systems.

Physical therapists restore, maintain, and promote optimal physical function as well as wellness, fitness, and quality of life (QOL) as it relates to movement and health. Physical therapy is a safe and effective alternative to opioids for the long-term treatment of chronic pain.

Physical therapists also prevent the onset, symptoms and progression of impairments, functional limitations, and disabilities that may result from diseases, disorders, conditions or injuries.

Physical therapists examine each individual and develop a specific treatment plan. Evidence-based services are used to decrease disability, reduce pain, improve function and independence, prevent illness, promote wellness and restore QOL.

### PHYSICAL THERAPY CREDENTIALS

Physical therapists are licensed healthcare professionals. Qualification for licensure includes passing the National Physical Therapy Exam (NPTE), administered by the Federation of State Boards of Physical Therapy.

Another important qualification for licensure is graduation from physical therapy education program accredited by the Commission on Accreditation in Physical Therapy Education (CAPTE) or a program that is deemed substantially equivalent to a CAPTE-accredited program. All physical therapists graduate with a doctoral degree.

### POPULATION SERVED BY PHYSICAL THERAPISTS

Physical therapists practice across the continuum of care, providing services in inpatient settings (including medical centers and community living centers), home health, outpatient clinics, and telerehabilitation.

Physical therapists are also key members of collaborative teams, which exist in the physical medicine and rehabilitation (PM&R) systems of care models (i.e., polytrauma and amputee systems of care).

Services may include:

- Pain management
- Manual intervention and joint mobilization

- Treatment of musculoskeletal disorders
- Strength and conditioning/therapeutic exercise
- Treatment of neurological diseases and stroke recovery
- Balance training/fall prevention
- Injury prevention
- Weight management program
- Wound care
- Pain management
- Women's health
- Telerehabilitation
- Home evaluations
- Adaptive mobility clinics

### PHYSICAL THERAPY STATISTICS

- Physical therapists are highly trained healthcare professionals. Entry-level education requirements include a professional doctoral degree in physical therapy.
- Many physical therapists have advanced skills, certification, and training in areas such as orthopedic, neurological, musculoskeletal, cardiovascular and pulmonary, women's health, electrophysiology, and vestibular rehabilitation (VR).

## Section 10.2 | **Occupational Therapy and Vocational Rehabilitation**

This section includes text excerpted from "Occupational Therapy Fact Sheet," U.S. Department of Veterans Affairs (VA), March 2018.

Occupational therapy (OT) involves the therapeutic use of everyday life activities (occupations) with individuals or groups for the purpose of participation in roles and situations in home, school, workplace, community, and other settings. OT provides services that promote health and wellness to those who have, or are at risk for developing, an injury, illness, disease or condition. OT evaluation and treatment supports patients' engagement in everyday life activities that affect health, well-being, and quality of life by addressing physical, cognitive, psycho-social, sensory, and other areas that could affect performance.

### PATIENT POPULATION

Occupational therapy personnel provide services within physical medicine and rehabilitation services (PM&RS), covering a population that ranges from children, young adult to geriatric.

### Comprehensive Multidisciplinary Team Approach

Occupational therapy services cover a wide spectrum of neurological, orthopedic, medical, surgical, and mental (behavioral) health conditions. Special populations treated include:

- Amputation
- Brain dysfunction or traumatic brain injury (TBI)
- Homelessness
- Posttraumatic stress disorder (PTSD)
- Spinal cord injury/disorders
- Stroke/neurological disorders
- Vision loss
- Home-based primary care

## TREATMENT SETTING

Occupational therapy personnel provide services in outpatient clinics, inpatient settings (including medical centers and community living centers), patients homes, and the expanding venue of telerehabilitation.

Occupational therapy services provided in physical medicine and rehabilitation (PM&R) and other clinics, include specialized programs for drivers training, polytrauma, telerehabilitation, and amputation care.

A full scope of services are available. In addition to addressing physical disabilities, occupational therapists also address the needs of patients with mental-health conditions and disorders.

## OCCUPATIONAL TRAINING AND CERTIFICATION

Occupational therapy service promotes an environment for clinical education.

The Office of Academic Affiliations (OAA) supports nearly 200 preprofessional occupational therapy students with stipends during their clinical training.

Many occupational therapists have advanced skills, certification, and training in areas, such as:

- Assistive technology
- Cognitive rehabilitation
- Drivers training
- Ergonomics
- Geriatric care
- Hand therapy
- Low vision
- Mental (behavioral) health
- Neurorehabilitation
- Pain management
- Seating and mobility, and
- Work hardening

## Section 10.3 | **Speech Therapy**

This section contains text excerpted from "Poststroke Rehabilitation," *Know Stroke*, National Institute of Neurological Disorders and Stroke (NINDS), September 2014. Reviewed November 2019.

Speech therapy helps individuals with aphasia to relearn how to use language or develop alternative means of communication. It also helps people improve their ability to swallow, and speech therapy works with patients to develop problem-solving and social skills needed to cope with the after-effects of a disability.

Many specialized therapeutic techniques have been developed to assist people with aphasia. Some forms of short-term therapy can improve comprehension rapidly. Intensive exercises such as repeating the therapist's words, practicing following directions, and doing reading or writing exercises form the cornerstone of language rehabilitation. Conversational coaching and rehearsal, as well as the development of prompts or cues to help people remember specific words, are sometimes beneficial. Speech therapies also help patients develop strategies for circumventing language disabilities. These strategies can include the use of symbol boards or sign language. Advances in computer technology have spurred the development of equipment to enhance communication.

Speech therapists use special types of imaging techniques to study swallowing patterns of individuals and identify the exact source of their impairment. Difficulties with swallowing have many possible causes, including a delayed swallowing reflex, an inability to manipulate food with the tongue, or an inability to detect food remaining lodged in the cheeks after swallowing. When the cause has been pinpointed, speech-language pathologists work with the individual to devise strategies to overcome or minimize the deficit. Sometimes, simply changing body position and improving posture during eating can bring about improvement. The texture of foods can be modified to make swallowing easier; for example, thin liquids, which often cause choking, can be thickened. Changing eating habits by taking small bites and chewing slowly can also help alleviate dysphagia.

## Section 10.4 | **Recreation Therapy and Creative Arts Therapy**

This section contains text excerpted from the following sources: Text under the heading "Recreation Therapy" is excerpted from "Why Recreation Therapy—Rehabilitation and Prosthetic Services," U.S. Department of Veteran Affairs (VA), January 22, 2019; Text under the heading "Population Served by Recreation Therapists" is excerpted from "Recreation Therapy Service Fact Sheet," U.S. Department of Veterans Affairs (VA), February 2019; Text under the heading "Creative Arts Therapy" is excerpted from "Why Creative Arts Therapy?—Rehabilitation and Prosthetic Services," U.S. Department of Veteran Affairs (VA), January 22, 2019; Text beginning with the heading "Creative Arts Therapists" is excerpted from "Creative Arts Therapies Fact Sheet," U.S. Department of Veteran Affairs (VA), February 2019.

### RECREATION THERAPY

Recreation therapy is a healthcare discipline designed to provide specialized application of therapeutic activities or interventions to assist in maintaining or improving the health status, functional capabilities, promoting recovery treatment, and ultimately the quality of life for patients with injuries, chronic illness, and disabling conditions. Recreation therapy treatment, education, and prevention or health promotion programs incorporate individualized and personalized interventions that are specifically designed to promote and reinforce healthy leisure lifestyle behaviors that will maintain or improve well-being or functioning. Recreation therapy utilizes traditional, contemporary, and state of the art technology such as telerehabilitation, virtual reality, assistive devices, and multisensory technologies to design an individualized and personalized opportunities to keep those with injuries, chronic illness, and disabling conditions active and integrated in their families and communities. Recreation therapy engages the individual, a family, a peer group, or other social groups to collaborate, cooperate, and solidify their efforts to accomplish individual and/or group goals or objectives.

Community management and reintegration enhance individuals ability to navigate through different kinds of environments, surfaces, and settings safely. Recreation therapist can help them function in their communities by breaking down tasks into smaller components. Some of the things we take for granted such as mobility, accessibility, money management, pedestrian safety, route finding etc., can be challenging. Community management and reintegration builds confidence in the individual's ability to transition back into their community and to function as independently as possible.

Recreation Therapy offers a unique nonpharmacological approach to managing various components of medical or mental-health issues such as behavior management, anger management, pain management, reality orientation, coping and adjustment, stress management and relaxation, and substance abuse. Recreation therapy can also make a significant contribution to those requiring hospice and/or palliative care utilizing comfort, relaxation, and sensory activities such as music, art, light touch, aroma, reminiscing, journaling, pet visits, etc.

## POPULATIONS SERVED BY RECREATION THERAPISTS

Recreation therapists practice across the continuum of care, providing services in inpatient settings, outpatient clinics, and telerehabilitation.

- Recreation therapists serve as key members of numerous interdisciplinary treatment teams;
- Recreation therapists construct appropriate and evidence-based recreation therapy interventions for treating patients with complex medical or mental-health issues such as polytrauma, traumatic brain injury (TBI); posttraumatic stress disorder (PTSD); spinal cord injury (SCI); substance-use disorder (SUD)/addictions; serious mental illness (SMI); and hospice/palliative care.
- Recreation therapists design individualized treatment interventions to reduce stress, anxiety and maladaptive behaviors, recover basic motor functioning and reasoning abilities, build confidence, and develop compensatory strategies to master critical life skills necessary for community reengagement.

## CREATIVE ARTS THERAPY

The creative arts therapies (art, dance, drama, music) offer unique and distinct opportunities for self-expression of each person's individual feelings, emotions, physical abilities, and self-identity, as well as one's relationships with others and the world in which they live. Thus, the creative arts therapies are uniquely able to promote functional rehabilitation in physical, emotional, psychological, and social domains, or to the palliation of symptoms-related to a terminal illness. As a primary expression of the individual person, the creative arts therapies provide the tools or the means through which a person can rehabilitate medical or psychological conditions.

The creative arts therapies offer a unique nonpharmacological approach to managing various components of medical or mental-health issues such as pain management, reality orientation, cognitive processing, and substance abuse.

The capacity to enjoy life and to maintain self-esteem is vital to the wellbeing of an individual particularly when recovery or adjustment is involved. Based on a core knowledge of human behavior and physiology, the goal of recreation therapy and creative arts therapies is to creatively develop an individual's potential for self-sufficiency, enrichment, and fulfillment.

## CREATIVE ARTS THERAPISTS

Creative arts therapists are human service professionals who use arts modalities and creative processes to promote wellness, recovery, rehabilitation through unique personal interactions.

Each creative arts therapy discipline has its own set of professional standards and requisite qualifications. Creative arts therapists are highly skilled, credentialed professionals have completed extensive coursework and clinical training.

## THERAPEUTIC INTERVENTIONS

Creative arts therapists use the techniques, tools, and materials of their unique discipline for therapeutic purposes that promote creative self-expression in order to treat chronic pain, facilitate relaxation, facilitated physical rehabilitation, encourage communication and socialization, and to facilitate cognitive retraining for patients with neurocognitive disorders or traumatic brain injury.

In the treatment of substance abuse, art-based techniques provide a unique opportunity to help patients break through barriers to the recovery process.

# Section 10.5 | **Prosthetists and Orthotists**

This section contains text excerpted from "Orthotists and Prosthetists," U.S. Bureau of Labor Statistics (BLS), U.S. Department of Labor (DOL), September 4, 2019.

## WHAT ORTHOTISTS AND PROSTHETISTS DO

Orthotists and prosthetists create devices that allow patients to regain or improve mobility and functionality. Orthotists and prosthetists design and fabricate medical supportive devices and measure and fit patients for them. These devices include artificial limbs (arms, hands, legs, and feet), braces, and other medical or surgical devices.

Orthotists and prosthetists typically do the following:

- Evaluate and interview patients to determine their needs
- Take measurements or impressions of the part of a patient's body that will be fitted with a brace or artificial limb
- Design and fabricate orthopedic and prosthetic devices based on physicians' prescriptions
- Select materials to be used for the orthotic or prosthetic device
- Instruct patients in how to use and care for their devices
- Adjust, repair, or replace prosthetic and orthotic devices
- Document care in patients' records

Orthotists and prosthetists may work in both orthotics and prosthetics, or they may choose to specialize in one area. Orthotists are specifically trained to work with medical supportive devices, such as spinal or knee braces. Prosthetists are specifically trained to work with prostheses, such as artificial limbs and other body parts.

**Table 10.1.** Percentage of Employment in Orthotists and Prosthetists

| | |
|---|---|
| Medical equipment and supplies manufacturing | 32% |
| Ambulatory healthcare services | 27% |
| Health and personal care stores | 16% |
| Hospitals; state, local, and private | 10% |
| Federal government, excluding postal service | 9% |

Some orthotists and prosthetists construct devices for their patients. Others supervise the construction of the orthotic or prosthetic devices by medical appliance technicians.

## WORK ENVIRONMENT OF ORTHOTISTS AND PROSTHETISTS

Orthotists and prosthetists held about 9,100 jobs in 2018. The largest employers of orthotists and prosthetists were as follows:

Orthotists and prosthetists who fabricate orthotics and prosthetics may be exposed to health or safety hazards when handling certain materials, but there is little risk of injury if workers follow proper procedures, such as wearing goggles, gloves, and masks.

# Section 10.6 | Other Rehabilitation Professionals

"Other Rehabilitation Professionals," © 2020 Omnigraphics. Reviewed November 2019.

## REHABILITATION NURSE

A rehabilitation nurse provides supervisory medical care that makes full use of the breadth of clinical skills through collaboration with an interdisciplinary team of medical professionals. This care makes a visible difference in a patient's life, irrespective of the environment.

The most important trait of a rehabilitation nurse is the ability to work well with all members of the patient's care team—including members of the interdisciplinary healthcare team, the patient, and the patient's caregivers and family—immediately after the onset of a disabling injury or chronic illness. The training that rehabilitation nurses receive allows them to closely supervise the patient's care and maintain or improve their functional abilities. These services align with the comprehensive-care plan that the rehabilitation nurse and other healthcare team members develop to help patients achieve their goals and reach their maximum potential.

Rehabilitation nurses:

- Promote health, successful living, and disability prevention through involvement in activities that will assist patients, families, and communities and encourage them to stay healthy
- Provide the highest-quality standard of care based on the best available scientific evidence to patients and families by continually updating their skills and training
- Collaborate effectively with a team of experts to ensure that patients and families are getting the highest-quality care during the rehabilitation process while simultaneously informing the team of experts on the progress of the patient

Rehabilitation nurses also advocate for funding and policy legislation that benefit people with disabilities and chronic illness; hold leadership positions in local, state, and federal agencies; and share their knowledge by researching, publishing, and disseminating information.

## CLINICAL SOCIAL WORKER

Clinical social workers are important members of the rehabilitation team. These professionals are licensed to provide mental-health services across the country and have extensive knowledge of social policy, the efficient delivery of social services, and how to optimally plan for the future. Their commitment to social-work ethics and values is evident as they apply their expertise about human behavior to the task of serving as liaison contact for the patient, family, and rehabilitation treatment team. Furthermore, clinical social workers share responsibility in coordinating with hospitals, insurance companies, and other related institutions to enhance a patient's social well-being and maximize their quality of life.

The experience, empathy, and knowledge of a clinical social worker are applied to their management of the physical, psychological, social, and economic aspects of their patients' lives. Clinical social workers provide or arrange for case management; group or individual therapy and family counseling; and advocate for jobs and housing needs, community resources, education, and other social issues affecting their patients.

## PSYCHIATRIST, PSYCHOLOGIST, OR NEUROPSYCHOLOGIST

Psychiatrists, psychologists, or neuropsychologists are trained healthcare professionals who serve patients undergoing rehabilitative treatment. They examine the cognitive function of patients to determine the patient's thinking and learning capacity and to provide a range of services accordingly. Psychiatrists, psychologists, or neuropsychologists also assist the patient and patient's family as they adjust to short-term, long-term, or permanent disability. Their expertise focuses on the psychological well-being of patients.

## REGISTERED DIETITIAN

Registered dietitians educate patients about nutritional requirements and diets that enhance their well-being. A registered dietitian has advanced knowledge about dietary and nutritional needs, and knows how to make adjustments to a patient's diet that will improve their overall health and recovery. Their knowledge allows them to assess a patient's eating abilities, determine their food preferences, and then apply this knowledge to planning an optimum diet that addresses a patient's medical needs while enhancing the patient's overall well-being.

## CASE MANAGER

A rehabilitation case manager provides and manages services and resources that benefit a patient who is on rehabilitation. They monitor and document a patient's progress, and are involved in planning, developing, and coordinating the documented preliminary and posttreatments services and resources.

## RESPIRATORY THERAPIST

Respiratory therapists assist in the function of human breathing for those with airway and breathing issues. Their specialized training is beneficial to patients with the following symptoms:

- Low oxygen levels
- Tracheostomy tubes (for those unable to breathe through their mouths and noses)
- Patients on ventilators who are unable to breathe on their own and depend on a machine to do the breathing for them
- People with chronic heart or lung problems who need breathing treatments and assistance

## CHAPLAIN

A chaplain is a specialist who can aid in a patient's rehabilitation. A chaplain advocates for physical, emotional, social, and spiritual balance by offering spiritual hope that can help a person with a disability cope and recover. Their spiritual counseling is often effective at energizing patients, their families, and healthcare staff members, particularly during periods of crisis, by reaffirming spiritual beliefs and offering themselves as a bridge to maintaining or establishing a relationship with a church or house of worship or spiritual path.

Chaplains serve in many hospital settings and rehabilitation units and make daily visits; they are also usually on call 24 hours a day. Usually, chaplains are ordained ministers or priests or someone with specialized training in hospital pastoral care or chaplaincy. Patients in hospitals or rehabilitation centers that do not employ a chaplain can rely on their own clergy or spiritual advisor to provide them with spiritual guidance.

## REHABILITATION ENGINEERING PROFESSIONALS

Rehabilitation engineering professionals are well-trained and include the rehabilitation engineer, rehabilitation technologist/assistive technologist, and rehabilitation technician.

**Rehabilitation engineer.** Pays attention to the innovative and methodical application of scientific knowledge and technology in designing and developing a device, system, or process that will meet the needs of a person with a disability.

**Rehabilitation technologist/assistive technologist.** Methodically combines scientific and engineering knowledge and methods with technical skills to complement engineering applications developed for a person with a disability.

**Rehabilitation technician.** Works under the direct supervision of a rehabilitation engineer or rehabilitation technologist/assistive technologist to mainly assemble and test parts of devices or systems that have been designed to meet the needs of a person with a disability.

### References

1. "Rehabilitation Nurses Play a Variety of Roles," Association of Rehabilitation Nurses, May 8, 2018.
2. "Overview of the PM&R Treatment Team," The Johns Hopkins University, John Hopkins Medicine, April 20, 2018.
3. "Rehabilitation Engineers, Technologists, and Technicians: Vital Members of the Assistive Technology Team," National Center for Biotechnology Information (NCBI), June 28, 2018.

# Chapter 11 | **Orthopedic and Musculoskeletal Rehabilitation**

**Chapter Contents**

## Section 11.1 | **Joint Replacements**

This section includes text excerpted from "Joint Replacement Surgery," National Institute of Arthritis and Musculoskeletal and Skin Diseases (NIAMS), August 2016. Reviewed November 2019.

### WHAT IS JOINT REPLACEMENT SURGERY?

Joint replacement surgery is removing a damaged joint and putting in a new one. The doctor may suggest a joint replacement to improve how you live. Replacing a joint can relieve pain and help you move and feel better.

Hips and knees are replaced most often. Other joints that can be replaced include the shoulders, fingers, ankles, and elbows.

The new joint can be made of plastic, metal, or ceramic parts. Sometimes, the surgeon will not remove the whole joint, but will only replace or fix the damaged parts. Types of new joints include:

- **Cemented joints:** Used more often in older people who do not move around as much and in people with "weak" bones. The cement holds the new joint to the bone.
- **Uncemented joints:** Often recommended for younger, more active people and those with good bone quality. It may take longer to heal, because it takes longer for bone to grow and attach to it.
- **Hybrid replacements:** Use both methods to keep the new joint in place.

### WHY MAY JOINT REPLACEMENT SURGERY BE NEEDED?

Pain, stiffness, and swelling may be due to joint damage caused by:

- Arthritis
- Years of use
- Disease

To see if you need a joint replaced, your doctor may:

- Look at your joint with an x-ray or another machine
- Put a small, lighted tube (arthroscope) into your joint to look for damage
- Take a small sample of your tissue for testing

After looking at your joint, the doctor may recommend:

- Exercise
- Walking aids, such as braces or canes
- Physical therapy
- Medicines and vitamin supplements

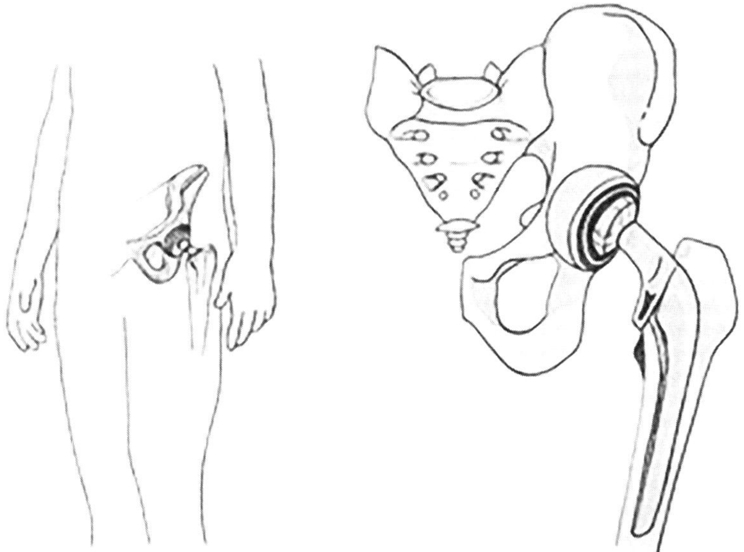

**Figure 11.1.** Hip Replacement

- Osteotomy, which involves cutting and lining up bone. This may be simpler than replacing a joint, but it may take longer to recover. However, this operation has become less common.

If you still have constant pain and have trouble with things such as walking, climbing stairs, and taking a bath, your doctor may recommend joint replacement.

## WHAT HAPPENS DURING JOINT REPLACEMENT SURGERY

During joint replacement your doctors will:

- Give you medicine so you will not feel pain. The medicine may block the pain only in one part of the body, or it may put your whole body to sleep.
- Replace the damaged joint with a new human-made joint.
- Move you to a recovery room until you are fully awake or the numbness goes away.

## WHAT CAN I EXPECT AFTER JOINT REPLACEMENT SURGERY?

With knee or hip surgery, you will probably need to stay in the hospital for a few days. If you are elderly or have additional disabilities, you may then need to spend several weeks in an intermediate-care facility before going home. You and your team of doctors will determine how long you stay in the hospital.

After hip or knee replacement, you will often stand or begin walking the day of surgery. At first, you will walk with a walker or crutches. You may have some temporary pain in the new joint because your muscles are weak from not being used. Also, your body is healing. The pain can be helped with medicines and should end in a few weeks or months.

Physical therapy can begin the day after surgery to help strengthen the muscles around the new joint and help you regain motion in the joint. If you have your shoulder joint replaced, you can usually begin exercising the same day of your surgery. A physical therapist will help you with gentle range-of-motion exercises. Before you leave the hospital, your therapist will show you how to use a pulley device to help bend and extend your arm.

## WHAT ARE THE COMPLICATIONS OF JOINT REPLACEMENT SURGERY?

New technology and advances in surgical techniques have greatly reduced the complications involved with joint replacements. When complications do occur, most are treatable. Possible complications include:

- **Infection.** Areas in the wound or around the new joint may get infected. It may happen while you're still in the hospital or after you go home. It may even occur years later. Minor infections in the wound are usually treated with drugs. Deep infections may need a second operation to treat the infection or replace the joint.
- **Blood clots.** If your blood moves too slowly, it may begin to form lumps of blood parts called "clots." If pain and swelling develop in your legs after hip or knee surgery, blood clots may be the cause. The doctor may suggest drugs to make your blood thin or special stockings, exercises, or boots to help your blood move faster. If swelling, redness, or pain occurs in your leg after you leave the hospital, contact your doctor right away.
- **Loosening.** The new joint may loosen, causing pain. If the loosening is bad, you may need another operation to reattach the joint to the bone.
- **Dislocation.** Sometimes after hip or other joint replacement, the ball of the prosthesis can come out of its socket. In most cases, the hip can be corrected without surgery. A brace may be worn for a while if a dislocation occurs.
- **Wear.** Some wear can be found in all joint replacements. Too much wear may help cause loosening. The doctor may need to operate again if the prosthesis comes loose. Sometimes, the plastic can wear thin, and the doctor may just replace the plastic and not the whole joint.
- **Nerve and blood vessel injury.** Nerves near the replaced joint may be damaged during surgery, but this does not happen often. Over time, the damage often improves and may disappear. Blood vessels may also be injured.

As you move your new joint and let your muscles grow strong again, pain will lessen, flexibility will increase, and movement will improve.

## Section 11.2 | **Amputations**

This section includes text excerpted from "Long-Term Care Following Traumatic Amputation," U.S. Department of Veterans Affairs (VA), May 7, 2014. Reviewed November 2019.

Individuals with traumatic amputations represent a population with wide-ranging medical and rehabilitation needs. These needs can include issues directly related to the amputation itself, issues related to traumatic injury of other body parts, as well as more long-term secondary complications. Individuals with trauma-related amputations typically sustain their injuries at a relatively young age and have a long life expectancy, emphasizing the need for longitudinal care considerations.

### AMPUTATION-SPECIFIC CONSIDERATIONS

#### Residual Limb Care

Following amputation, the residual limb undergoes a number of changes over time which can potentially result in secondary complications and result in a limited ability to wear a prosthesis for functional activities.

These changes and secondary complications include:

- Soft tissue and muscle atrophy
- Skin irritation and breakdown
- Joint contracture
- Infection (soft tissue and bone)
- Proximal osteoarthritis/musculoskeletal complications
- Heterotopic ossification
- Osteopenia and osteoporosis

#### Pain Management

Pain following amputation can generally be classified as residual limb pain or phantom limb pain.

Residual limb pain typically improves following amputation surgery, but can be persistent and associated with prosthetic use.

Phantom limb pain (pain perceived in the part of the body that is missing) can be chronic and severe enough to interfere with prosthetic use and functional abilities.

## OTHER TRAUMATIC INJURY CONSIDERATIONS

Amputations related to combat and other trauma are commonly associated with moderate to severe injury severity scores, and multiple comorbid injuries that require long-term management and care. These associated injuries have the potential to impact medical and rehabilitation outcomes such as functional independence, satisfaction, and quality of life (QOL).

Frequently associated injuries include:

- Traumatic brain injury (TBI)
- Fractures and other musculoskeletal injuries
- Soft tissue injuries and burns
- Peripheral nerve injuries
- Abdominal injuries
- Hearing loss and tinnitus
- Vision impairment or loss
- Genitourinary injuries (common with dismounted blast explosions)
- Mental-health conditions such as posttraumatic stress disorder (PTSD), depression, and adjustment disorder

## SECONDARY COMPLICATIONS

Amputation of one or more limbs has a longitudinal impact on many areas outside of the residual limb itself. The two areas most commonly affected are musculoskeletal and the cardiovascular systems. Many of the considerations in these areas gradually progress or worsen over time, whereas other conditions may be more intermittent. These conditions highlight the importance of comprehensive prevention strategies including proper nutrition, exercise, tobacco cessation, and wellness counseling for individuals with amputations. Wellness promotion and preventive measures should be part of one's lifestyle. Medical monitoring and education should be routine in amputation clinics and rehabilitation services.

### Musculoskeletal Considerations

Longitudinal considerations for musculoskeletal conditions include:

- Osteoarthritis in the nonamputated extremity
- Overuse syndromes
- Delayed amputation after initial limb salvage
- General musculoskeletal pain and low back pain

### Weight Gain/Obesity

Decreased activity levels and metabolic changes can result in weight gain and obesity. This weight gain can lead to a vicious cycle where weight gain makes prosthetic fitting and use more difficult, thus resulting in even greater declines inactivity.

### Cardiovascular Disease

The aging amputee population has significantly worse cardiovascular and metabolic issues that appear to be directly related to their traumatic amputation, and not accounted for by obesity, sedentary lifestyle, or tobacco use. Persons with traumatic amputations have been identified as having increased hypertension, ischemic heart disease, and diabetes mellitus.

## Section 11.3 | **Postpolio Syndrome**

This section includes text excerpted from "Postpolio Syndrome Fact Sheet," National Institute of Neurological Disorders and Stroke (NINDS), August 13, 2019.

### WHAT IS POSTPOLIO SYNDROME?

Polio, or poliomyelitis, is an infectious viral disease that can strike at any age and affects a person's nervous system. Between the late 1940s and early 1950s, polio crippled around 35,000 people each year in the United States alone, making it one of the most feared diseases of the twentieth century.

The polio vaccine was first introduced in 1955; its use since then has eradicated polio from the United States. The World Health Organization (WHO) reports polio cases have decreased by more than 99 percent since 1988, from an estimated 350,000 cases then, to 1,352 reported cases in 2010. As a result of the global effort to eradicate the disease, only three countries (Afghanistan, Nigeria, and Pakistan) remain polio-endemic as of February 2012, down from more than 125 in 1988.

Postpolio syndrome is a condition that affects polio survivors years after recovery from an initial acute attack of the poliomyelitis virus. Most often, polio survivors start to experience gradual new weakening in muscles that were previously affected by the polio infection. The most common symptoms include slowly progressive muscle weakness, fatigue (both generalized and muscular), and a gradual decrease in the size of muscles (muscle atrophy). Pain from joint degeneration and increasing skeletal deformities such as scoliosis (curvature of the spine) is common and may precede the weakness and muscle atrophy. Some individuals experience only minor symptoms while others develop visible muscle weakness and atrophy.

Postpolio syndrome is rarely life-threatening, but the symptoms can significantly interfere with an individual's ability to function independently. Respiratory muscle weakness, for instance, can result in trouble with proper breathing, affecting daytime functions and sleep. Weakness in swallowing muscles can result in aspiration of food and liquids into the lungs and lead to pneumonia.

## WHO IS AT RISK?

While polio is a contagious disease, postpolio syndrome cannot be caught from others having the disorder. Only a polio survivor can develop postpolio syndrome.

The severity of weakness and disability after recovery from poliomyelitis tends to predict the relative risk of developing postpolio syndrome. Individuals who had minimal symptoms from the original illness are more likely to experience only mild postpolio syndrome symptoms. A person who was more acutely affected by the poliovirus and who attained a greater recovery may experience a more severe case of postpolio syndrome, with greater loss of muscle function and more severe fatigue.

The exact incidence and prevalence of postpolio syndrome is unknown. The U.S. National Health Interview Survey (NHIS) in 1987 contained specific questions for persons given the diagnosis of poliomyelitis with or without paralysis. No survey since then has addressed the question. Results published from 1994 to 1995 estimated there were about one million polio survivors in the U.S., with 443,000 reporting to have had paralytic polio. Accurate statistics do not exist, as a percentage of polio survivors have died and new cases have been diagnosed. Researchers estimate that the condition affects 25 to 40 percent of polio survivors.

## HOW IS POSTPOLIO SYNDROME DIAGNOSED?

The diagnosis of postpolio syndrome relies nearly entirely on clinical information. There are no laboratory tests specific for this condition and symptoms vary greatly among individuals. Physicians diagnose postpolio syndrome after completing a comprehensive medical history and physical examination, and by excluding other disorders that could explain the symptoms.

Physicians look for the following criteria when diagnosing postpolio syndrome:

- Prior paralytic poliomyelitis with evidence of motor neuron loss. This is confirmed by the history of the acute paralytic illness, signs of residual weakness and atrophy of muscles on neuromuscular examination, and signs of motor neuron loss on electromyography (EMG). Rarely, people had subtle paralytic polio where there was no obvious deficit. In such cases, prior polio should be confirmed with an EMG study rather than a reported history of nonparalytic polio.
- A period of partial or complete functional recovery after acute paralytic poliomyelitis, followed by an interval (usually 15 years or more) of stable neuromuscular function
- Slowly progressive and persistent new muscle weakness or decreased endurance, with or without generalized fatigue, muscle atrophy, or muscle and joint pain. Onset may at times follow trauma, surgery, or a period of inactivity, and can appear to be sudden. Less commonly,

symptoms attributed to postpolio syndrome include new challenges involving breathing or swallowing.
- Symptoms that persist for at least a year
- Exclusion of other neuromuscular, medical, and skeletal abnormalities as causes of symptoms

Postpolio syndrome may be difficult to diagnose in some people because other medical conditions can complicate the evaluation. Depression, for example, is associated with fatigue and can be misinterpreted as postpolio syndrome. A number of conditions may cause health concerns in persons with polio that are not due to additional loss of motor neuron function.

Polio survivors with new symptoms resembling postpolio syndrome should consider seeking treatment from a physician trained in neuromuscular disorders. It is important to clearly establish the origin and potential causes for declining strength and to assess progression of weakness not explained by other health diagnoses. Magnetic resonance imaging (MRI) and computed tomography (CT) of the spinal cord, electrophysiological studies, and other tests are frequently used to investigate the course of decline in muscle strength and exclude other diseases that could be causing or contributing to the new progressive symptoms. A muscle biopsy or a spinal fluid analysis can be used to exclude other, possibly treatable, conditions that mimic postpolio syndrome. Polio survivors may acquire other illnesses and should always have regular check-ups and preventive diagnostic tests. However, there is no diagnostic test for postpolio syndrome, nor is there one that can identify which polio survivors are at greatest risk.

## HOW IS POSTPOLIO SYNDROME TREATED?

There are no effective pharmaceutical treatments that can stop deterioration or reverse the deficits caused by the syndrome itself. However, a number of controlled studies have demonstrated that nonfatiguing exercises may improve muscle strength and reduce tiredness. Most of the clinical trials in postpolio syndrome have focused on finding safe therapies that could reduce symptoms and improve quality of life.

Although there are no effective treatments, there are recommended management strategies. Patients should consider seeking medical advice from a physician experienced in treating neuromuscular disorders. Patients should also consider the judicious use of exercise, preferably under the supervision of an experienced health professional. Physicians often advise patients on the use of mobility aids, ventilation equipment, revising activities of daily living activities to avoid rapid muscle tiring and total body exhaustion, and avoiding activities that cause pain or fatigue lasting more than 10 minutes. Most importantly, patients should avoid the temptation to attribute all signs and symptoms to prior polio, thereby missing out on important treatments for concurrent conditions.

Learning about postpolio syndrome is important for polio survivors and their families. Managing postpolio syndrome can involve lifestyle changes. Support groups that encourage self-help, group participation, and positive action can be helpful. Counseling may be needed to help individuals and families adjust to the late effects of poliomyelitis. Experiencing new symptoms of weakness and using assistive devices may bring back distressing memories of the original illness.

## WHAT IS THE ROLE OF EXERCISE IN THE TREATMENT OF POSTPOLIO SYNDROME?

Pain, weakness, and fatigue can result from overuse of muscles and joints. These same symptoms also can result from disuse of muscles and joints. This fact has caused a misunderstanding about whether to encourage or discourage exercise for polio survivors or individuals with postpolio syndrome.

Exercise is safe and effective when carefully prescribed and monitored by experienced health professionals. Exercise is more likely to benefit those muscle groups that were least affected by polio. Cardiopulmonary endurance training is usually more effective than strengthening exercises, especially when activities are paced to allow for frequent breaks and strategies are used to conserve energy. Heavy or intense resistive exercise and weight-lifting using polio-affected muscles may be counterproductive, as this can further weaken rather than strengthen these muscles.

Exercise prescriptions should include:

- The specific muscle groups to be included
- The specific muscle groups to be excluded, and
- The type of exercise, together with frequency and duration

Exercise should be reduced or discontinued if it causes additional weakness, excessive fatigue, or unduly prolonged recovery time is noted by either the individual with postpolio syndrome or the professional monitoring the exercise. As a general rule, no muscle should be exercised to the point of causing pain, fatigue, or weakness.

## CAN POSTPOLIO SYNDROME BE PREVENTED?

Polio survivors often ask if there is a way to prevent the development of postpolio syndrome. Presently, no intervention has been found to stop the deterioration of surviving neurons. Physicians recommend that polio survivors get a good night's sleep, maintain a well-balanced diet, avoid unhealthy habits such as smoking and overeating, and follow a prescribed exercise program. Lifestyle changes, such as weight control, the use of assistive devices, and taking certain anti-inflammatory medications, may help with some of the symptoms of postpolio syndrome.

## Section 11.4 | Fractures and Rehabilitation



### FRACTURE AND ITS TYPES

A fracture is a broken bone. Fractures can range from a small crack to a complete break. Fractures usually occurs due to a blunt-force impact, stress, or other trauma.

There are two major types of fractures: acute fracture and stress fracture. An acute fracture is caused when there is a complete or partial break in the bone resulting from a direct blow on a part of the body. Acute fractures takes longer to heal and require rehabilitation and surgery in some cases. Stress fractures happen as a result of the overuse of muscles, which causes the body to transfer the excess weight onto the bones, causing small cracks in the bone. Athletes, who exert repeated physical stress on their bodies during training and exercise, are the most common victims of stress fractures.

### SYMPTOMS OF FRACTURES

The symptoms of a fracture differ based on the type of bone affected, the patient's age and overall health, and the extent of the injury. However, the following are the most common symptoms:

- Intense pain in a bone
- Deformity of a limb
- Bleeding or bruising
- Swelling or tenderness around the injury
- Numbness and tingling
- Limitation of joint motion

### DIAGNOSIS AND TREATMENT OF A FRACTURE

A physical examination is carried out by a doctor, who identifies the signs and symptoms that lead to a diagnose of the fracture. After the diagnosis, an x-ray is taken and, in severe cases, a computed tomography (CT) or magnetic resonance imaging (MRI) may be used to estimate the level of damage.

Fracture treatments vary based on whether it is an open or closed fracture. In a closed fracture, the skin is intact, so stabilization and immobilization are the primary form of treatment. Stabilization and immobilization can be accomplished by making use of a splint or cast that the injured patient uses during a natural healing process that will occur automatically.

In an open fracture, the bone is exposed, or a fracture has displaced or misaligned the bone. Surgery is required to reset the bone before the natural healing process can take over. The process of resetting the bone is called "fracture reduction." During a fracture reduction, the surgeon makes an incision in the affected area, which allows the doctor to identify and align the broken bone. In some cases, the surgeon also uses metal rods, screws, or wires to secure the fracture.

## POSTFRACTURE REHABILITATION

The major objectives of postfracture rehabilitation are the prevention of disuse atrophy and the mobilization and stabilization of the associated joints. Patients are typically referred to a physiotherapist for rehabilitation after a fracture. During the postfracture rehabilitation process, the physiotherapist analyzes the patient's condition and follows a customized protocol, or guide, that addresses patients' individual needs and varying medical conditions. The main objective of rehabilitation is to restore the patient's functional ability.

To restore the patient's muscle and bone strength to an optimal level, the rehabilitation may include, but not be restricted to, the following:

- Soft-tissue massage to control edema, muscle spasms, and swelling
- Stretching exercises to restore joint range of movement
- Recovering joint mobility
- Progressive strengthening and endurance training
- Balance control and gait training (walking practice)

Generally, a fracture heals within eight weeks, after which the physical therapist determines the appropriate treatment program based on an initial evaluation of the patient's general health. The rehabilitation program usually lasts six weeks and may be extended, depending on the amount of damage sustained and the effort required for the healing process.

Physical agents and modalities may be used to alleviate pain and swelling. To improve muscle recovery, electrical stimulation may be used. Scar massage and mobilization may be used to decrease scar adhesions and refine mobility around the surgical scar tissue. In the case of a leg or ankle fracture, weight-bearing restrictions may be prescribed. Similarly, for arm or shoulder fractures, lifting restrictions may be put into place. The physical therapist helps to maintain these restrictions and provides guidance on the proper way to lift things safely and also offers expert guidance on the appropriate use of a cane or walker.

For optimal recovery, rehabilitation is combined with orthopedics since both fields deal with bones, muscles, and ligaments.

### References


1. "What Is Post Surgical/Fracture Rehabilitation?" South Tees Hospitals NHS Foundation Trust, January 13, 2014.
2. "Fracture," Physiopedia, March 6, 2017.

3. "Postfracture Rehabilitation," Oakridge Physiotherapy Centre, July 13, 2015.
4. Wedro, Benjamin. "Broken Bone (Types of Bone Fractures)," MedicineNet, July 17, 2019.
5. "Fracture Rehabilitation," Circle Health, September 15, 2017.

## Section 11.5 | **Arthritis**

This section contains text excerpted from the following sources: Text beginning with the heading "What Is Arthritis?" is excerpted from "Frequently Asked Questions (FAQs) about Arthritis," Centers for Disease Control and Prevention (CDC), January 10, 2019; Text beginning with the heading "Why Is Physical Activity Important for People with Arthritis?" is excerpted from "Physical Activity for Arthritis," Centers for Disease Control and Prevention (CDC), November 8, 2010; Text under the heading "Assistive Devices Can Make Life with Arthritis Easier" is © 2016 Omnigraphics. Reviewed November 2019.

### WHAT IS ARTHRITIS?

Arthritis is a general term for conditions that affect the joints or tissues around the joint. There are more than 100 types of arthritis. Most types of arthritis cause pain and stiffness in and around the affected joint or joints. Some types of arthritis, such as rheumatoid arthritis (RA), also affect the immune system and some internal organs of the body.

### WHAT ARE THE MOST COMMON TYPES OF ARTHRITIS?

The most common form of arthritis in the United States is osteoarthritis. Other common types of arthritis include rheumatoid arthritis, gout, and fibromyalgia. Fibromyalgia is included in arthritis for public-health purposes.

### WHAT ARE THE SYMPTOMS OF ARTHRITIS?

Different types of arthritis have different symptoms. Pain and stiffness in and around one or more joints are common symptoms for most types of arthritis. Depending on the type of arthritis, symptoms can develop suddenly or gradually over time. Symptoms may come and go, or persist over time.

### WHY IS PHYSICAL ACTIVITY IMPORTANT FOR PEOPLE WITH ARTHRITIS?

If you have arthritis, participating in joint-friendly physical activity can improve your arthritis pain, function, mood, and quality of life. Joint-friendly physical activities are low-impact, which means they put less stress on the body, reducing the risk of injury. Examples of joint-friendly activities include walking, biking and swimming. Being physically active can also delay the onset of arthritis-related disability and help people with arthritis manage other chronic conditions such as diabetes, heart disease, and obesity.

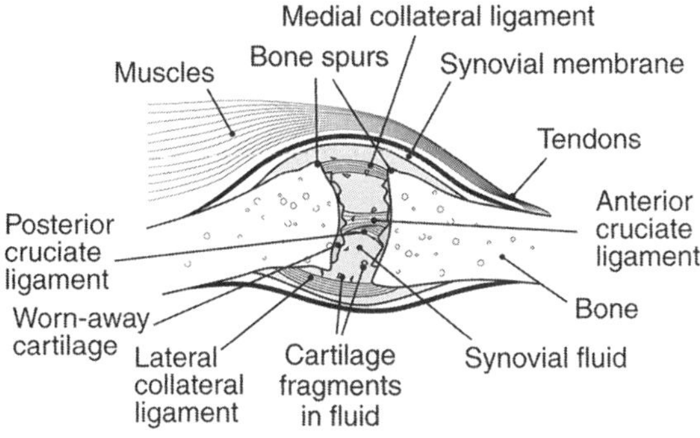


**Figure 11.2.** A Joint with Severe Osteoarthritis
*(Source: National Institute of Arthritis and Musculoskeletal and Skin Diseases (NIAMS).)*

## HOW DO I EXERCISE SAFELY WITH ARTHRITIS?

You can safely exercise and enjoy the benefits of increased physical activity with these S.M.A.R.T. tips.

- **S**tart low, go slow.
- **M**odify activity when arthritis symptoms increase, try to stay active.
- **A**ctivities should be "joint-friendly."
- **R**ecognize safe places and ways to be active.
- **T**alk to a health professional or certified exercise specialist.

### Start Low, and Go Slow

When starting or increasing physical activity, start slow and pay attention to how your body tolerates it. People with arthritis may take more time for their body to adjust to a new level of activity. If you are not active, start with a small amount of activity, for example, three to five minutes two times a day. Add activity a little at a time (such as 10 minutes at a time) and allow enough time for your body to adjust to the new level before adding more activity.

### Modify Activity When Arthritis Symptoms Increase, Try to Stay Active

Your arthritis symptoms, such as pain, stiffness, and fatigue, may come and go and you may have good days and bad days. Try to modify your activity to stay as active as possible without making your symptoms worse.

### Activities Should Be "Joint Friendly"

Choose activities that are easy on the joints such as walking, bicycling, water aerobics, or dancing. These activities have a low risk of injury and do not twist or "pound" the joints too much.

### Recognize Safe Places and Ways to Be Active

Safety is important for starting and maintaining an activity plan. If you are currently inactive or you are not sure how to start your own physical activity program, an exercise class may be a good option. If you plan and direct your own activity, find safe places to be active. For example, walk-in an area where the sidewalks or pathways are level and free of obstructions, are well-lit and are separated from heavy traffic.

### Talk to a Health Professional or Certified Exercise Specialist

Your doctor is a good source of information about physical activity. Healthcare professionals and certified exercise professionals can answer your questions about how much and what types of activity match your abilities and health goals.

## WHAT TYPES OF ACTIVITIES SHOULD I DO?

**Low-impact aerobic activities** do not put stress on the joints and include brisk walking, cycling, swimming, water aerobics, light gardening, group exercise classes, and dancing.

For major health benefits, do at least:

- 150 minutes (2 hours and 30 minutes) of moderate-intensity aerobic activity, such as cycling at less than 10 miles per hour, or
- 75 minutes (1 hour and 15 minutes) of vigorous-intensity aerobic activity, such as cycling at 10 mph or faster, each week. Another option is to do a combination of both. A rule of thumb is that one minute of vigorous-intensity activity is about the same as two minutes of moderate-intensity activity.

In addition to aerobic activity, you should also do muscle-strengthening activities that involve all major muscle groups two or more days a week.

**Muscle-strengthening exercises** include lifting weights, working with resistance bands, and yoga. These can be done at home, in an exercise class, or at a fitness center.

**Flexibility exercises** such as stretching and yoga are also important for people with arthritis. Many people with arthritis have joint stiffness that makes daily tasks difficult. Doing daily flexibility exercises helps maintain range of motion so you can keep doing everyday things such as household tasks, hobbies, and visiting with friends and family.

**Balance exercises** such as walking backward, standing on one foot, and tai chi are important for those who are at a risk of falling or have trouble walking. Do balance exercises three days per week if you are at risk of falling. Balance exercises are included in many group exercise classes.

## HOW HARD ARE YOU WORKING?

Measure the relative intensity of your activity with the talk test. In general, if you are doing a moderate activity you can talk, but not sing, during the activity. If you are doing vigorous activity, you will not be able to say more than a few words without pausing for breath.

## WHAT DO I DO IF I HAVE PAIN DURING OR AFTER EXERCISE?

It is normal to have some pain, stiffness, and swelling after starting a new physical activity program. It may take 6 to 8 weeks for your joints to get used to your new activity level, but sticking with your activity program will result in long-term pain relief.

Here are some tips to help you manage pain during and after physical activity so you can keep exercising:

- Until your pain improves, modify your physical activity program by exercising less frequently (fewer days per week) or for shorter periods of time (less time each session).
- Try a different type of exercise that puts less pressure on the joints—for example, switch from walking to water aerobics.
- Do proper warm-up and cool-down before and after exercise.
- Exercise at a comfortable pace—you should be able to carry on a conversation while exercising.
- Make sure you have good fitting, comfortable shoes.

See your doctor if you experience any of the following:

- Pain that is sharp, stabbing, and constant
- Pain that causes you to limp
- Pain that lasts more than two hours after exercise or gets worse at night
- Pain or swelling that does not get better with rest, medication, or hot or cold packs
- Large increases in swelling or your joints feel "hot" or are red

## ASSISTIVE DEVICES CAN MAKE LIFE WITH ARTHRITIS EASIER

The joint pain and stiffness associated with arthritis can make it difficult for people to accomplish everyday self-care tasks, such as bathing, dressing, cooking, cleaning, and moving around. A variety of assistive technologies and adaptive devices have been developed to help people to do these tasks with less pain and make it easier for them to live independently. Assistive technology can improve or conserve functional capabilities of people with arthritis, enabling them to perform tasks that were once difficult to accomplish. Self-help devices for arthritis can range from simple rubber grippers that help people open jars to sophisticated robots that can process sensory information and compensate for partial or total loss of function. Since arthritis is a lifelong condition, the most appropriate tools to help manage it may change over time.

## Recognizing the Need for Assistive Devices

As people with arthritis experience gradual changes in their ability levels, they sometimes give up their favorite activities. They may not be aware that using adaptive equipment could enable them to continue enjoying those activities they want to do. Arthritis affects every person differently, so the decision about when to use assistive devices depends upon each individual. The type of equipment required depends on the stage of the disease, the degree of disability, and the kind of task to be accomplished. Patients with rheumatoid arthritis, for instance, often find it difficult to perform tasks that require the joints to bear weight or oppose resistance. As a result, they tend to gain the functional capability from products that provide joint support, increase leverage for lifting, and extend range of motion.

## Acquiring Assistive Devices

The best place to begin the process of acquiring assistive devices may be the doctor's office. A general practitioner or a rheumatologist can provide a referral to an occupational therapist. These medical professionals specialize in helping people with arthritis or other forms of disability to perform day-to-day tasks and to live independently. Professionals evaluate a patient's environment and recommend changes or adaptive equipment that may aid the person's everyday life.

Many types of assistive devices and adaptive equipment can be purchased from hardware stores, medical supply companies, full-service pharmacies, or online retailers. Some stores provide additional training in the device usage or offer help with the equipment installation. Nonprofit organizations such as the Arthritis Foundation are another potential source of information about the range of devices available and the best places to get them. The U.S. Rehabilitation Services Administration also supports Centers for Independent Living (CIL) in many communities across the country. These centers employ technology specialists who can recommend assistive devices to fit an individual's level of disability and specific needs. They also offer demonstrations on how to use assistive devices.

## Types of Assistive Devices

Various types of assistive devices are available to help people with arthritis in order to perform the following.

- **Moving.** Common devices that can help people with arthritis stand and walk more easily include orthotic shoe inserts, braces and splints, a cane or crutch, and extenders for chair legs.

- **Cooking.** Assistive devices that can reduce joint strain in the kitchen include reach extenders, jar openers, lever-style faucets, large cabinet knobs, step stools, and labor-saving devices like electric can openers, food processors, dishwashers, and slow cookers.
- **Personal care.** Adaptive equipment to make bathing and grooming easier includes handrails in the tub or shower, long-handled brushes or bath mitts, elevated toilet seats, and electric toothbrushes and razors.
- **Dressing.** Devices designed to assist people with arthritic limitations in getting dressed include sock pullers, zipper hooks, buttoning aids, and shoehorns.
- **Working.** Many types of workplace modifications and accommodations can help people with arthritis perform the functions of employment, including hands-free headsets, adjustable work tables, ergonomic workstation designs, and accessible restrooms.
- **Driving.** In addition to special car adaptations like steering wheel knobs, swivel seats, and wheelchair hoists, cars can be fitted with panoramic mirrors, seatbelt aids, and keyless entry and ignition systems to make driving easier for people with arthritis.

## References

1. "Self-Help Arthritis Devices," Arthritis Foundation, n.d.
2. "Assistive Devices for Easier Living with RA," WebMD, 2014.
3. Brichford, Connie. "Assistive Devices for Rheumatoid Arthritis," Everyday Health, 2015.

## Section 11.6 | **Chronic Pain**

This section includes text excerpted from "Chronic Pain Information Page," National Institute of Neurological Disorders and Stroke (NINDS), March 27, 2019.

While acute pain is a normal sensation triggered in the nervous system to alert you to possible injury and the need to take care of yourself, chronic pain is different. Chronic pain persists. Pain signals keep firing in the nervous system for weeks, months, even years. There may have been an initial mishap such as a sprained back, serious infection, or there may be an ongoing cause of pain such as arthritis, cancer, ear infection, but some people suffer chronic pain in the absence of any past injury or evidence of body damage. Many chronic pain conditions affect older adults. Common chronic pain complaints include headache, low back pain, cancer pain, arthritis pain, neurogenic pain (pain resulting from damage to the peripheral nerves or to the central nervous system itself), psychogenic pain (pain not due to past disease or injury or any visible sign of damage inside or outside the nervous system). A person may have two or more co-existing chronic pain conditions. Such conditions can include chronic fatigue syndrome, endometriosis, fibromyalgia, inflammatory bowel disease, interstitial cystitis, temporomandibular joint dysfunction, and vulvodynia. It is not known whether these disorders share a common cause.

### TREATMENT OF CHRONIC PAIN

Medications, acupuncture, local electrical stimulation, and brain stimulation, as well as surgery, are some treatments for chronic pain. Some physicians use placebos, which in some cases has resulted in a lessening or elimination of pain. Psychotherapy, relaxation and medication therapies, biofeedback, and behavior modification may also be employed to treat chronic pain.

### PROGNOSIS OF CHRONIC PAIN

Many people with chronic pain can be helped if they understand all the causes of pain and the many and varied steps that can be taken to undo what chronic pain has done. Scientists believe that advances in neuroscience will lead to more and better treatments for chronic pain in the years to come.

## Section 11.7 | **Repetitive Stress Injury**

This section contains text excerpted from the following sources: Text in this section begins with excerpts from "Prevention of Job-Related Musculoskeletal Disorders Draws National Audience at Conference Hosted by NIOSH, OSHA," Centers for Disease Control and Prevention (CDC), July 22, 2015. Reviewed November 2019; Text beginning with the heading "Repetitive Motion Disorder" is excerpted from "Repetitive Motion Disorders Information Page," National Institute of Neurological Disorders and Stroke (NINDS), March 27, 2019; Text under the heading "Warning Signs" is excerpted from "Repetitive Stress Injuries and Warning Signs," Lawerence Berkley National Laboratory, U.S. Department of Energy (DOE), April 26, 2019.

One of the fastest-growing threats to workplace safety and health—musculoskeletal disorders, which include conditions also known as "repetitive stress injuries" (RSIs) or "repetitive motion disorders" (RMDs)—is the subject of a major concern.

"By eliminating repetitive stress injuries, American companies could save $20 billion each year in workers' compensation," U.S. Labor Secretary Robert B. Reich said. Musculoskeletal disorders are the country's most costly category of workplace injuries and illnesses. In addition to spending $20 billion annually on workers' compensation costs due to RSIs, the U.S. spends another $100 billion on lost productivity, employee turnover, and other indirect expenses.

## REPETITIVE MOTION DISORDER

Repetitive motion disorders are a family of muscular conditions that result from repeated motions performed in the course of normal work or daily activities. RMDs include carpal tunnel syndrome, bursitis, tendonitis, epicondylitis, ganglion cyst, tenosynovitis, and trigger finger. RMDs are caused by too many uninterrupted repetitions of an activity or motion, unnatural or awkward motions such as twisting the arm or wrist, overexertion, incorrect posture, or muscle fatigue. RMDs occur most commonly in the hands, wrists, elbows, and shoulders, but can also happen in the neck, back, hips, knees, feet, legs, and ankles. The disorders are characterized by pain, tingling, numbness, visible swelling or redness of the affected area, and the loss of flexibility and strength. For some individuals, there may be no visible sign of injury, although they may find it hard to perform easy tasks Over time, RMDs can cause temporary or permanent damage to the soft tissues in the body—such as the muscles, nerves, tendons, and ligaments—and compression of nerves or tissue. Generally, RMDs affect individuals who perform repetitive tasks such as assembly line work, meatpacking, sewing, playing musical instruments, and computer work. The disorders may also affect individuals who engage in activities such as carpentry, gardening, and tennis.

## PROGNOSIS

Most individuals with RMDs recover completely and can avoid re-injury by changing the way they perform repetitive movements, the frequency with which they perform them, and the amount of time they rest between movements. Without treatment, RMDs may result in permanent injury and complete loss of function in the affected area.

## TREATMENT

Treatment for RMDs usually includes reducing or stopping the motions that cause symptoms. Options include taking breaks to give the affected area time to rest, and adopting stretching and relaxation exercises. Applying ice to the affected area and using medications such as pain relievers, cortisone, and anti-inflammatory drugs can reduce pain and swelling. Splints may be able to relieve pressure on the muscles and nerves. Physical therapy may relieve the soreness and pain in the muscles and joints. In rare cases, surgery may be required to relieve symptoms and prevent permanent damage. Some employers have developed ergonomic programs to help workers adjust their pace of work and arrange office equipment to minimize harm.

## WARNING SIGNS

Employees injured at work must report to Health Services in Building 26 for evaluation, treatment, and/or referral. Repetitive stress injuries are included in this policy.

If you experience tingling, numbness, swelling, or pain in your hand or wrist for several hours or more than one day, do not wait—report it. By their nature, repetitive stress injuries such as carpal tunnel syndrome become more serious over time. Early detection, evaluation, and treatment are essential to prevent serious injury.

Employees at risk for cumulative trauma disorders (CTDs) may experience some of the following symptoms:

- Numbness or a burning sensation in the arm, hand, or fingers, especially fingertips at night
- Reduced grip strength in the hand
- Swelling or stiffness in the joints, or decreased range of joint motion
- Pain from movement or pressure, in wrists, forearms, elbows, neck, or back
- Reduced range of motion in the shoulder, neck, or back
- Dry, itchy, or sore eyes
- Blurred or double vision
- Aching or tingling; cramping

After you report an ergonomic-related injury, a workstation evaluation by environmental health and safety (EH&S) management will be requested automatically by Health Services.

## Section 11.8 | Repetitive Stress Injuries in Teens

"Repetitive Stress Injuries in Teens," © 2018 Omnigraphics. Reviewed November 2019.

### WHAT ARE REPETITIVE STRESS INJURIES?

Repetitive stress injuries (RSIs) happen when undue pressure is placed on a part of the body repeatedly over an extended period of time. RSIs can cause pain, swelling, inflammation, muscle strains, spinal discs problems, and tendon or nerve damages. Sometimes, an RSI is also known as cumulative trauma disorder (CTD). These injuries are most often linked to work-related activities; however, in teens, they tend to occur while playing sports or during the regular use of computers, phones, and tablets.

Sports-related injuries may be referred to as overuse injuries, which frequently happen at growth plates—the area at the end of bones—as the bone cells multiply rapidly. When there is repeated stress for a long time in a particular area of the body, the joints and surrounding tissues get inflamed leading to an injury. The elbows, knees, shoulders, and heels are areas that are often affected by RSIs.

## CAUSES OF REPETITIVE STRESS INJURIES

Many activities can result in RSIs; however, some of the most common causes in teens can include:

- Typing, holding a mouse, or using a keyboard for a long period of time.
- Sports, such as tennis or football, that involve repetitive, forceful motions
- Playing video games and texting frequently
- Playing a musical instrument
- Working in cold temperatures
- Poorly designed equipment or tools
- Awkward posture
- Heavy lifting

## SYMPTOMS OF REPETITIVE STRESS INJURIES

An RSI is caused by physical stress; however, mental stress can worsen the condition. Some typical symptoms of RSI include:

- Weakness or tiredness in the hands or arms
- Stiffness or soreness in the neck and back area
- Pulsating or throbbing sensation in the muscles or joints
- Numbness, pain, or tingling in the affected area

If these symptoms are present, a healthcare provider needs to be consulted immediately. Even though these symptoms may tend to be intermittent, ignoring them can lead to even more serious issues.

## TYPES OF REPETITIVE STRESS INJURIES THAT AFFECT TEENS

There are more than 100 different types of RSIs. Some of them affect teens most often include:

- **Stress fractures.** When a bone undergoes repeated strain from walking, running, or jumping, tiny cracks can develop on the surface of the bone due to rhythmic and repetitive overloading. These are called "stress fractures."
- **Tendonitis.** Tendons are bands that connect muscles to bones. When the tendons become inflamed, the condition is known as tendonitis.
- **Bursitis.** A bursa is a sac filled with fluid that acts as a cushion for the joints. An inflammation or swelling of the bursa is known as bursitis.
- **Carpal tunnel syndrome.** The median nerve and a number of ligaments run through a space in the wrist called the "carpal tunnel." When swelling occurs in this area, the result is a disorder called "carpal tunnel syndrome."

Some other RSIs that can affect teens include Osgood-Schlatter disease in childhood, shin splints, patellofemoral syndrome, and epicondylitis.

## DIAGNOSIS AND TREATMENT OF REPETITIVE STRESS INJURIES

In order to diagnose RSI, a healthcare provider will generally begin by asking a series of questions about daily activities, repeated tasks, types of discomfort, and when and how pain is experienced. A doctor may order blood tests and x-rays to aid in the diagnosis. If RSI is not treated, it can become severe and possibly have permanent consequences.

Treatment is based on the type of RSI diagnosed; but in all cases, it's important to stop the repetitive motion and rest the affected area. Some types of commonly used treatments include:

- **Physical therapy.** Exercises or manual therapy under the direction of trained professional can help improve joint movement.
- **Bracing or splinting.** These can help protect the injury by immobilizing it and giving it time to heal.
- **Heat or cold treatment.** Warm or cold packs on the affected area can help bring relief.
- **Medications.** Anti-inflammatory painkillers and muscle relaxers may be prescribed by healthcare providers. In some cases, antidepressants or sleep aids might also be recommended.
- **Steroid injections.** These may be required to reduce inflammation, but only if it is severe, as adverse effects are possible.
- **Surgery.** If the condition is extremely serious and can't be treated by other means, surgery may be necessary.

## PREVENTION OF REPETITIVE STRESS INJURIES

Growing bodies are more prone to RSIs because of their rapid growth spurts. And modern teens tend to spend a lot of time on computers and phones, as well as engaging in sports and other physical activities, which make them particularly susceptible to RSIs. Below are some ways to help minimize the risk.

For computer-related injuries:

- Make sure the top of the computer screen is aligned to the forehead of the user.
- Sit upright in the chair with feet touching the ground and back resting on the back of the seat.
- Avoid slouching, since this can cause unnecessary strain on the neck, back, and spine.
- Ensure that fingers and wrists are aligned at the same level while typing.
- Avoid excessive texting.
- Take a break about every 30 minutes.

## Orthopedic and Musculoskeletal Rehabilitation

For sports-related injuries:

- Warm up and cool down before and after a workout or playing a game.
- Uses properly fitted sports gear.
- Alternate between different activities to avoid repetitive stress.

## References

1. Gavin, Mary L., MD. "Repetitive Stress Injuries," The Nemours Foundation/KidsHealth®, January 2014.
2. Newman, Tim. "Repetitive Strain Injury (RSI): Diagnosis, Symptoms, and Treatment," Medical News Today, September 8, 2017.
3. Pitchford, Keith, MD. "Your Teenager and Repetitive Stress Injuries," Great Lakes Orthopedics & Sports Medicine, December 16, 2016.
4. "Repetitive Stress Injuries Handbook," National Education Association (NEA), October 2004.
5. "Teen RSI—Repetitive Stress Injuries," Parentingteens.com, October 30, 2010.

# Chapter 12 | Neurorehabilitation

**Chapter Contents**

## Section 12.1 | **Spinal Cord Injury**

This section contains text excerpted from the following sources: Text beginning with the heading "What Is Spinal Cord Injury?" is excerpted from "Spinal Cord Injury Information Page," National Institute of Neurological Disorders and Stroke (NINDS), March 27, 2019; Text under the heading "How Does Rehabilitation Help People Recover from Spinal Cord Injuries?" is excerpted from "Spinal Cord Injury: Hope through Research," National Institute of Neurological Disorders and Stroke (NINDS), August 13, 2019.

### WHAT IS SPINAL CORD INJURY?

A spinal cord injury (SCI) usually begins with a sudden, traumatic blow to the spine that fractures or dislocates vertebrae. The damage begins at the moment of injury when displaced bone fragments, disc material, or ligaments bruise or tear into spinal cord tissue. Most injuries to the spinal cord do not completely sever it. Instead, an injury is more likely to cause fractures and compression of the vertebrae, which then crush and destroy axons—extensions of nerve cells that carry signals up and down the spinal cord between the brain and the rest of the body. An injury to the spinal cord can damage a few, many, or almost all of these axons. Some injuries will allow almost complete recovery. Others will result in complete paralysis.

### TREATMENT OF SPINAL CORD INJURY

Improved emergency care for people with spinal cord injuries and aggressive treatment and rehabilitation can minimize damage to the nervous system and even restore limited abilities. Respiratory complications are often an indication of the severity of spinal cord injury About one-third of those with injury to the neck area will need help with breathing and require respiratory support. The steroid drug methylprednisolone appears to reduce the damage to nerve cells if it is given within the first eight hours after injury. Rehabilitation programs combine physical therapies with skill-building activities and counseling to provide social and emotional support. Electrical simulation of nerves by neural prosthetic devices may restore specific functions, including bladder, breathing, cough, and arm or leg movements, though eligibility for use of these devices depends on the level and type of the spinal cord injury.

### PROGNOSIS OF SPINAL CORD INJURY

Spinal cord injuries are classified as either complete or incomplete. An incomplete injury means that the ability of the spinal cord to convey messages to or from the brain is not completely lost. People with incomplete injuries retain some motor or sensory function below the injury. A complete injury is indicated by a total lack of sensory and motor function below the level of injury. People who survive a SCI will most likely have medical complications such as chronic pain and bladder and bowel dysfunction, along with an increased susceptibility

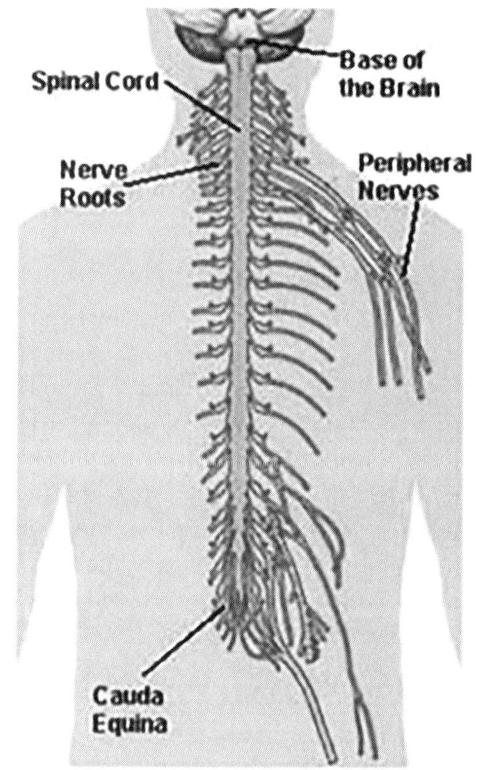


**Figure 12.1.** Anatomy of Spinal Cord
*(Source: National Institute of Cancer (NCI).)*

to respiratory and heart problems. Successful recovery depends upon how well these chronic conditions are handled day-to-day.

Surgery to relieve compression of the spinal tissue by surrounding bones broken or dislocated by the injury is often necessary, through timing of such surgery may vary widely.

## HOW DOES REHABILITATION HELP PEOPLE RECOVER FROM SPINAL CORD INJURIES?

No two people will experience the same emotions after surviving a spinal cord injury, but almost everyone will feel frightened, anxious, or confused about what has happened. It is common for people to have very mixed feelings: relief that they are still alive, but disbelief at the nature of their disabilities.

Rehabilitation programs combine physical therapies with skill-building activities and counseling to provide social and emotional support. The education and active involvement of the newly injured person and her or his family and friends is crucial.

## Neurorehabilitation

A rehabilitation team is usually led by a doctor specializing in physical medicine and rehabilitation (called a "physiatrist"), and often includes social workers, physical and occupational therapists, recreational therapists, rehabilitation nurses, rehabilitation psychologists, vocational counselors, nutritionists, a case worker, and other specialists.

In the initial phase of rehabilitation, therapists emphasize regaining communication skills and leg and arm strength. For some individuals, mobility will only be possible with the assistance of devices such as a walker, leg braces, or a wheelchair. Communication skills such as writing, typing, and using the telephone may also require adaptive devices for some people with tetraplegia.

Physical therapy includes exercise programs geared toward muscle strengthening. Occupational therapy helps redevelop fine motor skills, particularly those needed to perform activities of daily living such as getting in and out of a bed, self-grooming, and eating. Bladder and bowel management programs teach basic toileting routines. People acquire coping strategies for recurring episodes of spasticity, autonomic dysreflexia, and neurogenic pain.

Vocational rehabilitation includes identifying the person's basic work skills and physical and cognitive capabilities to determine the likelihood for employment; identifying potential workplaces and any assistive equipment that will be needed; and arranging for a user-friendly workplace. If necessary, educational training is provided to develop skills for a new line of work that may be less dependent upon physical abilities and more dependent upon computer or communication skills. Individuals with disabilities that prevent them from returning to the workforce are encouraged to maintain productivity by participating in activities that provide a sense of satisfaction and self-esteem, such as educational classes, hobbies, memberships in special interest groups, and participation in family and community events.

Recreation therapy encourages people with SCI to participate in recreational sports or activities at their level of mobility, as well as achieve a more balanced and normal lifestyle that provides opportunities for socialization and self-expression.

Adaptive devices also may help people with spinal cord injury to regain independence and improve mobility and quality of life. Such devices may include a wheelchair, electronic stimulators, assisted gait training, neural prostheses, computer adaptations, and other computer-assisted technology.

## Section 12.2 | **Traumatic Brain Injury**

This section contains text excerpted from the following sources: Text in this section begins with excerpts from "TBI: Get the Facts," Centers for Disease Control and Prevention (CDC), March 11, 2019; Text under the heading "Rehabilitation Therapies" is excerpted from "What Are the Treatments for TBI?" *Eunice Kennedy Shriver* National Institute of Child Health and Human Development (NICHD), December 1, 2016. Reviewed November 2019.

Traumatic brain injury (TBI) is a major cause of death and disability in the United States. From 2006 to 2014, the number of TBI-related emergency department visits, hospitalizations, and deaths increased by 53 percent. In 2014, an average of 155 people in the United States died each day from injuries that include a TBI. Those who survive a TBI can face effects that last a few days, or the rest of their lives. Effects of TBI can include impairments related to thinking or memory, movement, sensation (e.g., vision or hearing), or emotional functioning (e.g., personality changes, depression). These issues not only affect individuals but also can have lasting effects on families and communities.

### WHAT IS A TRAUMATIC BRAIN INJURY?

A TBI is caused by a bump, blow, or jolt to the head that disrupts the normal function of the brain. Not all blows or jolts to the head result in a TBI. The severity of a TBI may range from "mild" (i.e., a brief change in mental status or consciousness) to "severe" (i.e., an extended period of unconsciousness or memory loss after the injury). Most TBIs that occur each year are mild, commonly called "concussions."

### WHAT ARE THE LEADING CAUSES OF TRAUMATIC BRAIN INJURY?

- In 2014, falls were the leading cause of TBI. Falls accounted for almost half (48%) of all TBI-related emergency department (ED) visits. Falls disproportionately affect children and older adults:
  - Almost half (49%) of TBI-related ED visits among children 0 to 17 years were caused by falls.
  - Nearly 4 in 5 (81%) TBI-related ED visits in older adults aged 65 years and older were caused by falls.
- Being struck by or against an object was the second leading cause of TBI-related ED visits, accounting for about 17 percent of all TBI-related ED visits in the United States in 2014.
- Over 1 in 4 (28%) TBI-related ED visits in children less than 17 years of age or less were caused by being struck by or against an object.
- Falls and motor vehicle crashes were the first and second leading causes of all TBI-related hospitalizations (52% and 20%, respectively).
- Intentional self-harm was the first leading cause of TBI-related deaths (33%) in 2014.

**Table 12.1.** Categories of Symptoms

| Thinking Remembering | Physical | Emotional Mood | Sleep |
|---|---|---|---|
| Difficulty thinking clearly | Headache<br>Fuzzy or blurry vision | Irritability | Sleeping more than usual |
| Feeling slowed down | Nausea or vomiting (early on)<br>Dizziness | Sadness | Sleep less than usual |
| Difficulty concentrating | Sensitivity to noise or light<br>Balance problems | More emotional | Trouble falling asleep |
| Difficulty remembering new information | Feeling tired, having no energy | Nervousness or anxiety | |

## SYMPTOMS OF TRAUMATIC BRAIN INJURY

Most people with a TBI recover well from symptoms experienced at the time of the injury. Most TBIs that occur each year are mild, commonly called "concussions" which is a mild TBI. But, for some people, symptoms can last for days, weeks, or longer. In general, recovery may be slower among older adults, young children, and teens. Those who have had a TBI in the past are also at risk of having another one. Some people may also find that it takes longer to recover if they have another TBI.

Some of these symptoms may appear right away. Others may not be noticed for days or months after the injury, or until the person resumes their everyday life. Sometimes, people do not recognize or admit that they are having problems. Others may not understand their problems and how the symptoms they are experiencing impact their daily activities.

The signs and symptoms of a concussion can be difficult to sort out. Early on, problems may be overlooked by the person with the concussion, family members, or doctors. People may look fine even though they are acting or feeling differently.

## POTENTIAL EFFECTS OF SEVERE TRAUMATIC BRAIN INJURY

The long-term effects of a TBI have been described as being similar to the effects of a chronic disease. Individuals who experience mild TBI are more likely to recover from their initial injury symptoms, although some individuals experience longer-term effects. Individuals who experience more severe TBI are more likely to have lasting effects from the injury.

A TBI may lead to a wide range of short- or long-term issues affecting:

- Cognitive function (attention and memory)
- Motor function (extremity weakness, impaired coordination and balance)

- Sensation (hearing, vision, impaired perception and touch)
- Behavior (emotional regulation, depression, anxiety, aggression, impairments in behavioral control, personality changes)

A severe TBI may lead to death, or result in an extended period of unconsciousness (coma) or amnesia. Individuals may experience significant changes in thinking and behavior. Moderate-to-severe TBI may also result in a reduced lifespan.

The consequences of severe TBI can affect all aspects of an individual's life, including relationships with family and friends, the ability to progress at school or work, doing household tasks, driving, or participating in other daily activities.

## REHABILITATION THERAPIES

Therapies can help someone with TBI relearn skills such as walking or cooking, or develop strategies for self-care, such as making lists of the steps involved in getting dressed. Rehabilitation can include several different kinds of therapy for physical, emotional, and cognitive difficulties. Depending on the injury, these treatments may be needed only briefly after the injury, occasionally throughout a person's life, or on an ongoing basis.

### Types of Therapies for Traumatic Brain Injury

Most people with moderate to severe brain injury will need some type of rehabilitation therapy to address physical, emotional, and cognitive issues from the TBI. Therapies will likely include relearning old skills or learning new ways to make up for lost skills. A treatment program should be designed to meet each person's specific needs and to strengthen her or his ability to function at home and in the community.

Therapy usually begins in the hospital and can continue in a number of possible settings, including in a skilled nursing facility, at home, in school, and in an outpatient program at a clinic. Therapy can be brief or long-term, depending on the type of injury, and it may need to change over time. Rehabilitation generally involves a number of healthcare specialists, the person's family, and a person who manages the team. When devising a long-term treatment plan, patients, their families, and their providers should be aware that moderate and severe TBI impairs patients' ability to make sound medical decisions even a month after injury.

Types of rehabilitation therapy may include:

- **Physical therapy**. This treatment works to build physical strength, coordination, and flexibility.
- **Occupational therapy**. An occupational therapist helps a person learn or relearn how to perform daily tasks, such as getting dressed, cooking, and bathing.

- **Speech therapy**. This therapy works on the ability to form words and other communication skills as well as how to use special communication devices if necessary. Speech therapy can also include evaluation and treatment of swallowing disorders (dysphagia).
- **Psychological counseling**. A counselor can help a person learn coping skills, work on relationships, and improve general emotional well-being.
- **Vocational counseling**. This type of rehabilitation focuses on a person's ability to return to work, find appropriate opportunities, and deal with workplace challenges.
- **Cognitive therapy**. This includes activities designed to improve memory, attention, perception, learning, planning, and judgment. For many people with TBI, cognitive therapy is among the most common types of rehabilitation.

## Section 12.3 | **Stroke**

This section contains text excerpted from the following sources: Text under the heading "What Is Stroke?" is excerpted from "Stroke: Hope through Research," National Institute of Neurological Disorders and Stroke (NINDS), August 13, 2019; Text beginning with the heading "What Is Poststroke Rehabilitation?" is excerpted from "Poststroke Rehabilitation Fact Sheet," National Institute of Neurological Disorders and Stroke (NINDS), August 13, 2019; Text under the heading "Preventing Another Stroke" is excerpted from "Recovering from Stroke," Centers for Disease Control and Prevention (CDC), March 27, 2018.

### WHAT IS STROKE?

A stroke occurs when the blood supply to part of the brain is suddenly interrupted or when a blood vessel in the brain bursts, spilling blood into the spaces surrounding brain cells. In the same way that a person suffering a loss of blood flow to the heart is said to be having a heart attack, a person with a loss of blood flow to the brain or sudden bleeding in the brain can be said to be having a "brain attack."

Brain cells die when they no longer receive oxygen and nutrients from the blood or when they are damaged by sudden bleeding into or around the brain. Ischemia is the term used to describe the loss of oxygen and nutrients for brain cells when there is inadequate blood flow. Ischemia ultimately leads to infarction, the death of brain cells which are eventually replaced by a fluid-filled cavity (or infarct) in the injured brain.

When blood flow to the brain is interrupted, some brain cells die immediately, while others remain at risk for death. These damaged cells make up the ischemic

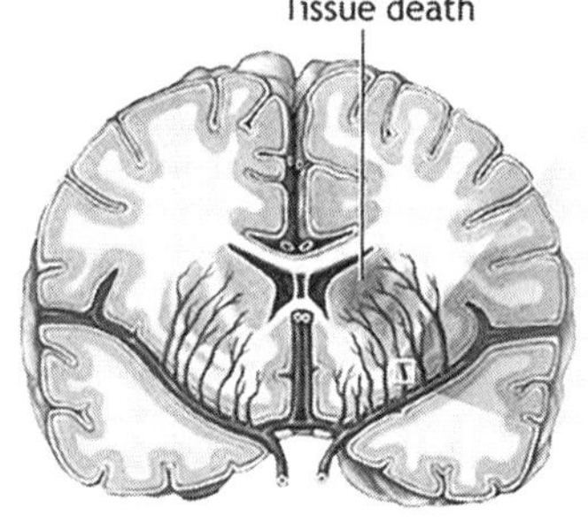


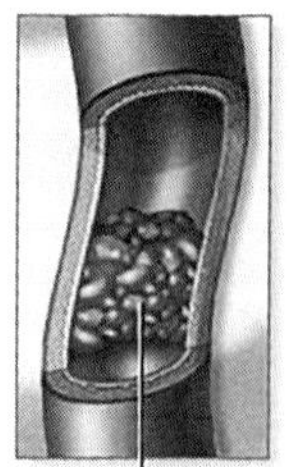


**Figure 12.2.** An Example of Stroke *(Source: Centers for Disease Control and Prevention (CDC).)*

penumbra and can linger in a compromised state for several hours. With timely treatment these cells can be saved.

Even though a stroke occurs in the unseen reaches of the brain, the symptoms of a stroke are easy to spot. They include sudden numbness or weakness, especially on one side of the body; sudden confusion or trouble speaking or understanding speech; sudden trouble seeing in one or both eyes; sudden trouble walking, dizziness, or loss of balance or coordination; or sudden severe headache with no known cause. All of the symptoms of stroke appear suddenly, and often there is more than one symptom at the same time. Therefore, stroke can usually be distinguished from other causes of dizziness or headache. These symptoms may indicate that a stroke has occurred and that medical attention is needed immediately.

## WHAT IS POSTSTROKE REHABILITATION?

Rehabilitation helps stroke survivors relearn skills that are lost when part of the brain is damaged. For example, these skills can include coordinating leg movements in order to walk or carrying out the steps involved in any complex activity. Rehabilitation also teaches survivors new ways of performing tasks to circumvent or compensate for any residual disabilities. Individuals may need to learn how to bathe and dress using only one hand, or how to communicate effectively when their ability to use language has been compromised. There is a strong consensus among rehabilitation experts that the most important element in any rehabilitation program is carefully directed, well-focused, repetitive practice—the same kind of practice used by all people when they learn a new skill, such as playing the piano or pitching a baseball.

Rehabilitative therapy begins in the acute-care hospital after the person's overall condition has been stabilized, often within 24 to 48 hours after the stroke. The first steps involve promoting independent movement because many individuals are paralyzed or seriously weakened. Patients are prompted to change positions frequently while lying in bed and to engage in passive or active range of motion exercises to strengthen their stroke-impaired limbs. ("Passive" range-of-motion exercises are those in which the therapist actively helps the patient move a limb repeatedly, whereas "active" exercises are performed by the patient with no physical assistance from the therapist.) Depending on many factors—including the extent of the initial injury—patients may progress from sitting up and being moved between the bed and a chair to standing, bearing their own weight, and walking, with or without assistance. Rehabilitation nurses and therapists help patients who are able to perform progressively more complex and demanding tasks, such as bathing, dressing, and using the toilet, and they encourage patients to begin using their stroke-impaired limbs while engaging in those tasks. Beginning to reacquire the ability to carry out these basic activities of daily living represents the first stage in a stroke survivor's return to independence.

For some stroke survivors, rehabilitation will be an ongoing process to maintain and refine skills and could involve working with specialists for months or years after the stroke.

## WHAT DISABILITIES CAN RESULT FROM A STROKE?

The types and degrees of disability that follow a stroke depend upon which area of the brain is damaged. Generally, stroke can cause five types of disabilities: paralysis or problems controlling movement; sensory disturbances including pain; problems using or understanding language; challenges involving thinking and memory; and emotional disturbances.

### Paralysis or Problems Controlling Movement (Motor Control)

Paralysis is one of the most common disabilities resulting from stroke. The paralysis is usually on the side of the body opposite the side of the brain damaged by stroke, and may affect the face, an arm, a leg, or the entire side of the body. This one-sided paralysis is called "hemiplegia" (one-sided weakness is called "hemiparesis"). Stroke patients with hemiparesis or hemiplegia may have difficulty with everyday activities such as walking or grasping objects. Some stroke patients have challenges involving swallowing, called "dysphagia," due to damage to the part of the brain that controls the muscles for swallowing. Damage to a lower part of the brain, the cerebellum, can affect the body's ability to coordinate movement, a disability called "ataxia," leading to challenges involving body posture, walking, and balance.

### Sensory Disturbances Including Pain

Stroke patients may lose the ability to feel touch, pain, temperature, or position. Sensory deficits may also hinder the ability to recognize objects that patients are holding and can even be severe enough to cause loss of recognition of one's own limb. Some stroke patients experience pain, numbness or odd sensations of tingling or prickling in paralyzed or weakened limbs, a symptom known as "paresthesias."

The loss of urinary continence is fairly common immediately after a stroke and often results from a combination of sensory and motor deficits. Stroke survivors may lose the ability to sense the need to urinate or the ability to control bladder muscles. Some may lack enough mobility to reach a toilet in time. Loss of bowel control or constipation also may occur. Permanent incontinence after a stroke is uncommon, but even a temporary loss of bowel or bladder control can be emotionally difficult for stroke survivors.

Stroke survivors frequently have a variety of chronic pain syndromes resulting from stroke-induced damage to the nervous system (neuropathic pain). In some stroke patients, pathways for sensation in the brain are damaged, causing the transmission of false signals that result in the sensation of pain in a limb or side of the body that has the sensory deficit. The most common of these pain syndromes is called "thalamic pain syndrome" (caused by a stroke to the thalamus, which processes sensory information from the body to the brain), which can be difficult to treat even with medications. Finally, some pain that occurs after stroke is not due to nervous system damage, but rather to mechanical problems caused by the weakness from the stroke. Patients who have a seriously weakened or paralyzed arm commonly experience moderate to severe pain that radiates outward from the shoulder. Most often, the pain results from lack of movement in a joint that has been immobilized for a prolonged period of time (such as having your arm or shoulder in a cast for weeks) and the tendons and ligaments around the joint become fixed in one position. This is commonly called a "frozen" joint. Passive movement (the joint is gently moved or flexed by a therapist or caregiver rather than by the individual) at the joint in a paralyzed limb is essential to prevent painful "freezing" and to allow easy movement if and when voluntary motor strength returns.

## Problems Using or Understanding Language (Aphasia)

At least one-fourth of all stroke survivors experience language impairments, involving the ability to speak, write, and understand spoken and written language. A stroke-induced injury to any of the brain's language-control centers can severely impair verbal communication. The dominant centers for language are in the left side of the brain for right-handed individuals and many left-handers as well. Damage to a language center located on the dominant side of the brain, known as "Broca's area," causes expressive aphasia. People with this type of aphasia have difficulty conveying their thoughts through words or writing. They lose the ability to speak the words they are thinking and to put words together in coherent, grammatically correct sentences. In contrast, damage to a language center located in a rear portion of the brain, called "Wernicke's area," results in receptive aphasia. People with this condition have difficulty understanding spoken or written language and often have incoherent speech. Although they can form grammatically correct sentences, their utterances are often devoid of meaning. The most severe form of aphasia, global aphasia, is caused by extensive damage to several areas of the brain involved in language function. People with global aphasia lose nearly all their linguistic abilities; they cannot understand language or use it to convey thought.

### Challenges Involving Thinking and Memory

Stroke can cause damage to parts of the brain responsible for memory, learning, and awareness. Stroke survivors may have dramatically shortened attention spans or may experience deficits in short-term memory. Individuals also may lose their ability to make plans, comprehend meaning, learn new tasks, or engage in other complex mental activities. Two fairly common deficits resulting from stroke are anosognosia, an inability to acknowledge the reality of the physical impairments resulting from stroke, and neglect, the loss of the ability to respond to objects or sensory stimuli located on the stroke-impaired side. Stroke survivors who develop apraxia (loss of ability to carry out learned purposeful movement) cannot plan the steps involved in a complex task and act on them in the proper sequence. Stroke survivors with apraxia may also have problems following a set of instructions. Apraxia appears to be caused by a disruption of the subtle connections that exist between thought and action.

### Emotional Disturbances

Many people who survive a stroke feel fear, anxiety, frustration, anger, sadness, and a sense of grief for their physical and mental losses. These feelings are a natural response to the psychological trauma of stroke. Some emotional disturbances and personality changes are caused by the physical effects of brain damage. Clinical depression, which is a sense of hopelessness that disrupts an individual's ability to function, appears to be the emotional disorder most commonly experienced by stroke survivors. Signs of clinical depression include sleep disturbances, a radical change in eating patterns that may lead to sudden weight loss or gain, lethargy, social withdrawal, irritability, fatigue, self-loathing, and suicidal thoughts. Poststroke depression can be treated with antidepressant medications and psychological counseling.

## WHAT MEDICAL PROFESSIONALS SPECIALIZE IN POSTSTROKE REHABILITATION?

Poststroke rehabilitation involves physicians; rehabilitation nurses; physical, occupational, recreational, speech-language, and vocational therapists; and mental-health professionals.

### Physicians

Physicians have the primary responsibility for managing and coordinating the long-term care of stroke survivors, including recommending which rehabilitation programs will best address individual needs. Physicians also are responsible for caring for the stroke survivor's general health and providing guidance aimed at preventing a second stroke, such as controlling high blood pressure or diabetes and eliminating risk factors such as cigarette smoking, excessive weight, a high-cholesterol diet, and high alcohol consumption.

Neurologists usually lead acute-care stroke teams and direct patient care during hospitalization. They sometimes participate on the long-term rehabilitation team. Other subspecialists often lead the rehabilitation stage of care, especially physiatrists, who specialize in physical medicine and rehabilitation.

### Rehabilitation Nurses

Nurses specializing in rehabilitation help survivors relearn how to carry out the basic activities of daily living. They also educate survivors about routine healthcare, such as how to follow a medication schedule, how to care for the skin, how to move out of bed and into a wheelchair, and special needs for people with diabetes. Rehabilitation nurses also work with survivors to reduce risk factors that may lead to a second stroke, and provide training for caregivers.

Nurses are closely involved in helping stroke survivors manage personal care issues, such as bathing and controlling incontinence. Most stroke survivors regain their ability to maintain continence, often with the help of strategies learned during rehabilitation. These strategies include strengthening pelvic muscles through special exercises and following a timed voiding schedule. If challenges involving incontinence continue, nurses can help caregivers learn to insert and manage catheters and to take special hygienic measures to prevent other incontinence-related health problems from developing.

### Physical Therapists

Physical therapists specialize in treating disabilities related to motor and sensory impairments. They are trained in all aspects of anatomy and physiology related to normal function, with an emphasis on movement. They assess the stroke survivor's strength, endurance, range of motion, gait abnormalities, and sensory deficits to design individualized rehabilitation programs aimed at regaining control over motor functions.

Physical therapists help survivors regain the use of stroke-impaired limbs, teach compensatory strategies to reduce the effect of remaining deficits, and establish ongoing exercise programs to help people retain their newly learned skills. People with a disability tend to avoid using impaired limbs, a behavior called "learned nonuse." However, the repetitive use of impaired limbs encourages brain plasticity and helps reduce disabilities.

### Neurorehabilitation

Strategies used by physical therapists to encourage the use of impaired limbs include selective sensory stimulation such as tapping or stroking, active and passive range-of-motion exercises, and temporary restraint of healthy limbs while practicing motor tasks.

In general, physical therapy emphasizes practicing isolated movements, repeatedly changing from one kind of movement to another, and rehearsing complex movements that require a great deal of coordination and balance, such as walking up or downstairs or moving safely between obstacles. People too weak to bear their own weight can still practice repetitive movements during hydrotherapy (in which water provides sensory stimulation as well as weight support) or while being partially supported by a harness. A trend in physical therapy emphasizes the effectiveness of engaging in goal-directed activities, such as playing games, to promote coordination. Physical therapists frequently employ selective sensory stimulation to encourage the use of impaired limbs and to help survivors with neglect regain awareness of stimuli on the neglected side of the body.

## Occupational and Recreational Therapists

Occupational therapists are concerned with improving motor and sensory abilities, and ensuring patient safety in the poststroke period. They help survivors relearn skills needed for performing self-directed activities (also called "occupations") such as personal grooming, preparing meals, and house cleaning. Therapists can teach some survivors how to adapt to driving and provide on-road training. They often teach people to divide a complex activity into its component parts, practice each part, and then perform the whole sequence of actions. This strategy can improve coordination and may help people with apraxia relearn how to carry out planned actions.

Occupational therapists also teach people how to develop compensatory strategies and change elements of their environment that limit activities of daily living. For example, people with the use of only one hand can substitute hook and loop fasteners (such as Velcro) for buttons on clothing. Occupational therapists also help people make changes in their homes to increase safety, remove barriers, and facilitate physical functioning, such as installing grab bars in bathrooms.

Recreational therapists help people with a variety of disabilities to develop and use their leisure time to enhance their health, independence, and quality of life.

## Speech-Language Pathologists

Speech-language pathologists help stroke survivors with aphasia relearn how to use language or develop alternative means of communication. They also help people improve their ability to swallow, and they work with patients to develop problem-solving and social skills needed to cope with the after-effects of a stroke.

Many specialized therapeutic techniques have been developed to assist people with aphasia. Some forms of short-term therapy can improve comprehension rapidly. Intensive exercises such as repeating the therapist's words, practicing following directions, and doing reading or writing exercises form the cornerstone of language rehabilitation. Conversational coaching and rehearsal, as well as the development of prompts or cues to help people remember specific words, are sometimes beneficial. Speech-language pathologists also help stroke survivors develop strategies for circumventing language disabilities. These strategies can include the use of symbol boards or sign language. Advances in computer technology have spurred the development of new types of equipment to enhance communication.

Speech-language pathologists use special types of imaging techniques to study swallowing patterns of stroke survivors and identify the exact source of their impairment. Difficulties with swallowing have many possible causes, including a delayed swallowing reflex, an inability to manipulate food with the tongue, or an inability to detect food remaining lodged in the cheeks after swallowing. When the cause has been pinpointed, speech-language pathologists work with the individual to devise strategies to overcome or minimize the deficit. Sometimes, simply changing body position and improving posture during eating can bring about improvement. The texture of foods can be modified to make swallowing easier; for example, thin liquids, which often cause choking, can be thickened. Changing eating habits by taking small bites and chewing slowly can also help alleviate dysphagia.

### Vocational Therapists

Approximately one-fourth of all strokes occur in people between the ages of 45 and 65. For most people in this age group, returning to work is a major concern. Vocational therapists perform many of the same functions that ordinary career counselors do. They can help people with residual disabilities identify vocational strengths and develop résumés that highlight those strengths. They also can help identify potential employers, assist in specific job searches, and provide referrals to stroke vocational rehabilitation agencies.

Most important, vocational therapists educate individuals with a disability about their rights and protections as defined by the Americans with Disabilities Act of 1990. This law requires employers to make "reasonable accommodations" for employees with disabilities. Vocational therapists frequently act as mediators between employers and employees to negotiate the provision of reasonable accommodations in the workplace.

## WHEN CAN A STROKE PATIENT BEGIN REHABILITATION?

Rehabilitation should begin as soon as a stroke patient is stable, sometimes within 24 to 48 hours after a stroke. This first stage of rehabilitation can occur within an acute-care hospital; however, it is very dependent on the unique circumstances of the individual patient.

The largest stroke rehabilitation study in the United States, researchers compared two common techniques to help stroke patients improve their walking. Both methods—training on a body-weight supported treadmill or working on strength and balance exercises at home with a physical therapist—resulted in equal improvements in the individual's ability to walk by the end of one year. Researchers found that functional improvements could be seen as late as one year after the stroke, which goes against the conventional wisdom that most recovery is complete by six months. The trial showed that 52 percent of the participants made significant improvements in walking, everyday function and quality of life, regardless of how severe their impairment was, or whether they started training at 2 or 6 months after the stroke.

## WHERE CAN A STROKE PATIENT GET REHABILITATION?

At the time of discharge from the hospital, the stroke patient and family coordinate with hospital social workers to locate a suitable living arrangement. Many stroke survivors return home, but some move into some type of medical facility.

### Inpatient Rehabilitation Units

Inpatient facilities may be freestanding or part of larger hospital complexes. Patients stay in the facility, usually for 2 to 3 weeks, and engage in a coordinated, intensive program of rehabilitation. Such programs often involve at least 3 hours of active therapy a day, 5 or 6 days a week. Inpatient facilities offer a comprehensive range of medical services, including full-time physician supervision and access to the full range of therapists specializing in poststroke rehabilitation.

### Outpatient Units

Outpatient facilities are often part of a larger hospital complex and provide access to physicians and the full range of therapists specializing in stroke rehabilitation. Patients typically spend several hours, often three days each week at the facility taking part in coordinated therapy sessions and return home at night. Comprehensive outpatient facilities frequently offer treatment programs as intense as those of inpatient facilities, but they also can offer less demanding regimens, depending on the patient's physical capacity.

### Nursing Facilities

Rehabilitative services available at nursing facilities are more variable than are those at inpatient and outpatient units. Skilled nursing facilities usually place a greater emphasis on rehabilitation, whereas traditional nursing homes emphasize residential care. In addition, fewer hours of therapy are offered compared to outpatient and inpatient rehabilitation units.

### Home-Based Rehabilitation Programs

Home rehabilitation allows for great flexibility so that patients can tailor their program of rehabilitation and follow individual schedules. Stroke survivors may participate in an intensive level of therapy several hours per week or follow a less demanding regimen. These arrangements are often best suited for people who require treatment by only one type of rehabilitation therapist. Patients dependent on Medicare coverage for their rehabilitation must meet Medicare's "homebound" requirements to qualify for such services; at this time lack of transportation is not a valid reason for home therapy. The major disadvantage of home-based rehabilitation programs is the lack of specialized equipment. However, undergoing treatment at home gives people the advantage of practicing skills and developing compensatory strategies in the context of their own living environment. In the stroke rehabilitation trial, intensive balance and strength rehabilitation in the home was equivalent to treadmill training at a rehabilitation facility in improving walking.

## PREVENTING ANOTHER STROKE

If you have had a stroke, you are at high risk for another stroke:

- One in four strokes each year are recurrent.
- The chance of stroke within 90 days of a transient ischemic attack (TIA) may be as high as 17 percent, with the greatest risk during the first week.

That is why it is important to treat the causes of stroke, including heart disease, high blood pressure, atrial fibrillation (fast, irregular heartbeat), high cholesterol, and diabetes. Your doctor may prescribe you medicine or tell you to change your diet, exercise, or adopt other healthy lifestyle habits. Surgery may also be helpful in some cases.

# Section 12.4 | Guillain-Barré Syndrome

This section includes text excerpted from "Guillain-Barré Syndrome Fact Sheet," National Institute of Neurological Disorders and Stroke (NINDS), August 13, 2019.

## WHAT IS GUILLAIN-BARRÉ SYNDROME?

Guillain-Barré syndrome (GBS) is a rare neurological disorder in which the body's immune system mistakenly attacks part of its peripheral nervous system—the network of nerves located outside of the brain and spinal cord. GBS can range from a very mild case with brief weakness to nearly devastating paralysis, leaving the person unable to breathe independently. Fortunately, most people eventually recover from even the most severe cases of GBS. After recovery, some people will continue to have some degree of weakness.

Guillain-Barré syndrome can affect anyone. It can strike at any age (although it is more frequent in adults and older people) and both sexes are equally prone to the disorder. GBS is estimated to affect about one person in 100,000 each year.

## WHAT CAUSES GUILLAIN-BARRÉ SYNDROME

The exact cause of GBS is not known. Researchers do not know why it strikes some people and not others. It is not contagious or inherited.

What they do know is that the affected person's immune system begins to attack the body itself. It is thought that, at least in some cases, this immune attack is initiated to fight an infection and that some chemicals on infecting bacteria and viruses resemble those on nerve cells, which, in turn, also become targets of attack. Since the body's own immune system does the damage, GBS is called an "autoimmune disease" ("auto" meaning "self"). Normally the immune system uses antibodies (molecules produced in an immune response) and special white blood cells to protect us by attacking infecting microorganisms (bacteria and viruses). In Guillain-Barré syndrome, however, the immune system mistakenly attacks the healthy nerves.

Most cases usually start a few days or weeks following a respiratory or gastrointestinal viral infection. Occasionally surgery will trigger the syndrome. In rare cases vaccinations may increase the risk of GBS. Some countries worldwide reported an increased incidence of GBS following infection with the Zika virus.

## WHAT ARE THE SYMPTOMS OF GUILLAIN-BARRÉ SYNDROME?

Unexplained sensations often occur first, such as tingling in the feet or hands, or even pain (especially in children), often starting in the legs or back. Children will also show symptoms with difficulty walking and may refuse to walk. These sensations tend to disappear before the major, longer-term symptoms appear. Weakness on both sides of the body is the major symptom that prompts most people to seek medical attention. The weakness may first appear as difficulty climbing stairs or walking. Symptoms often affect the arms, breathing muscles, and even the face, reflecting more widespread nerve damage. Occasionally symptoms start in the upper body and move down to the legs and feet.

Most people reach the greatest stage of weakness within the first two weeks after symptoms appear; by the third, week 90 percent of affected individuals are at their weakest.

In addition to muscle weakness, symptoms may include:

- Difficulty with eye muscles and vision
- Difficulty swallowing, speaking, or chewing
- Pricking or pins and needles sensations in the hands and feet

- Pain that can be severe, particularly at night
- Coordination problems and unsteadiness
- Abnormal heartbeat/rate or blood pressure
- Challenges involving digestion and/or bladder control

These symptoms can increase in intensity over a period of hours, days, or weeks until certain muscles cannot be used at all and, when severe, the person is almost totally paralyzed. In these cases, the disorder is life-threatening—potentially interfering with breathing and, at times, with blood pressure or heart rate.

## WHAT HAPPENS IN GUILLAIN-BARRÉ SYNDROME

Many of the body's nerves are similar to household wires. There is a central conducting core in the nerves called the "axon" that carries an electric signal. The axon (an extension of a nerve cell) is surrounded by a covering, such as insulation, called "myelin." The myelin sheath surrounding the axon speeds up the transmission of nerve signals and allows the transmission of signals over long distances.

### Weakness

When we move, for example, an electric signal from the brain travels through and out of the spinal cord to peripheral nerves along muscles of the legs, arms, and elsewhere—called "motor nerves." In most cases of GBS, the immune system damages the myelin sheath that surrounds the axons of many peripheral nerves; however, it also may also damage the axons themselves. As a result, the nerves cannot transmit signals efficiently and the muscles begin to lose their ability to respond to the brain's commands. This causes weakness.

The weakness seen in GBS usually comes on quickly and worsens over hours or days. Symptoms are usually equal on both sides of the body. In addition to weak limbs, muscles controlling breathing can weaken to the point that the person must be attached to a machine to help support breathing.

### Sensation Changes

Since nerves are damaged in GBS, the brain may receive abnormal sensory signals from the rest of the body. This results in unexplained, spontaneous sensations, called "paresthesias," that may be experienced as tingling, a sense of insects crawling under the skin (called "formications"), and pain. Deep muscular pain may be experienced in the back and/or legs.

## REHABILITATIVE CARE

As individuals begin to improve, they are usually transferred from the acute care hospital to a rehabilitation setting. Here, they can regain strength, receive physical rehabilitation and other therapy to resume activities of daily living, and prepare to return to their preillness life.

Complications in GBS can affect several parts of the body. Often, even before recovery begins, caregivers may use several methods to prevent or treat complications. For example, a therapist may be instructed to manually move and position the person's limbs to help keep the muscles flexible and prevent muscle shortening. Injections of blood thinners can help prevent dangerous blood clots from forming in leg veins. Inflatable cuffs may also be placed around the legs to provide intermittent compression. All or any of these methods helps prevent blood stagnation and sludging (the buildup of red blood cells in veins, which could lead to reduced blood flow) in the leg veins. Muscle strength may not return uniformly; some muscles that get stronger faster may tend to take over a function that weaker muscles normally perform—called "substitution." The therapist should select specific exercises to improve the strength of the weaker muscles so their original function can be regained.

Occupational and vocational therapy help individuals learn new ways to handle everyday functions that may be affected by the disease, as well as work demands and the need for assistive devices and other adaptive equipment and technology.

## Section 12.5 | **Multiple Sclerosis**

This section includes text excerpted from "Multiple Sclerosis: Hope through Research," National Institute of Neurological Disorders and Stroke (NINDS), August 13, 2019.

Multiple sclerosis (MS) is the most common disabling neurological disease of young adults. It most often appears when people are between 20 to 40 years old. However, it can also affect children and older people.

The course of MS is unpredictable. A small number of those with MS will have a mild course with little to no disability, while another smaller group will have a steadily worsening disease that leads to increased disability over time. Most people with MS, however, will have short periods of symptoms followed by long stretches of relative relief, with partial or full recovery. There is no way to predict, at the beginning, how an individual person's disease will progress.

### WHAT IS MULTIPLE SCLEROSIS?

Multiple sclerosis is a neuroinflammatory disease that affects myelin, a substance that makes up the membrane (called the "myelin sheath") that wraps around nerve fibers (axons). Myelinated axons are commonly called "white

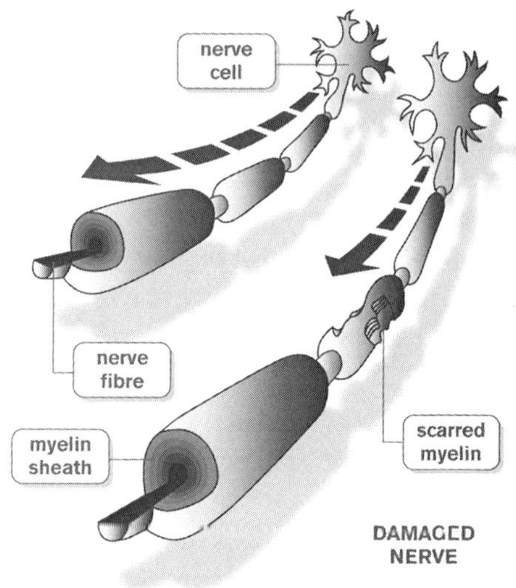


**Figure 12.3.** A Healthy Nerve and A Damaged Nerve
*(Source: U.S. Department of Veterans Affairs (VA).)*

matter." Researchers have learned that MS also damages the nerve cell bodies, which are found in the brain's gray matter, as well as the axons themselves in the brain, spinal cord, and optic nerve (the nerve that transmits visual information from the eye to the brain). As the disease progresses, the brain's cortex shrinks (cortical atrophy).

The term multiple sclerosis refers to the distinctive areas of scar tissue (sclerosis or plaques) that are visible in the white matter of people who have MS. Plaques can be as small as a pinhead or as large as the size of a golf ball. Doctors can see these areas by examining the brain and spinal cord using a type of brain scan called "magnetic resonance imaging" (MRI).

While MS sometimes causes severe disability, it is only rarely fatal and most people with MS have a normal life expectancy.

## WHAT ARE THE SIGNS AND SYMPTOMS OF MULTIPLE SCLEROSIS?

The symptoms of MS usually begin over one to several days, but in some forms, they may develop more slowly. They may be mild or severe and may go away quickly or last for months. Sometimes the initial symptoms of MS are overlooked because they disappear in a day or so and normal function returns. Because symptoms come and go in the majority of people with MS, the presence of symptoms is called an "attack," or in medical terms, an exacerbation. Recovery from symptoms is referred to as remission, while a return of symptoms is called "a relapse." This form of MS is, therefore, called "relapsing-remitting MS," in contrast to a more slowly developing form called "primary progressive MS." Progressive MS can also be a second stage of the illness that follows years of relapsing-remitting symptoms.

A diagnosis of MS is often delayed because MS shares symptoms with other neurological conditions and diseases.

The first symptoms of MS often include:

- Vision problems such as blurred or double vision or optic neuritis, which causes pain in the eye and a rapid loss of vision
- Weak, stiff muscles, often with painful muscle spasms
- Tingling or numbness in the arms, legs, trunk of the body, or face
- Clumsiness, particularly difficulty staying balanced when walking
- Bladder control problems, either inability to control the bladder or urgency
- Dizziness that does not go away

Multiple sclerosis may also cause later symptoms such as:

- Mental or physical fatigue which accompanies the above symptoms during an attack
- Mood changes such as depression or euphoria
- Changes in the ability to concentrate or to multitask effectively
- Difficulty making decisions, planning, or prioritizing at work or in private life

Some people with MS develop transverse myelitis, a condition caused by inflammation in the spinal cord. Transverse myelitis causes loss of spinal cord function over a period of time lasting from several hours to several weeks. It usually begins as a sudden onset of lower back pain, muscle weakness, or abnormal sensations in the toes and feet, and can rapidly progress to more severe symptoms, including paralysis. In most cases of transverse myelitis, people recover at least some function within the first 12 weeks after an attack begins. Transverse myelitis can also result from viral infections, arteriovenous malformations, or neuroinflammatory problems unrelated to MS. In such instances, there are no plaques in the brain that suggest previous MS attacks.

Neuromyelitis optica is a disorder associated with transverse myelitis as well as optic nerve inflammation. Patients with this disorder usually have antibodies against a particular protein in their spinal cord, called the "aquaporin channel." These patients respond differently to treatment than most people with MS.

Most individuals with MS have muscle weakness, often in their hands and legs. Muscle stiffness and spasms can also be a problem. These symptoms may be severe enough to affect walking or standing. In some cases, MS leads to partial or complete paralysis. Many people with MS find that weakness and fatigue are worse when they have a fever or when they are exposed to heat. MS exacerbations may occur following common infections.

Tingling and burning sensations are common, as well as the opposite, numbness and loss of sensation. Moving the neck from side to side or flexing it back and forth may cause While it is rare for pain to be the first sign of MS, pain often occurs with optic neuritis and trigeminal neuralgia, a neurological disorder that affects one of the nerves that runs across the jaw, cheek, and face. Painful spasms of the limbs and sharp pain shooting down the legs or around the abdomen can also be symptoms of MS.

Most individuals with MS experience difficulties with coordination and balance at some time during the course of the disease. Some may have a continuous trembling of the head, limbs, and body, especially during movement, although such trembling is more common with other disorders such as Parkinson disease.

Fatigue is common, especially during exacerbations of MS. A person with MS may be tired all the time or may be easily fatigued from mental or physical exertion.

Urinary symptoms, including loss of bladder control and sudden attacks of urgency, are common as MS progresses. People with MS sometimes also develop constipation or sexual problems.

Depression is a common feature of MS. A small number of individuals with MS may develop more severe psychiatric disorders such as bipolar disorder and paranoia, or experience inappropriate episodes of high spirits, known as "euphoria."

People with MS, especially those who have had the disease for a long time, can experience difficulty with thinking, learning, memory, and judgment. The first signs of what doctors call cognitive dysfunction may be subtle. The person may have problems finding the right words to say, or trouble remembering how to do routine tasks on the job or at home. Day-to-day decisions that once came easily may now be made more slowly and show poor judgment. Changes may be so small or happen so slowly that it takes a family member or friend to point them out.

## HOW DO DOCTORS TREAT THE SYMPTOMS OF MULTIPLE SCLEROSIS?

Multiple sclerosis causes a variety of symptoms that can interfere with daily activities but which can usually be treated or managed to reduce their impact. Many of these issues are best treated by neurologists who have advanced training in the treatment of MS and who can prescribe specific medications to treat the problems.

### Vision Restrictions

Eye and vision restrictions are common in people with MS but rarely result in permanent blindness. Inflammation of the optic nerve or damage to the myelin that covers the optic nerve and other nerve fibers can cause a number of symptoms, including blurring or graying of vision, blindness in one eye, loss of normal color vision, depth perception, or a dark spot in the center of the visual field (scotoma).

Uncontrolled horizontal or vertical eye movements (nystagmus) and "jumping vision" (opsoclonus) are common to MS, and can be either mild or severe enough to impair vision.

Double vision (diplopia) occurs when the two eyes are not perfectly aligned. This occurs commonly in MS when a pair of muscles that control a specific eye movement are not coordinated due to weakness in one or both muscles. Double vision may increase with fatigue or as the result of spending too much time reading or on the computer. Periodically resting the eyes may be helpful.

## Weak Muscles, Stiff Muscles, Painful Muscle Spasms, and Weak Reflexes

Muscle weakness is common in MS, along with muscle spasticity. "Spasticity" refers to muscles that are stiff or that go into spasms without any warning. Spasticity in MS can be as mild as a feeling of tightness in the muscles or so severe that it causes painful, uncontrolled spasms. It can also cause pain or tightness in and around the joints. It also frequently affects walking, reducing the normal flexibility or "bounce" involved in taking steps.

## Tremor

People with MS sometimes develop tremor, or uncontrollable shaking, often triggered by movement. Tremor can be very disabling. Assistive devices and weights attached to limbs are sometimes helpful for people with tremor. Deep brain stimulation and drugs such as clonazepam may be useful.

## Challenges Involving Walking and Balance

Many people with MS experience difficulty walking. In fact, studies indicate that half of those with relapsing-remitting MS will need some kind of help walking within 15 years of their diagnosis if they remain untreated. The most common walking problem in people with MS experience is ataxia—unsteady, uncoordinated movements—due to damage with the areas of the brain that coordinate movement of muscles. People with severe ataxia generally benefit from the use of a cane, walker, or other assistive device. Physical therapy can also reduce walking problems in many cases.

In 2010, the U.S. Food and Drug Administration (FDA) approved the drug dalfampridine to improve walking in patients with MS. It is the first drug approved for this use. Clinical trials showed that patients treated with dalfampridine had faster walking speeds than those treated with a placebo pill.

## Fatigue

Fatigue is a common symptom of MS and may be both physical (for example, tiredness in the legs) and psychological (due to depression). Probably the most important measures people with MS can take to counter physical fatigue are to avoid excessive activity and to stay out of the heat, which often aggravates MS symptoms. On the other hand, daily physical activity programs of mild to moderate intensity can significantly reduce fatigue. An antidepressant such as fluoxetine may be prescribed if the fatigue is caused by depression. Other drugs that may reduce fatigue in some individuals include amantadine and modafinil.

Fatigue may be reduced if the person receives occupational therapy to simplify tasks and/or physical therapy to learn how to walk in a way that saves physical energy or that takes advantage of an assistive device. Some people benefit from stress management programs, relaxation training, membership in an MS support group, or individual psychotherapy. Treating sleep problems and MS symptoms that interfere with sleep (such as spastic muscles) may also help.

## Pain

People with MS may experience several types of pain during the course of the disease.

Trigeminal neuralgia is a sharp, stabbing, facial pain caused by MS affecting the trigeminal nerve as it exits the brainstem on its way to the jaw and cheek. It can be treated with anticonvulsant or antispasmodic drugs, alcohol injections, or surgery.

People with MS occasionally develop central pain, a syndrome caused by damage to the brain and/or spinal cord. Drugs such as gabapentin and nortriptiline sometimes help to reduce central pain.

Burning, tingling, and prickling (commonly called "pins and needles") are sensations that happen in the absence of any stimulation. The medical term for them is "dysesthesias" They are often chronic and hard to treat.

Chronic back or other musculoskeletal pain may be caused by walking problems or by using assistive aids incorrectly. Treatments may include heat, massage, ultrasound treatments, and physical therapy to correct faulty posture and strengthen and stretch muscles.

## Challenges Involving Bladder Control and Constipation

The most common bladder control problems encountered by people with MS are urinary frequency, urgency, or the loss of bladder control. The same spasticity that causes spasms in legs can also affect the bladder. A small number of individuals will have the opposite problem—retaining large amounts of urine. Urologists can help with treatment of bladder-related problems. A number of medical treatments are available. Constipation is also common and can be treated with a high-fiber diet, laxatives, and other measures.

### Sexual Issues

People with MS sometimes experience sexual problems. Sexual arousal begins in the central nervous system, as the brain sends messages to the sex organs along nerves running through the spinal cord. If MS damages these nerve pathways, sexual response—including arousal and orgasm—can be directly affected. Sexual problems may also stem from MS symptoms such as fatigue, cramped or spastic muscles, and psychological factors related to lowered self-esteem or depression. Some of these problems can be corrected with medications. Psychological counseling also may be helpful.

### Depression

Studies indicate that clinical depression is more frequent among people with MS than it is in the general population or in persons with many other chronic, disabling conditions. MS may cause depression as part of the disease process, since it damages myelin and nerve fibers inside the brain. If the plaques are in parts of the brain that are involved in emotional expression and control, a variety of behavioral changes can result, including depression. Depression can intensify symptoms of fatigue, pain, and sexual dysfunction. It is most often treated with selective serotonin reuptake inhibitor (SSRI) antidepressant medications, which are less likely than other antidepressant medications to cause fatigue.

### Inappropriate Laughing or Crying

MS is sometimes associated with a condition called "pseudobulbar affect" that causes inappropriate and involuntary expressions of laughter, crying, or anger. These expressions are often unrelated to mood; for example, the person may cry when they are actually very happy, or laugh when they are not especially happy. In 2010, the FDA approved the first treatment specifically for pseudobulbar affect, a combination of the drugs dextromethorphan and quinidine. The condition can also be treated with other drugs such as amitriptyline or citalopram.

### Cognitive Changes

Half- to three-quarters of people with MS experience "cognitive impairment," which is a phrase doctors use to describe a decline in the ability to think quickly and clearly and to remember easily. These cognitive changes may appear at the same time as the physical symptoms or they may develop gradually over time. Some individuals with MS may feel as if they are thinking more slowly, are easily distracted, have trouble remembering, or are losing their way with words. The right word may often seem to be on the tip of their tongue.

Some experts believe that it is more likely to be cognitive decline, rather than physical impairment, that causes people with MS to eventually withdraw from the workforce. A number of neuropsychological tests have been developed to evaluate the cognitive status of individuals with MS. Based on the outcomes of these tests, a neuropsychologist can determine the extent of strengths and weaknesses in different cognitive areas.

## Section 12.6 | **Parkinson Disease and Alzheimer Disease**

This section contains text excerpted from the following sources: Text beginning with the heading "What Is Parkinson Disease?" is excerpted from "Parkinson Disease," National Institute on Aging (NIA), National Institutes of Health (NIH), May 16, 2017; Text under the heading "Parkinson Disease and Exercise" is excerpted from "Parkinson Disease," Rehabilitation Research & Development Service (RR&D), U.S. Department of Veterans Affairs (VA), October 14, 2016. Reviewed November 2019; Text beginning with the heading "What Is Alzheimer Disease?" is excerpted from "Alzheimer Disease," Centers for Disease Control and Prevention (CDC), September 20, 2019.

### WHAT IS PARKINSON DISEASE?

Parkinson disease (PD) is a brain disorder that leads to shaking, stiffness, and difficulty with walking, balance, and coordination. Parkinson symptoms usually begin gradually and get worse over time. As the disease progresses, people may have difficulty walking and talking. They may also have mental and behavioral changes, sleep problems, depression, memory difficulties, and fatigue.

Both men and women can have PD. However, the disease affects about 50 percent more men than women.

One clear risk factor for PD is age. Although most people with Parkinson first develop the disease at about age 60, about 5 to 10 percent of people with Parkinson have "early-onset" disease, which begins before the age of 50. Early-onset forms of Parkinson are often, but not always, inherited, and some forms have been linked to specific gene mutations.

### WHAT CAUSES PARKINSON DISEASE

Parkinson disease occurs when nerve cells, or neurons, in an area of the brain that controls movement become impaired and/or die. Normally, these neurons produce an important brain chemical known as "dopamine." When the neurons die or become impaired, they produce less dopamine, which causes the movement problems of Parkinson. Scientists still do not know what causes cells that produce dopamine to die.

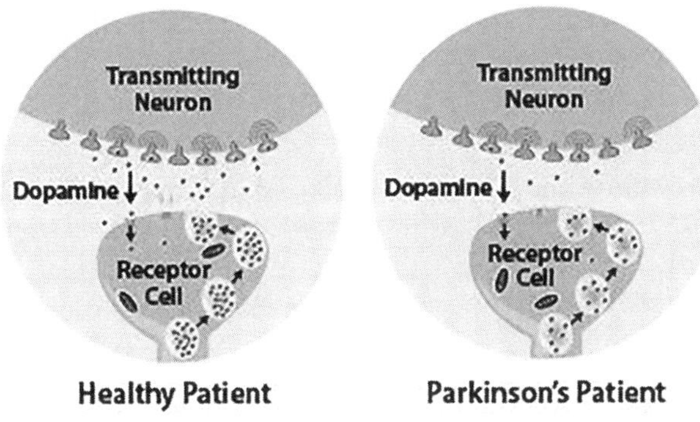


**Figure 12.4.** Parkinson Patients Has Less Dopamine *(Source: National Institute of Environmental Health Sciences (NIEHS).)*

People with Parkinson also lose the nerve endings that produce norepinephrine, the main chemical messenger of the sympathetic nervous system, which controls many automatic functions of the body, such as heart rate and blood pressure. The loss of norepinephrine might help explain some of the nonmovement features of Parkinson, such as fatigue, irregular blood pressure, decreased movement of food through the digestive tract, and sudden drop in blood pressure when a person stands up from a sitting or lying-down position.

Many brain cells of people with Parkinson contain Lewy bodies, unusual clumps of the protein alpha-synuclein. Scientists are trying to better understand the normal and abnormal functions of alpha-synuclein and its relationship to genetic mutations that impact PD and Lewy body dementia.

Although some cases of Parkinson appear to be hereditary, and a few can be traced to specific genetic mutations, in most cases the disease occurs randomly and does not seem to run in families. Many researchers now believe that PD results from a combination of genetic factors and environmental factors such as exposure to toxins.

## SYMPTOMS OF PARKINSON DISEASE

Parkinson disease has four main symptoms:

- Tremor (trembling) in hands, arms, legs, jaw, or head
- Stiffness of the limbs and trunk
- Slowness of movement
- Impaired balance and coordination, sometimes leading to falls

Other symptoms may include depression and other emotional changes; difficulty swallowing, chewing, and speaking; urinary problems or constipation; skin problems; and sleep disruptions.

Symptoms of Parkinson and the rate of progression differ among individuals. Sometimes people dismiss early symptoms of Parkinson as the effects of normal aging. In most cases, there are no medical tests to definitively detect the disease, so it can be difficult to diagnose accurately.

Early symptoms of PD are subtle and occur gradually. For example, affected people may feel mild tremors or have difficulty getting out of a chair. They may notice that they speak too softly, or that their handwriting is slow and looks cramped or small. Friends or family members may be the first to notice changes in someone with early Parkinson. They may see that the person's face lacks expression and animation, or that the person does not move an arm or leg normally.

People with Parkinson often develop a parkinsonian gait that includes a tendency to lean forward, small quick steps as if hurrying forward, and reduced swinging of the arms. They also may have trouble initiating or continuing movement.

Symptoms often begin on one side of the body or even in one limb on one side of the body. As the disease progresses, it eventually affects both sides. However, the symptoms may still be more severe on one side than on the other.

Many people with Parkinson note that prior to experiencing stiffness and tremor, they had sleep problems, constipation, decreased the ability to smell, and restless legs.

## DIAGNOSIS OF PARKINSON DISEASE

A number of disorders can cause symptoms similar to those of PD. People with Parkinson-like symptoms that result from other causes are sometimes said to have parkinsonism. While these disorders initially may be misdiagnosed as Parkinson, certain medical tests, as well as response to drug treatment, may help to distinguish them from Parkinson. Since many other diseases have similar features but require different treatments, it is important to make an exact diagnosis as soon as possible.

There are no blood or laboratory tests to diagnose nongenetic cases of PD. Diagnosis is based on a person's medical history and a neurological examination. Improvement after initiating medication is another important hallmark of PD.

## TREATMENT OF PARKINSON DISEASE

Although there is no cure for PD, medicines, surgical treatment, and other therapies can often relieve some symptoms.

### Medicines for Parkinson Disease

Medicines prescribed for Parkinson include:

- Drugs that increase the level of dopamine in the brain

- Drugs that affect other brain chemicals in the body
- Drugs that help control nonmotor symptoms

The main therapy for Parkinson is levodopa, also called "L-dopa." Nerve cells use levodopa to make dopamine to replenish the brain's dwindling supply. Usually, people take levodopa along with another medication called "carbidopa." Carbidopa prevents or reduces some of the side effects of levodopa therapy—such as nausea, vomiting, low blood pressure, and restlessness—and reduces the amount of levodopa needed to improve symptoms.

People with Parkinson should never stop taking levodopa without telling their doctor. Suddenly stopping the drug may have serious side effects, such as being unable to move or having difficulty breathing.

Other medicines used to treat Parkinson symptoms include:

- Dopamine agonists to mimic the role of dopamine in the brain
- MAO-B inhibitors to slow down an enzyme that breaks down dopamine in the brain
- COMT inhibitors to help break down dopamine
- Amantadine, an old antiviral drug, to reduce involuntary movements
- Anticholinergic drugs to reduce tremors and muscle rigidity

### Deep Brain Stimulation

For people with Parkinson who do not respond well to medications, deep brain stimulation, or DBS, may be appropriate. DBS is a surgical procedure that surgically implants electrodes into part of the brain and connects them to a small electrical device implanted in the chest. The device and electrodes painlessly stimulate the brain in a way that helps to stop many of the movement-related symptoms of Parkinson, such as tremor, slowness of movement, and rigidity.

### Other Therapies

Other therapies may be used to help with PD symptoms. They include physical, occupational, and speech therapies, which help with gait and voice disorders, tremors and rigidity, and decline in mental functions. Other supportive therapies include a healthy diet and exercises to strengthen muscles and improve balance.

## PARKINSON DISEASE AND EXERCISE

Research has demonstrated the great benefits of exercise for patients with PD. Not only have exercise programs been shown to improve motor function and reduce the risk of falls, but they also improve the overall quality of life and possibly slow down the course of the disease.

- **Walking improves PD symptoms**—A 2014 study led by researchers with the Iowa City VA Health Care System and the University of Iowa found that patients who walked briskly for 45 minutes, three times a week, showed improvements in their Parkinson symptoms. They were also less depressed and less tired. Walking provides a safe and easily accessible way of improving the symptoms of PD.
- **Low-intensity workouts improve mobility**—Researchers studying 67 patients with PD at the VA Maryland Health Care System learned, in 2013, that low-intensity workouts, stretching, and resistance exercise all improved the mobility of patients with Parkinson disease. Those who walked on a treadmill at a comfortable pace for nearly an hour showed the most consistent improvement in gait and mobility.
- **Home-based exercise programs**—A home-based approach to exercises provides the benefits of a safe exercise program to people with PD. The exercise program will be centered on remote, real-time instruction and supervision. This will make the benefits of exercise available to PD patients who cannot travel to exercise locations and rehabilitation centers.

## WHAT IS ALZHEIMER DISEASE?

- The most common type of dementia.
- A progressive disease beginning with mild memory loss possibly leading to loss of the ability to carry on a conversation and respond to the environment.
- Involves parts of the brain that controls thought, memory, and language.
- Can seriously affect a person's ability to carry out daily activities.

## WHO HAS ALZHEIMER DISEASE

- In 2014, as many as 5 million Americans were living with Alzheimer disease (AD).
- The symptoms of the disease can first appear after age 60 and the risk increases with age.
- Younger people may get AD, but it is less common.
- The number of people living with the disease doubles every 5 years beyond age 65.
- This number is projected to nearly triple to 14 million people by 2060

## WHAT IS KNOWN ABOUT ALZHEIMER DISEASE?

Scientists do not yet fully understand what causes AD. There probably is not one single cause, but several factors that affect each person differently.

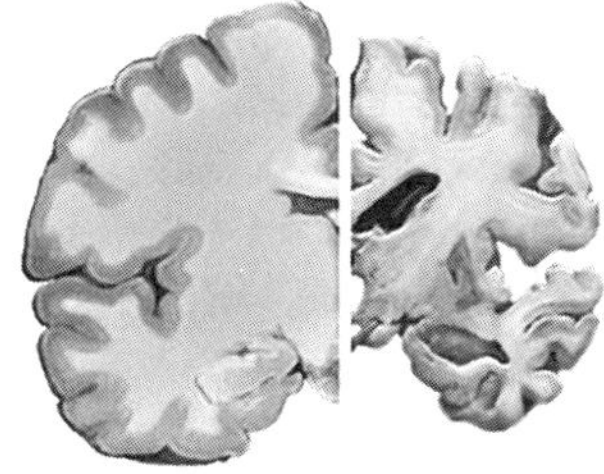


**Figure 12.5.** How a Brain of a Person with Alzheimer Disease Looks When Compared with a Healthy Brain *(Source: National Institute of Aging (NIA).)*

- Age is the best known risk factor for AD.
- Family history—researchers believe that genetics may play a role in developing AD.
- Changes in the brain can begin years before the first symptoms appear.
- Researchers are studying whether education, diet, and environment play a role in developing AD.
- Scientists are finding more evidence that some of the risk factors for heart disease and stroke, such as high blood pressure and high cholesterol may also increase the risk of AD.
- There is growing evidence that physical, mental, and social activities may reduce the risk of AD.

## HOW DO I KNOW IF IT IS ALZHEIMER DISEASE?

Alzheimer disease is not a normal part of aging.

Memory problems are typically one of the first warning signs of cognitive loss.

According to the National Institute on Aging, in addition to memory problems, someone with AD may experience one or more of the following signs:

- Memory loss that disrupts daily life, such as getting lost in a familiar place or repeating questions.
- Trouble handling money and paying bills.
- Difficulty completing familiar tasks at home, at work or at leisure.
- Decreased or poor judgment.
- Misplaces things and being unable to retrace steps to find them.
- Changes in mood, personality, or behavioral.

If you or someone you know has several or even most of the signs listed above, it does not mean that you or they have AD. It is important to consult a healthcare provider when you or someone you know has concerns about memory loss, thinking skills, or behavioral changes.

- Some causes for symptoms, such as depression and drug interactions, are reversible. However, they can be serious and should be identified and treated by a healthcare provider as soon as possible.

- Early and accurate diagnosis provides opportunities for you and your family to consider or review financial planning, develop advance directives, enroll in clinical trials, and anticipate care needs.

## HOW IS ALZHEIMER DISEASE TREATED?

Medical management can improve the quality of life for individuals living with AD and their caregivers. There is no known cure for AD.

Treatment addresses several different areas:

- Helping people maintain mental function.
- Managing behavioral symptoms.
- Slowing or delaying the symptoms of the disease.

### Support for Family and Friends

Many people living with AD are cared for at home by family members.

Caregiving can have positive aspects for the caregiver as well as the person being cared for. It may bring personal fulfillment to the caregiver, such as satisfaction from helping a family member or friend, and lead to the development of new skills and improved family relationships.

Although most people willingly provide care to their loved ones and friends, caring for a person with AD at home can be a difficult task and might become overwhelming at times. Each day brings new challenges as the caregiver copes with changing levels of ability and new patterns of behavior. As the disease gets worse, people living with AD often need more intensive care.

# Chapter 13 | Cardiovascular and Pulmonary Rehabilitation

**Chapter Contents**

## Section 13.1 | **Cardiac Rehabilitation**

This section contains text excerpted from the following sources: Text in this section begins with excerpts from "How Cardiac Rehabilitation Can Help Heal Your Heart," Centers for Disease Control and Prevention (CDC), July 10, 2017; Text under the heading "Treatment of Obesity in Cardiac Rehabilitation" is excerpted from "The Treatment of Obesity in Cardiac Rehabilitation," U.S. Department of Health and Human Services (HHS), September 1, 2011. Reviewed November 2019.

If you have a heart attack or other heart problem, cardiac rehabilitation (rehab) is an important part of your recovery. Cardiac rehab can help prevent another, perhaps more serious, heart attack and can help you build heart-healthy habits. Learn more about who needs cardiac rehab and how it can help your recovery.

Nearly 800,000 people in the United States have a heart attack every year. About 1 in 4 of those people had already had a heart attack. Cardiac rehab not only can help a person recover from a heart problem, but it can also prevent another heart problem in the future.

### WHAT IS CARDIAC REHABILITATION?

Cardiac rehab is an important program for anyone recovering from a heart attack, heart failure, or other heart problems that required surgery or medical care.

Cardiac rehab is a supervised program that includes:

- Physical activity
- Education about healthy living, including healthy eating, taking medicine as prescribed, and ways to help you quit smoking
- Counseling to find ways to relieve stress and improve mental health

A team of people may help you through cardiac rehab, including your healthcare team, exercise and nutrition specialists, physical therapists, and counselors or mental-health professionals.

### WHO NEEDS CARDIAC REHABILITATION

Anyone who has had a heart problem, such as a heart attack, heart failure, or heart surgery, can benefit from cardiac rehab. Studies have found that cardiac rehab helps men and women, people of all ages, and people with mild, moderate, and severe heart problems.

But, certain people are less likely to go to or finish a cardiac rehab program. These include:

- **Women.** Studies show that women, especially minority women, are less likely than men to go to or complete a cardiac rehab program. This may be because doctors may be less likely to suggest cardiac rehab to women.

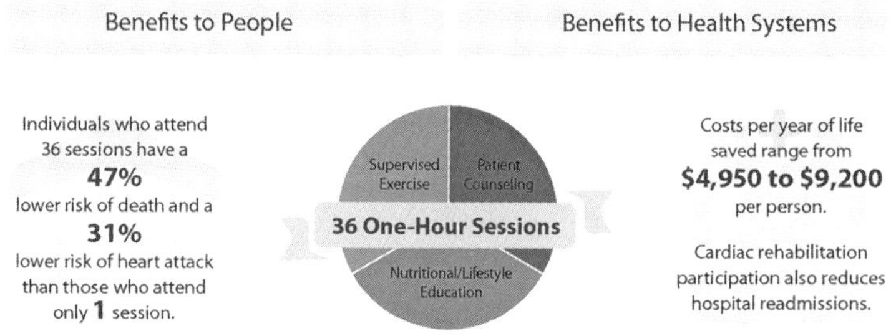


**Figure 13.1.** Cardiac Rehabilitation Benefits *(Source: "Cardiac Rehabilitation Communications Toolkit," Million Hearts, U.S. Department of Health and Human Services (HHS).)*

- **Older adults.** Older adults are also less likely to join a cardiac rehab program following a heart problem. They may think they are unable to do the physical activity because of their age, or they may have other conditions that can make exercising harder, such as arthritis. This makes cardiac rehabilitation especially useful for older adults, since it can improve strength and mobility to help make daily tasks easier.

## HOW DOES CARDIAC REHABILITATION HELP?

Cardiac rehab can have many benefits to your health in both the short and long-term, including:

- Strengthening your heart and body after a heart attack.
- Relieving symptoms of heart problems, such as chest pain.
- Building healthier habits, including getting more physical activity, quitting smoking, and eating a heart-healthy diet. A nutritionist or dietitian may work with you to help you limit foods with unhealthy fats and eat more fruits and vegetables that are high in vitamins, minerals, and fiber.
- Reducing stress
- Improving your mood. People are more likely to feel depressed after a heart attack. Cardiac rehab can help prevent and lessen depression.
- Increasing your energy and strength, making daily activities easier, such as carrying groceries and climbing stairs
- Making you more likely to take your prescribed medicines that help lower your risk for future heart problems
- Preventing future heart problems and death. Studies have found that cardiac rehab decreases the chances you will die in the five years following a heart attack or bypass surgery by around 20 to 30 percent.

## TREATMENT OF OBESITY IN CARDIAC REHABILITATION

Obesity is an independent risk factor for the development of coronary heart disease (CHD). At entry into cardiac rehabilitation (CR) over 80 percent of patients are overweight and over 50 percent have metabolic syndrome. Yet, CR programs do not generally include weight loss programs as a programmatic component and weight loss outcomes in CR have been abysmal. A recently published study outlines a template for weight reduction based upon a combination of behavioral weight-loss counseling and an approach to exercise that maximized exercise-related caloric expenditure. This approach to exercise optimally includes walking as the primary exercise modality and eventually requires almost daily longer distance exercise to maximize caloric expenditure. Additionally, lifestyle exercises such as stair climbing and avoidance of energy-saving devices should be incorporated into the daily routine. Risk factor benefits of weight loss and exercise training in overweight patients with coronary heart disease are broad and compelling. Improvements in insulin resistance, lipid profiles, blood pressure, clotting abnormalities, endothelial-dependent vasodilatory capacity, and measures of inflammation such as C-reactive protein have all been demonstrated. CR/secondary prevention programs can no longer ignore the challenge of obesity management in patients with CHD. Individual programs need to develop clinically effective and culturally sensitive approaches to weight control. Finally, multicenter randomized clinical trials of weight loss in CHD patients with assessment of long-term clinical outcomes need to be performed.

# Section 13.2 | **Pulmonary Rehabilitation**

This section includes text excerpted from "Pulmonary Rehabilitation," MedlinePlus, National Institutes of Health (NIH), August 30, 2019.

## WHAT IS PULMONARY REHABILITATION?

Pulmonary rehabilitation, also known as "pulmonary rehab" or "(PR)," is a program for people who have chronic (ongoing) breathing problems. It can help improve your ability to function and quality of life. PR does not replace your medical treatment. Instead, you use them together.

Pulmonary rehabilitation is often an outpatient program that you do in a hospital or clinic. Some people have PR in their homes. You work with a team of healthcare providers to find ways to lessen your symptoms, increase your ability to exercise and make it easier to do your daily activities.

## WHO NEEDS PULMONARY REHABILITATION

Your healthcare provider may recommend pulmonary rehabilitation (PR) if you have a chronic lung disease or another condition that makes it hard for you to breathe and limits your activities. For example, PR may help you if you:

- **Have chronic obstructive pulmonary disease (COPD).** The two main types are emphysema and chronic bronchitis. In COPD, your airways (tubes that carry air in and out of your lungs) are partially blocked. This makes it hard to get air in and out.
- **Have an interstitial lung disease such as sarcoidosis and pulmonary fibrosis.** These diseases cause scarring of the lungs over time. This makes it hard to get enough oxygen.
- **Have cystic fibrosis (CF).** CF is an inherited disease that causes thick, sticky mucus to collect in the lungs and block the airways.
- **Need lung surgery.** You may have PR before and after lung surgery to help you prepare for and recover from the surgery.
- **Have a muscle-wasting disorder that affects the muscles used for breathing.** An example is muscular dystrophy.

Pulmonary rehabilitation works best if you start it before your disease is severe. However, even people who have advanced lung disease can benefit from PR.

## WHAT DOES PULMONARY REHABILITATION INCLUDE?

When you first start pulmonary rehabilitation (PR), your team of healthcare providers will want to know about your health. You will have lung function, exercise, and possibly blood tests. Your team will go over your medical history and treatments. They may check on your mental health and ask about your diet. Then they will work together to create a plan that is right for you. It may include

- **Exercise training.** Your team will come up with an exercise plan to improve your endurance and muscle strength. You will likely have exercises for both your arms and legs. You might use a treadmill, stationary bike, or weights. You may need to start slowly and increase your exercise as you get stronger.
- **Nutritional counseling.** Being either overweight or underweight can affect your breathing. A nutritious eating plan can help you work towards a healthy weight.
- **Education about your disease and how to manage it.** This includes learning how to avoid situations that make your symptoms worse, how to avoid infections, and how/when to take your medicines.
- **Techniques you can use to save your energy.** Your team may teach you easier ways to do daily tasks. For example, you may learn ways to avoid reaching, lifting, or bending. Those movements make it harder

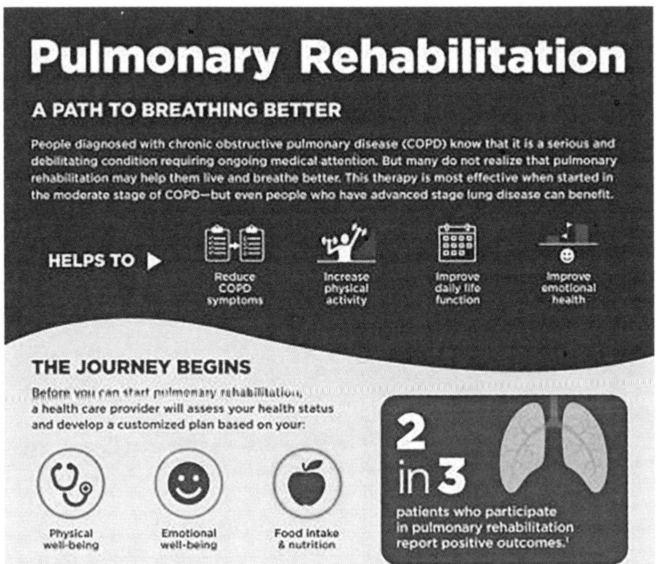


**Figure 13.2.** Pulmonary Rehabilitation: A Path to Breathing Better
*(Source: National Heart, Lung, and Blood Institute (NHLBI).)*

to breathe, since they use up energy and make you tighten your abdominal muscles. You may also learn how to better deal with stress, since stress can also take up energy and affect your breathing.

- **Breathing strategies.** You will learn techniques to improve your breathing. These techniques may increase your oxygen levels, decrease how often you take breaths, and keep your airways open longer.
- **Psychological counseling and/or group support.** It can feel scary to have trouble breathing. If you have a chronic lung disease, you are more likely to have depression, anxiety, or other emotional problems. Many PR programs include counseling and/or support groups. If not, your PR team may be able to refer you to an organization that offers them.

# Chapter 14 | Pediatric Rehabilitation

**Chapter Contents**

# Section 14.1 | Cerebral Palsy

This section contains text excerpted from the following sources: Text beginning with the heading "What Is Cerebral Palsy?" is excerpted from "What Is Cerebral Palsy?" Centers for Disease Control and Prevention (CDC), April 30, 2019; Text under the heading "Treatment of Cerebral Palsy" is excerpted from "What Are Common Treatments for Cerebral Palsy?" *Eunice Kennedy Shriver* National Institute of Child Health and Human Development (NICHD), December 1, 2016. Reviewed November 2019.

## WHAT IS CEREBRAL PALSY?

Cerebral palsy (CP) is a group of disorders that affect a person's ability to move and maintain balance and posture. CP is the most common motor disability in childhood. Cerebral means having to do with the brain. Palsy means weakness or problems with using the muscles. CP is caused by abnormal brain development or damage to the developing brain that affects a person's ability to control her or his muscles. The symptoms of CP vary from person to person.

A person with severe CP might need to use special equipment to be able to walk, or might not be able to walk at all and might need lifelong care. A person with mild CP, on the other hand, might walk a little awkwardly, but might not need any special help. CP does not get worse over time, though the exact symptoms can change over a person's lifetime.

All people with CP have challenges involving movement and posture. Many also have related conditions such as intellectual disability; seizures; challenges involving vision, hearing, or speech; changes in the spine (such as scoliosis); or joint problems (such as contractures).

## TYPES OF CEREBRAL PALSY

Doctors classify CP according to the main type of movement disorder involved. Depending on which areas of the brain are affected, one or more of the following movement disorders can occur:

- Stiff muscles (spasticity)
- Uncontrollable movements (dyskinesia)
- Poor balance and coordination (ataxia)

There are four main types of CP. They are as follows:

### Spastic Cerebral Palsy

The most common type of CP is spastic CP. Spastic CP affects about 80 percent of people with CP. People with spastic CP have increased muscle tone. This means their muscles are stiff and, as a result, their movements can be awkward. Spastic CP usually is described by what parts of the body are affected:

- Spastic diplegia/diparesis—In this type of CP, muscle stiffness is mainly in the legs, with the arms less affected or not affected at all. People with spastic diplegia might have difficulty walking because tight hip and leg muscles cause their legs to pull together, turn inward, and cross at the knees (also known as "scissoring").
- Spastic hemiplegia/hemiparesis—This type of CP affects only one side of a person's body; usually, the arm is more affected than the leg.
- Spastic quadriplegia/quadriparesis—Spastic quadriplegia is the most severe form of spastic CP and affects all four limbs, the trunk, and the face. People with spastic quadriparesis usually cannot walk and often have other developmental disabilities such as intellectual disability; seizures; or challenges involving vision, hearing, or speech.

### Dyskinetic Cerebral Palsy (Also Includes Athetoid, Choreoathetoid, and Dystonic Cerebral Palsies)

People with dyskinetic CP have problems controlling the movement of their hands, arms, feet, and legs, making it difficult to sit and walk. The movements are uncontrollable and can be slow and writhing or rapid and jerky. Sometimes the face and tongue are affected and the person has a hard time sucking, swallowing, and talking. A person with dyskinetic CP has muscle tone that can change (varying from too tight to too loose) not only from day to day but, even during a single day.

### Ataxic Cerebral Palsy

People with ataxic CP have challenges involving balance and coordination. They might be unsteady when they walk. They might have a hard time with quick movements or movements that need a lot of control, such as writing. They might have a hard time controlling their hands or arms when they reach for something.

### Mixed Cerebral Palsy

Some people have symptoms of more than one type of CP. The most common type of mixed CP is spastic-dyskinetic CP.

## EARLY SIGNS OF CEREBRAL PALSY

The signs of CP vary greatly because there are many different types and levels of disability. The main sign that a child might have CP is a delay reaching motor or movement milestones (such as rolling over, sitting, standing, or walking). Following are some other signs of possible CP. It is important to note that some children without CP also might have some of these signs.

### In a Baby Younger than 6 Months of Age

- His head lags when you pick him up while he is lying on his back

- He feels stiff
- He feels floppy
- When held cradled in your arms, he seems to overextend his back and neck, constantly acting as if he is pushing away from you
- When you pick him up, his legs get stiff and they cross or scissor

### In a Baby Older than 6 Months of Age

- She does not roll over in either direction
- She cannot bring her hands together
- She has difficulty bringing her hands to her mouth
- She reaches out with only one hand while keeping the other fisted

### In a Baby Older than 10 Months of Age

- He crawls in a lopsided manner, pushing off with one hand and leg while dragging the opposite hand and leg
- He scoots around on his buttocks or hops on his knees but does not crawl on all fours

Tell your child's doctor or nurse if you notice any of these signs.

## SCREENING AND DIAGNOSIS OF CEREBRAL PALSY

Diagnosing CP at an early age is important to the well-being of children and their families. Diagnosing CP can take several steps:

### Developmental Monitoring

Developmental monitoring (also called "surveillance") means tracking a child's growth and development over time. If any concerns about the child's development are raised during monitoring, then a developmental screening test should be given as soon as possible.

### Developmental Screening

During the developmental screening a short test is given to see if the child has specific developmental delays, such as motor or movement delays. If the results of the screening test are cause for concern, then the doctor will make referrals for developmental and medical evaluations.

### Developmental and Medical Evaluations

The goal of the developmental evaluation is to diagnose the specific type of disorder that affects a child.

## TREATMENT OF CEREBRAL PALSY

A child may need one or several different types of treatment depending on how severe the symptoms are and what parts of the body are affected. The treatment differs from person to person, depending on each one's specific needs. Although the initial damage of cerebral palsy in the brain cannot be reversed, earlier and aggressive treatments may help to improve function and adjustments for the young nervous system and musculoskeletal system. Families may also work with their healthcare providers and, during the school years, school staff to develop individual care and treatment programs.

Common types of treatment for cerebral palsy:

- **Physical therapy and rehabilitation**. A child with cerebral palsy usually starts these therapies in the first few years of life or soon after being diagnosed. Physical therapy is one of the most important parts of treatment. It involves exercises and activities that can maintain or improve muscle strength, balance, and movement. A physical therapist helps the child learn skills such as sitting, walking, or using a wheelchair.
  - **Occupational therapy**. This type of therapy helps a child learn to do everyday activities such as dressing and going to school.
  - **Recreational therapy.** Participating in art programs, cultural activities, and sports can help improve a child's physical and intellectual skills.
  - **Speech and language therapy.** A speech therapist can help a child learn to speak more clearly, help with swallowing problems, and teach new ways to communicate, such as by using sign language or a special communication device.
- **Orthotic devices.** Braces, splints, and casts can be placed on the affected limbs and can improve movement and balance. Other devices that can help with movement and posture include wheelchairs, rolling walkers, and powered scooters.
- **Assistive devices and technologies.** These include special computer-based communication machines, Velcro-fastened shoes, or crutches, which can help make daily life easier.
- **Medication.** Certain medications can relax stiff or overactive muscles and reduce abnormal movement. They may be taken by mouth, injected into affected muscles, or infused into the fluid surrounding the spinal cord through a pump implanted near the spinal cord. For children who have cerebral palsy and epilepsy (seizures), standard epileptic medications should be considered, but these medications may also have negative effects on the developing brain.
- **Surgery**. A child may need surgery if symptoms are severe. For instance, surgery can lengthen stiff, tightly contracted muscles. A surgeon can also place arms or legs in better positions or correct or improve an abnormally curved spine. Sometimes, if other treatments

have not worked, a surgeon can cut certain nerves to treat abnormal, spastic movements. Before conducting surgery, it is important for a healthcare provider to assess the procedure's benefits by carefully analyzing the biomechanics of the joints and muscles.

Not all therapies are appropriate for everyone with cerebral palsy. It is important for parents, patients, and healthcare providers to work together to come up with the best treatment plan for the patient.

## Section 14.2 | Muscular Dystrophies

This section contains text excerpted from the following sources: Text beginning with the heading "What Is Muscular Dystrophy?" is excerpted from "What Is Muscular Dystrophy?" Centers for Disease Control and Prevention (CDC), July 5, 2019; Text beginning with the heading "What Causes Muscular Dystrophy" is excerpted from "Muscular Dystrophy: Hope through Research," National Institute of Neurological Disorders and Stroke (NINDS), August 13, 2019; Text under the heading "What Are the Treatments for Muscular Dystrophy?" is excerpted from "What Are the Treatments for Muscular Dystrophy?" *Eunice Kennedy Shriver* National Institute of Child Health and Human Development (NICHD), December 1, 2016. Reviewed November 2019.

### WHAT IS MUSCULAR DYSTROPHY?

Muscular dystrophies (MDs) are a group of muscle diseases caused by mutations in a person's genes. Over time, muscle weakness decreases mobility, making everyday tasks difficult. There are many kinds of MD, each affecting specific muscle groups, with signs and symptoms appearing at different ages, and varying in severity. MD can run in families, or a person can be the first in their family to have a MD. There may be several different genetic types within each kind of MD, and people with the same kind of MD may experience different symptoms.

Muscular dystrophies are rare, with little data on how many people are affected. The Centers for Disease Control and Prevention (CDC) is working to estimate the number of people with each major kind of MD in the United States.

### TYPES OF MUSCULAR DYSTROPHY

#### Duchenne/Becker

Duchenne muscular dystrophy (DMD) and Becker muscular dystrophy (BMD) can have the same symptoms and are caused by mutations in the same gene. BMD symptoms can begin later in life and be less severe than DMD. However, because these two kinds are very similar, they are often studied and referred to together (DBMD).

#### How Many People Are Affected?

About 14 in 100,000 males 5 to 24 years of age

#### Who Is More Likely to Be Affected: Males or Females?

Males

#### When Does Muscle Weakness Typically Begin?

Duchenne muscular dystrophy symptoms usually begin before 5 years of age. In BMD, symptoms usually appear later, even into adulthood.

#### Which Parts of the Body Show Weakness First?

Upper legs and upper arms

#### What Other Parts of the Body Can Be Affected?

Heart, lungs, throat, stomach, intestines, and spine

### Myotonic

#### How Many People Are Affected?

About 8 in 100,000 people of all ages are affected

#### Who Is More Likely to Be Affected: Males or Females?

Males and females equally

#### When Does Muscle Weakness Typically Begin?

Usually between 10 to 30 years of age, but ranges from birth to 70 years old.

#### Which Parts of the Body Show Weakness First?

Face, neck, arms, hands, hips, and lower legs

#### What Other Parts of the Body Can Be Affected?

Heart, lungs, stomach, intestines, brain, eyes, and hormone-producing organs

### Limb-Girdle

#### How Many People Are Affected?

About 2 in 100,000 people of all ages

#### Who Is More Likely to Be Affected: Males or Females?

Males and females equally

#### When Does Muscle Weakness Typically Begin?

Childhood or adulthood, depending on the type of Limb-Girdle (LGMD)

#### Which Parts of the Body Show Weakness First?

Upper arms, upper legs

#### What Other Parts of the Body Can Be Affected?

Heart, spine, hips, calves, and trunk

## Facioscapulohumeral

### How Many People Are Affected?

About 4 in 100,000 people of all ages

### Who Is More Likely to Be Affected: Males or Females?

Males and females equally

### When Does Muscle Weakness Typically Begin?

Young adulthood

### Which Parts of the Body Show Weakness First?

Face, shoulders, and upper arms

### What Other Parts of the Body Can Be Affected?

Eyes, ears, and lower legs

## Congenital

### How Many People Are Affected?

About 1 in 100,000 people of all ages

### Who Is More Likely to Be Affected: Males or Females?

Males and females equally

### When Does Muscle Weakness Typically Begin?

At birth or in early infancy

### Which Parts of the Body Show Weakness First?

Neck, upper arms, upper legs, and lungs

### What Other Parts of the Body Can Be Affected?

Brain, heart, and spine

## Distal

### How Many People Are Affected?

Less than 1 in 100,000 people

### Who Is More Likely to Be Affected: Males or Females?

Males and females equally

### When Does Muscle Weakness Typically Begin?

Adulthood

### Which Parts of the Body Show Weakness First?

Feet, hands, lower legs, and lower arms

### What Other Parts of the Body Can Be Affected?

Heart, arms, and legs

## WHAT CAUSES MUSCULAR DYSTROPHY

All of the muscular dystrophies are inherited and involve a mutation in one of the thousands of genes that program proteins critical to muscle integrity. The body's cells don't work properly when a protein is altered or produced in insufficient quantity (or sometimes missing completely). Many cases of MD occur from spontaneous mutations that are not found in the genes of either parent, and this defect can be passed to the next generation.

Genes are like blueprints: they contain coded messages that determine a person's characteristics or traits. They are arranged along 23 rod-like pairs of chromosomes, with one half of each pair being inherited from each parent. Each half of a chromosome pair is similar to the other, except for one pair, which determines the sex of the individual. Muscular dystrophies can be inherited in three ways:

- Autosomal dominant inheritance occurs when a child receives a normal gene from one parent and a defective gene from the other parent. Autosomal means the genetic mutation can occur on any of the 22 nonsex chromosomes in each of the body's cells. Dominant means only one parent needs to pass along the abnormal gene in order to produce the disorder. In families where one parent carries a defective gene, each child has a 50 percent chance of inheriting the gene and, therefore, the disorder. Males and females are equally at risk and the severity of the disorder can differ from person to person.
- Autosomal recessive inheritance means that both parents must carry and pass on the faulty gene. The parents each have one defective gene but are not affected by the disorder. Children in these families have a 25 percent chance of inheriting both copies of the defective gene and a 50 percent chance of inheriting one gene and, therefore, becoming a carrier, able to pass along the defect to their children. Children of either sex can be affected by this pattern of inheritance.
- X-linked (or sex-linked) recessive inheritance occurs when a mother carries the affected gene on one of her two X chromosomes and passes it to her son (males always inherit an X chromosome from their mother and a Y chromosome from their father, while daughters inherit an X chromosome from each parent). Sons of carrier mothers have a 50 percent chance of inheriting the disorder. Daughters also have a 50 percent chance of inheriting the defective gene but usually are not affected, since the healthy X chromosome they receive from their father can offset the faulty one received from their mother. Affected fathers cannot pass an X-linked disorder to their sons but their daughters will be carriers of that disorder. Carrier females occasionally can exhibit milder symptoms of MD.

## HOW DOES MUSCULAR DYSTROPHY AFFECT MUSCLES?

Muscles are made up of thousands of muscle fibers. Each fiber is actually a number of individual cells that have joined together during development and are encased by an outer membrane. Muscle fibers that make up individual muscles are bound together by connective tissue.

Muscles are activated when an impulse, or signal, is sent from the brain through the spinal cord and peripheral nerves (nerves that connect the central nervous system to sensory organs and muscles) to the neuromuscular junction (the space between the nerve fiber and the muscle it activates). There, a release of the chemical acetylcholine triggers a series of events that cause the muscle to contract.

The muscle fiber membrane contains a group of proteins—called the "dystrophin-glycoprotein complex"—which prevents damage as muscle fibers contract and relax. When this protective membrane is damaged, muscle fibers begin to leak the protein creatine kinase (needed for the chemical reactions that produce energy for muscle contractions) and take on excess calcium, which causes further harm. Affected muscle fibers eventually die from this damage, leading to progressive muscle degeneration.

Although MD can affect several body tissues and organs, it most prominently affects the integrity of muscle fibers. The disease causes muscle degeneration, progressive weakness, fiber death, fiber branching and splitting, phagocytosis (in which muscle fiber material is broken down and destroyed by scavenger cells), and, in some cases, chronic or permanent shortening of tendons and muscles. Also, overall muscle strength and tendon reflexes are usually lessened or lost due to replacement of muscle by connective tissue and fat.

## ARE THERE OTHER MUSCULAR DYSTROPHY-LIKE CONDITIONS?

There are many other heritable diseases that affect the muscles, the nerves, or the neuromuscular junction. Such diseases as inflammatory myopathy, progressive muscle weakness, and cardiomyopathy (heart muscle weakness that interferes with pumping ability) may produce symptoms that are very similar to those found in some forms of MD), but they are caused by different genetic defects. The differential diagnosis for people with similar symptoms includes congenital myopathy, spinal muscular atrophy, and congenital myasthenic syndromes. The sharing of symptoms among multiple neuromuscular diseases, and the prevalence of sporadic cases in families not previously affected by MD, often makes it difficult for people with MD to obtain a quick diagnosis. Gene testing can provide a definitive diagnosis for many types of MD, but not all genes have been discovered that are responsible for some types of MD. Some individuals may have signs of MD, but carry none of the currently recognized genetic mutations. Studies of other related muscle diseases may, however, contribute to what we know about MD.

## WHAT ARE THE TREATMENTS FOR MUSCULAR DYSTROPHY?

No treatment is currently available to stop or reverse any form of MD. Instead, certain therapies and medications aim to treat the various problems that result from MD and improve the quality of life for patients. These include the following:

### Physical Therapy

Beginning physical therapy early can help keep muscles flexible and strong. A combination of physical activity and stretching exercises may be recommended.

### Respiratory Therapy

Many people with MD do not realize they have little respiratory strength until they have difficulty coughing or an infection leads to pneumonia. Regular visits to a specialist early in the diagnosis of MD can help guide treatment before a respiratory problem occurs. Eventually, many MD patients require assisted ventilation.

### Speech Therapy

MD patients who experience weakness in the facial and throat muscles may benefit from learning to slow the pace of their speech by pausing between breaths and by using special communication equipment.

### Occupational Therapy

As physical abilities change, occupational therapy can help patients with MD relearn these movements and abilities. Occupational therapy also teaches patients to use assistive devices such as wheelchairs and utensils.

### Corrective Surgery

At various times and depending on the form of MD, many patients require surgery to treat the conditions that result from MD. People with myotonic MD may need a pacemaker to treat heart problems or surgery to remove cataracts, a clouding of the lens of the eye that blocks light from entering the eye.

### Drug Therapy

Certain medications can help slow or control the symptoms of MD. These include the following:

- **Glucocorticoids, such as prednisone.** Studies show that daily treatment with prednisone can increase muscle strength, ability, and respiratory function and slow the progression of weakness. Side effects may include weight gain. Long-term use may result in brittle bones, cataracts, and high blood pressure.
- **Anticonvulsants.** Typically taken for epilepsy, these drugs may help control seizures and some muscle spasms.

- **Immunosuppressants.** Commonly given to treat autoimmune diseases such as lupus and eczema, immunosuppressive drugs may help delay some damage to dying muscle cells.
- Antibiotics to treat respiratory infections.

## Section 14.3 | Spina Bifida

This section includes text excerpted from "What Is Spina Bifida?" Centers for Disease Control and Prevention (CDC), September 3, 2019.

Spina bifida is a condition that affects the spine and is usually apparent at birth. It is a type of neural tube defect (NTD).

Spina bifida can happen anywhere along the spine if the neural tube does not close all the way. When the neural tube does not close all the way, the backbone that protects the spinal cord does not form and close as it should. This often results in damage to the spinal cord and nerves.

Spina bifida might cause physical and intellectual disabilities that range from mild to severe. The severity depends on:

- The size and location of the opening in the spine.
- Whether part of the spinal cord and nerves are affected.

### TYPES OF SPINA BIFIDA

The three most common types of spina bifida are:

**Myelomeningocele.** When people talk about spina bifida, most often they are referring to myelomeningocele. Myelomeningocele is the most serious type of spina bifida. With this condition, a sac of fluid comes through an opening in the baby's back. Part of the spinal cord and nerves are in this sac and are damaged. This type of spina bifida causes moderate to severe disabilities, such as problems affecting how the person goes to the bathroom, loss of feeling in the person's legs or feet, and not being able to move the legs.

**Meningocele.** Another type of spina bifida is meningocele. With meningocele, a sac of fluid comes through an opening in the baby's back. But, the spinal cord is not in this sac. There is usually little or no nerve damage. This type of spina bifida can cause minor disabilities.

**Spina bifida occulta.** Spina bifida occulta is the mildest type of spina bifida. It is sometimes called "hidden" spina bifida. With it, there is a small gap in the spine, but no opening or sac on the back. The spinal cord and the nerves usually are normal. Many times, spina bifida occulta is not discovered until late childhood or adulthood. This type of spina bifida usually does not cause any disabilities.

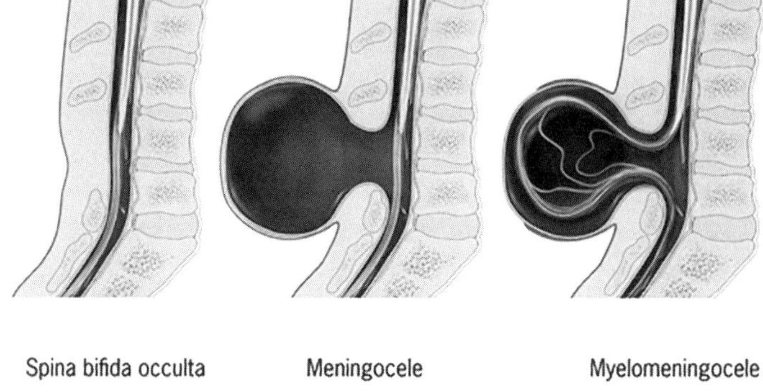


**Figure 14.1.** Types of Spina Bifida

## LIVING WITH SPINA BIFIDA: INFANTS

Having a new baby is an exciting and challenging time. New parents often feel many different emotions? such as love, joy, happiness, worry, and exhaustion. The same is true for parents who have a child affected by spina bifida. However, in addition to adjusting to life with a new baby, parents of a child with spina bifida also need to learn as much as possible about the condition to prepare for the needs of their child.

### Learning about Spina Bifida

When parents find out they are going to have a child with spina bifida, it can be overwhelming. It is important that they know that most children born with spina bifida reach their full potential.

It is very important for parents to take an active role in managing their child's care. Parents need to know about spina bifida and understand the health issues and treatment options to make the best possible choices for the health and happiness of their child.

- Parents should talk with a healthcare provider about any questions or concerns they have.
- Parents can start learning about spina bifida by reading The Centers for Disease Control and Prevention's (CDC) Basics and Health Issues and Treatments spina bifida pages.
- The Spina Bifida Association provides information on spina bifida and can be helpful in recommending clinics or healthcare providers who are experts in the care of children and adults with spina bifida.

### Physical Health

No two babies with spina bifida are exactly alike. Health issues will be different for each baby. Some babies have issues that are more severe than other babies.

## Pediatric Rehabilitation

With the right care, babies born with spina bifida will grow up to reach their full potential.

### Open Spina Bifida

When a baby is born with open spina bifida, in which the spinal cord is exposed (myelomeningocele), doctors will perform surgery to close it before birth or within the first few days of the baby's life.

### Hydrocephalus

Many babies born with spina bifida get hydrocephalus (often called "water on the brain"). This means that there is extra fluid in and around the brain. The extra fluid can cause the spaces in the brain, called "ventricles," to become too large and the head can swell. Hydrocephalus needs to be followed closely and treated properly to prevent brain injury.

If a baby with spina bifida has hydrocephalus, a surgeon can put in a shunt. A shunt is a small hollow tube that will help drain the fluid from the baby's brain and protect it from too much pressure. Additional surgery might be needed to change the shunt as the child grows up or if it becomes clogged or infected.

### Mobility and Physical Activity

People affected by spina bifida get around in different ways. These include walking without any aids or assistance; walking with braces, crutches or walkers; and using wheelchairs.

People with spina bifida higher on the spine (near the head) might have paralyzed legs and use wheelchairs. Those with spina bifida lower on the spine (near the hips) might have more use of their legs and use crutches, braces, or walkers, or they might be able to walk without these devices.

Doctors can start treatment for movement problems soon after a baby with spina bifida is born. A physical therapist can work with parents and caregivers to teach them how to exercise a baby's legs to increase strength, flexibility, and movement.

Regular physical activity is important for all babies, especially for those with conditions that affect movement, such as spina bifida. There are many ways for babies with spina bifida to be active. For example, they can:

- Play with toys, such as activity mats.
- Enjoy parks and recreation areas.
- Participate in community programs, such as the Early Intervention Program for Infants and Toddlers with Disabilities, which is a free program in many communities.
- Do exercises recommended by a physical therapist.

## LIVING WITH SPINA BIFIDA: TODDLERS AND PRESCHOOLERS

Life with a toddler or preschooler is both fun and challenging. These young children experience huge mental, social, and emotional changes. They have a lot of energy and enthusiasm for exploring and learning about their world and becoming independent. Developing independence can be especially challenging for children with spina bifida. Parents should start helping their child develop independence early in childhood.

### Encouraging Independence

For toddlers and preschoolers with spina bifida, there are many ways that parents and other caregivers can help them become more active and independent, such as:

- Teaching the child about her or his body and about spina bifida
- Encouraging the child to make choices, such as between two items of clothing
- Asking the child to help with daily tasks, such as putting away toys

Children with spina bifida might need extra help at times. But, it is very important that children be given the opportunity to complete a task before help is given. It is also important that parents give only the help that is needed rather than helping with the entire task. Parents must learn the difficult balance between giving the right amount of help to increase their child's independence and confidence, while at the same time being careful not to give the child tasks that cannot reasonably be completed—which might decrease their child's confidence.

### Physical Health

No two children with spina bifida are exactly alike. Health issues will be different for each child. Some children have issues that are more severe than other children. With the right care, children born with spina bifida will grow up to reach their full potential.

#### Mobility and Physical Activity

Children affected by spina bifida get around in different ways. These include walking without any aids or assistance; walking with braces, crutches or walkers; and using wheelchairs.

Children with spina bifida higher on the spine (near the head) might have paralyzed legs and use wheelchairs. Those with spina bifida lower on the spine (near the hips) might have more use of their legs and use crutches, braces, or walkers, or they might be able to walk without these devices.

A physical therapist can work with children, parents, and caregivers to teach them how to exercise the child's legs to increase strength, flexibility, and movement.

## Pediatric Rehabilitation

Regular physical activity is important for all children, but especially for those with conditions that affect movement, such as spina bifida. There are many ways for children with spina bifida to be active. For example, they can:

- Engage in active play with friends.
- Roll or walk in the neighborhood.
- Enjoy parks and recreation areas with playgrounds that are accessible for those with disabilities.
- Participate in community programs, such as the Early Intervention Program for Infants and Toddlers with Disabilities and Special Education Services for Preschoolers with Disabilities, which are free programs in many communities.
- Do exercises recommended by a physical therapist.

## Safety

Safety is an important issue for children with spina bifida. They can be at higher risk for injuries and abuse. It is important for parents and other family members to teach them how to stay safe and what to do if they feel threatened or have been hurt in any way.

## LIVING WITH SPINA BIFIDA: SCHOOL-AGED CHILDREN

Starting school brings children into regular contact with the larger world. Friendships become important and physical, social, and mental skills develop rapidly during this time. Children who feel good about themselves are more able to resist negative peer pressure and make better choices.

This is an important time for children to become more responsible and independent. This is also a good time to start exploring potential lifetime interests such as hobbies, music, or sports. Developing independence can be challenging for people affected by spina bifida. It is important to begin working on this process early in childhood.

## School

Many children with spina bifida do well in school. But, some can experience difficulties, especially children with shunts that are used to treat hydrocephalus. These children often have challenges involving learning. They might have difficulty paying attention or work slowly, be restless, or lose things. They also might have trouble making decisions. There are activities that children can do at home and at school to help with these problems. Healthcare professionals can provide information about these activities.

### Individualized Education Plan

An Individualized Education Plan (IEP) is important because it will help children develop skills at school. Children who participate in special education classes will have an IEP. An IEP is a legal document that lets the school know what kinds of assistance will be needed by a child during the school day. An IEP is created by parents and school personnel, such as a psychologist, teachers, a school nurse, and a physical education teacher, as well as any other professionals that parents think might be helpful.

#### 504 Plan

If a child does not qualify for an IEP, parents can request a 504 Plan be developed for their child at school. Usually, a 504 Plan is used by a general education student who is not eligible for special education services. By law, children may be eligible to have a 504 Plan which lists accommodations related to a child's disability. The 504 Plan accommodations may be needed to give the child an opportunity to perform at the same level as their peers. For example, a 504 Plan may include the child's assistive technology needs, such as using a tablet or laptop computer to take notes, and making sure they have a wheelchair accessible environment at school.

## Physical Health

No two children with spina bifida are exactly alike. Health issues will be different for each child. Some children have issues that are more severe than other children. With the right care, children born with spina bifida will grow up to reach their full potential.

#### Mobility and Physical Activity

Children with spina bifida higher on the spine (near the head) might have paralyzed legs and use wheelchairs. Those with spina bifida lower on the spine (near the hips) might have more use of their legs and use crutches, braces, or walkers, or they might be able to walk without these devices.

A physical therapist can work with children, parents, and caregivers to teach them how to exercise the child's legs to increase strength, flexibility, and movement.

Regular physical activity is important for all children, but especially for those with conditions that affect movement, such as spina bifida. CDC recommends 60 minutes of physical activity a day. There are many ways for children with spina bifida to be active. For example, they can:

- Engage in active play with friends.
- Roll or walk in the neighborhood.
- Enjoy parks and recreation areas with playgrounds that are accessible for those with disabilities.
- Attend summer camps and recreational facilities that are accessible for those with disabilities.
- Participate in sports activities (for example, swimming) and teams for people with or without disabilities.

#### Safety

Safety is an important issue for children with spina bifida. They can be at higher risk for injuries and abuse. As these children become more independent, it is important for their parents and other family members to teach them how to stay safe and what to do if they feel threatened or have been hurt in any way.

## LIVING WITH SPINA BIFIDA: ADOLESCENTS AND TEENS

Many physical, mental, emotional, and social changes are associated with the adolescent and teen years. Teens and adolescents develop their own personalities and interests and want to become more independent.

This transition period can be challenging, especially for people affected by spina bifida. It is important for parents and caregivers of adolescents and teens with spina bifida to take active steps toward making them independent starting in childhood, so that by the time they are older they can develop the necessary skills to help them reach their full potential.

### Physical Health

As people with spina bifida mature, they will perform more and more activities themselves. Most teens will dress and bathe themselves, manage their bathroom plans, and move about independently in their homes and communities. They might begin to make their own doctor appointments and continue to participate in updating their own Individualized Education Plan (IEP) or 504 Plan, if they have one. They also should participate in a seating or wheelchair evaluation at least once each year if they use a wheelchair. This evaluation will make sure the wheelchair fits correctly and makes moving as easy as possible.

#### Mobility and Physical Activity

People with spina bifida higher on the spine (near the head) might have paralyzed legs and use wheelchairs. Those with spina bifida lower on the spine (near the hips) might have more use of their legs and use crutches, braces, or walkers, or they might be able to walk without these devices.

A physical therapist can work with adolescents and teens to teach them how to exercise their legs to increase strength, flexibility, and movement.

Regular physical activity is important for all teens and adolescents, but especially for those with conditions that affect movement, such as spina bifida. CDC recommends 60 minutes of physical activity a day. There are many ways for teens and adolescents with spina bifida to be active. For example, they can:

- Engage in physical activities with friends.
- Roll or walk in the neighborhood.
- Lift weights.
- Participate in sports activities (for example, swimming) and on teams for people with and without disabilities.

- Attend summer camps and recreational facilities that are accessible for those with disabilities.

## Section 14.4 | Juvenile Rheumatoid Arthritis

This section includes text excerpted from "Juvenile Arthritis," National Institute of Arthritis and Musculoskeletal and Skin Diseases (NIAMS), June 2015. Reviewed November 2019.

### WHAT IS JUVENILE ARTHRITIS?

"Juvenile arthritis" is the term used to describe arthritis in children. Children can get arthritis just like adults. Arthritis is caused by inflammation of the joints. A joint is where two or more bones are joined together. Arthritis causes:

- Pain
- Swelling
- Stiffness
- Loss of motion

The most common type of arthritis in children is called "juvenile idiopathic arthritis" (idiopathic means "from unknown causes"). There are several other forms of arthritis affecting children.

Juvenile arthritis is a rheumatic disease or one that causes loss of function due to an inflamed supporting structure or structures of the body. Some rheumatic diseases also can involve internal organs.

### WHO GETS JUVENILE ARTHRITIS

Juvenile arthritis affects children of all ages and ethnic backgrounds. About 294,000 American children under age 18 have arthritis or other rheumatic conditions.

### WHAT ARE THE TYPES OF JUVENILE ARTHRITIS?

There are seven separate subtypes of juvenile idiopathic arthritis, each with distinct symptoms. However, with every subtype, a child will have arthritis symptoms of joint pain, swelling, tenderness, warmth, or stiffness that last for more than 6 continuous weeks.

The subtypes are:

- **Systemic juvenile idiopathic arthritis (formerly known as "systemic juvenile rheumatoid arthritis").** Systemic means the arthritis can affect the whole body, rather than just a specific organ or joint. A child has arthritis with, or that was preceded by, a fever that has lasted for at least 2 weeks. The fever has come and gone, but spiked, or hit its highest temperature, for at least 3 days. The fever occurs with at least one or more of the following:

- Generalized enlargement of the lymph nodes
- Enlargement of the liver or spleen
- Inflammation of the lining of the heart (pericarditis) or the lungs (pleuritis)
- The characteristic rheumatoid rash, which is flat, pale, pink, and generally not itchy. The individual spots of the rash are usually the size of a quarter or smaller. They are present for a few minutes to a few hours, and then disappear without any changes in the skin. The rash may move from one part of the body to another.

- **Oligoarticular juvenile idiopathic arthritis (formerly known as "pauciarticular juvenile rheumatoid arthritis").** A child has arthritis affecting one to four joints during the first 6 months of disease. Two subcategories of this type are:
  - Persistent oligoarthritis, which means the child never has more than four joints involved throughout the disease course
  - Extended oligoarthritis, which means that more than four joints are involved after the first 6 months of the disease
- **Polyarticular juvenile idiopathic arthritis—rheumatoid factor negative (formerly known as "polyarticular juvenile rheumatoid arthritis"—"rheumatoid factor negative").** A child has arthritis in five or more joints during the first 6 months of disease, and all tests for rheumatoid factor (proteins produced by the immune system that can attack healthy tissue, which are commonly found in rheumatoid arthritis and juvenile arthritis) are negative.
- **Polyarticular juvenile idiopathic arthritis—rheumatoid factor positive (formerly known as "polyarticular rheumatoid arthritis"—"rheumatoid factor positive").** A child has arthritis in five or more joints during the first 6 months of the disease. Also, at least two tests for rheumatoid factor, at least 3 months apart, are positive.
- **Psoriatic juvenile idiopathic arthritis.** A child has both arthritis and psoriasis (a skin disease), or has arthritis and at least two of the following:
  - Inflammation and swelling of an entire finger or toe (this is called "dactylitis")
  - Nail pitting or splitting
  - A first-degree relative with psoriasis
- **Enthesitis-related juvenile idiopathic arthritis.** The enthesis is the point at which a ligament, tendon, or joint capsule attaches to the bone.

If this point becomes inflamed, it can be tender, swollen, and painful with use. The most common locations are around the knee and at the Achilles tendon on the back of the ankle. A child is diagnosed with this condition if she or he has both arthritis and inflammation of an enthesitis site, or has either arthritis or enthesitis with at least two of the following:

- Inflammation of the sacroiliac joints (at the bottom of the back) or pain and stiffness in the lumbosacral area (in the lower back)
- A positive blood test for the human leukocyte antigen (HLA) *B27* gene
- Onset of arthritis in males after age 6 years
- A first-degree relative diagnosed with ankylosing spondylitis, enthesitis-related arthritis, or inflammation of the sacroiliac joint in association with inflammatory bowel disease or acute inflammation of the eye

- **Undifferentiated arthritis.** A child is said to have this condition if the signs and symptoms of the arthritis do not fulfill the criteria for one of the other six categories or if they fulfill the criteria for more than one category.

## WHAT ARE THE SYMPTOMS OF JUVENILE ARTHRITIS?

The most common symptom of all types of juvenile arthritis is persistent joint swelling, pain, and stiffness that is typically worse in the morning or after a nap. The pain may limit movement of the affected joint, although many children, especially younger ones, will not complain of pain.

One of the earliest signs of juvenile arthritis may be limping in the morning because of an affected knee.

Besides joint symptoms, children with systemic juvenile arthritis may have:

- A high fever that may appear and disappear very quickly
- A skin rash that may appear and disappear very quickly
- Swollen lymph nodes located in the neck and other parts of the body
- Inflammation of internal organs, including the heart (fewer than half of the cases) and the lungs (very rarely)

## WHAT CAUSES JUVENILE ARTHRITIS

Most forms of juvenile arthritis are autoimmune disorders in which the body's immune system—which normally helps to fight off bacteria or viruses—mistakenly attacks some of its own healthy cells and tissues. The result is inflammation, marked by redness, heat, pain, and swelling. Inflammation can cause joint damage.

Doctors do not know why the immune system attacks healthy tissues in children who develop juvenile arthritis. Scientists suspect that it is a two-step process. First, something in a child's genetic makeup gives her or him a tendency to develop juvenile arthritis; then an environmental factor, such as a virus, triggers the development of the disease.

Not all cases of juvenile arthritis are autoimmune, however. Recent research has shown that some people, such as many with systemic arthritis, have what is called an "autoinflammatory condition." Although the two terms sound similar, the disease processes behind autoimmune and autoinflammatory disorders are different.

### Autoimmune Disorders

When the immune system is working properly, foreign invaders such as bacteria and viruses provoke the body to produce proteins called "antibodies." Antibodies attach to these invaders so the immune system can recognize and destroy them. In an autoimmune reaction, the antibodies attach to the body's own healthy tissues by mistake, signaling the body to attack them. Because they target the self, these proteins are called "autoantibodies."

### Autoinflammatory Disorders

Like autoimmune disorders, autoinflammatory conditions also cause inflammation. And like autoimmune disorders, they also involve an overactive immune system. However, autoinflammation is not caused by autoantibodies. Instead, autoinflammation involves a more primitive part of the immune system that, in healthy people, causes white blood cells to destroy harmful substances. When this system goes awry, it causes inflammation for unknown reasons. Besides inflammation, autoinflammatory diseases often cause fever and rashes.

## IS THERE A TEST FOR JUVENILE ARTHRITIS?

There is no easy way a doctor can tell if a child has juvenile arthritis. Doctors usually suspect arthritis when a child has symptoms of:

- Constant joint pain or swelling
- Skin rashes that cannot be explained
- Fever along with swelling of lymph nodes or inflammation in the body's organs

To be sure that it is juvenile arthritis, doctors may:

- Perform a physical exam
- Ask about family health history
- Order lab or blood tests
- Order x-rays

## HOW IS JUVENILE ARTHRITIS TREATED?

The main goals of treatment are to:

- Preserve a high level of physical and social functioning
- Maintain a good quality of life

To achieve these goals, doctors recommend treatments that:

- Reduce swelling
- Maintain full movement in the affected joints
- Relieve pain
- Prevent, identify, and treat complications
- Most children with juvenile arthritis need a combination of medication and other treatments to reach these goals

## Medications

- **Nonsteroidal anti-inflammatory drugs (NSAIDs).** Aspirin, ibuprofen, naproxen, and naproxen sodium are examples of NSAIDs. They are often the first type of medication doctors prescribe for juvenile arthritis. All NSAIDs work similarly by blocking substances called "prostaglandins" that add to inflammation and pain. However, each NSAID is a different chemical, and each has a slightly different effect on the body. For unknown reasons, some children seem to respond better to one NSAID than another. NSAIDs should only be used at the lowest dose possible for the shortest time needed.

  You can buy some NSAIDs over the counter, while several others, including a subclass called "COX-2 inhibitors," need a prescription. All NSAIDs can have significant side effects, so consult your child's doctor before giving any of them. Your child's doctor should monitor your child if she or he takes NSAIDs regularly to control juvenile arthritis.

  Side effects of NSAIDs include stomach problems; skin rashes; high blood pressure; fluid retention; and liver, kidney, and heart problems. The longer a person uses NSAIDs, the more likely she or he is to have side effects, ranging from mild to serious. Many other medicines cannot be taken when a person is taking NSAIDs because NSAIDs alter the way the body uses or eliminates these other medicines.
- **Disease-modifying antirheumatic drugs (DMARDs).** If NSAIDs do not relieve symptoms of your child's juvenile arthritis, the doctor may prescribe this type of medication. DMARDs slow the progression of juvenile arthritis, but because they may take weeks or months to relieve symptoms, they often are taken with an NSAID. Although there are many different types of DMARDs, many doctors prescribe one called "methotrexate."

  Researchers have learned that methotrexate is safe and effective for some children with juvenile arthritis whose symptoms are not relieved by other medications. Because children only need small doses of methotrexate for relief of arthritis symptoms, potentially dangerous side effects rarely occur. The most serious complication can be liver damage, which a doctor can help prevent with regular blood tests and check-ups. Careful monitoring for side effects is important for people taking methotrexate. When side effects are noticed early, the doctor can reduce the dose and eliminate the side effects.

- **Corticosteroids.** If your child has very severe juvenile arthritis, stronger medicines may be needed to stop serious symptoms, such as inflammation of the sac around the heart (pericarditis). Corticosteroids, such as prednisone, may be added to the treatment plan to control severe symptoms. This medication can be given by IV (intravenous), mouth, or injection directly into a joint. Corticosteroids are powerful anti-inflammatory medicines. Corticosteroids can interfere with your child's normal growth and can cause other side effects, such as a round face, weakened bones, and an increased chance of having infections. Once the medication controls severe symptoms, the doctor will reduce the dose gradually and, in time, stop it completely. It can be dangerous to stop taking corticosteroids suddenly. Carefully follow the doctor's instructions about how to take or reduce the dose. For inflammation in one or just a few joints, injecting a corticosteroid compound into the affected joint or joints can often bring quick relief without the systemic side effects of oral or IV medication.
- **Biologic agents.** If your child has received little relief from other medications, she or he may be given one of a newer class of medications called "biologic response modifiers," or "biologic agents." These are based on compounds made by living cells. Tumor necrosis factor (TNF) inhibitors are biologic agents that work by blocking the actions of TNF, a naturally occurring protein in the body that helps cause inflammation. Other biologic agents block other inflammatory proteins, such as interleukin-1 or immune cells called "T cells."

  Different biologics tend to work better for the different subtypes of the disease.

## Other Treatments

- **Physical therapy.** A regular, general exercise program is an important part of a child's treatment plan. Exercise can help to maintain muscle tone and preserve and recover the range of motion of the joints. A physiatrist (rehabilitation specialist) or a physical therapist can design an appropriate exercise program for your child. The specialist also may recommend using splints and other devices to help maintain normal bone and joint growth.

- **Complementary and alternative therapies.** Many adults seek alternative ways of treating arthritis, such as special diets, supplements, acupuncture, massage, or even magnetic jewelry or mattress pads. Research shows that increasing numbers of children are using alternative and complementary therapies as well.

  Although there is little research to support many alternative treatments, some people seem to benefit from them. If your child's doctor feels the approach has value and is not harmful, you can incorporate it into the treatment plan. However, do not neglect regular healthcare or treatment of serious symptoms.

## WHO TREATS JUVENILE ARTHRITIS

A team approach is the best way to treat juvenile arthritis. It is best if a doctor trained to treat these types of diseases in children called a "pediatric rheumatologist" manages your child's care. However, many children's doctors and "adult" rheumatologists also treat children with arthritis.

Other members of your child's healthcare team may include:

- Physical therapist
- Occupational therapist
- Counselor or psychologist
- Eye doctor
- Dentist and orthodontist
- Bone surgeon
- Dietitian
- Pharmacist
- Social worker
- Rheumatology nurse
- School nurse

## EXERCISE IS KEY TO REDUCING SYMPTOMS OF JUVENILE ARTHRITIS

Pain sometimes limits what children with juvenile arthritis can do. However, exercise is key to reducing the symptoms of arthritis and maintaining function and range of motion of the joints. Ask your child's healthcare team for exercise guidelines.

Most children with arthritis can take part in physical activities and certain sports when their symptoms are under control. Swimming is a good activity because it uses many joints and muscles without putting weight on the joints.

During a disease flare, your child's doctor may advise your child to limit certain activities. It will depend on the joints involved. Once the flare is over, your child can return to her or his normal activities.

## Section 14.5 | Upper- and Lower-Limb Reduction Defects

This section includes text excerpted from "Facts about Upper- and Lower-Limb Reduction Defects," Centers for Disease Control and Prevention (CDC), November 1, 2018.

Upper- and lower-limb reduction defects occur when a part of or the entire arm (upper limb) or leg (lower limb) of a fetus fails to form completely during pregnancy. The defect is referred to as a "limb reduction" because a limb is reduced from its normal size or is missing.

### WHAT WE KNOW ABOUT UPPER- AND LOWER-LIMB REDUCTION DEFECTS

#### How Often Do Limb Reduction Defects Occur?

The Centers for Disease Control and Prevention (CDC) estimates that each year about 1,500 babies in the United States are born with upper limb reductions and about 750 are born with lower limb reductions. In other words, each year about 4 out of every 10,000 babies will have upper limb reductions and about 2 out of every 10,000 babies will have lower limb reductions. Some of these babies will have both upper- and lower-limb reduction defects.

#### What Problems Do Children with Limb Reduction Defects Have?

Babies and children with limb reduction defects will face various issues and difficulties, but the extent of these will depend on the location and size of the reduction. Some potential difficulties and problems include:

- Difficulties with normal development such as motor skills
- Needing assistance with daily activities such as self-care
- Limitations with certain movements, sports, or activities
- Potential emotional and social issues because of physical appearance

Specific treatment for limb reduction defects will be determined by the child's doctor, based on things such as the child's age, the extent and type of defect, and the child's tolerance for certain medications, procedures, and therapies.

The overall goal for treatment of limb reduction defects is to provide the child with a limb that has proper function and appearance. Treatment can vary for each child. Potential treatments include:

- Prosthetics (artificial limbs)
- Orthotics (splints or braces)
- Surgery
- Rehabilitation (physical or occupational therapy)

It is important to remember that some babies and children with limb reductions will have some difficulties and limitations throughout life, but with proper treatment and care they can live long, healthy, and productive lives.

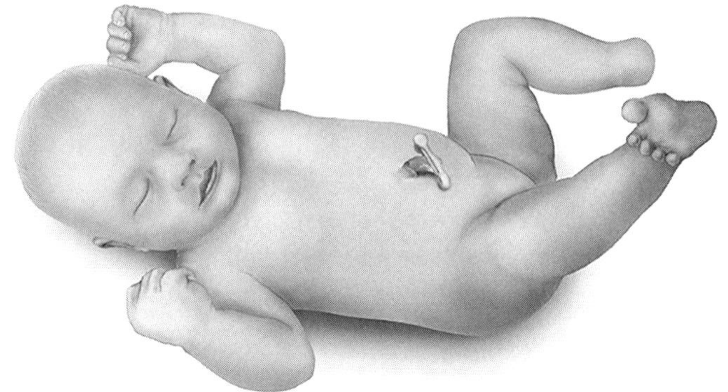

**Figure 14.2.** Congenital Absence of Foot and Toes

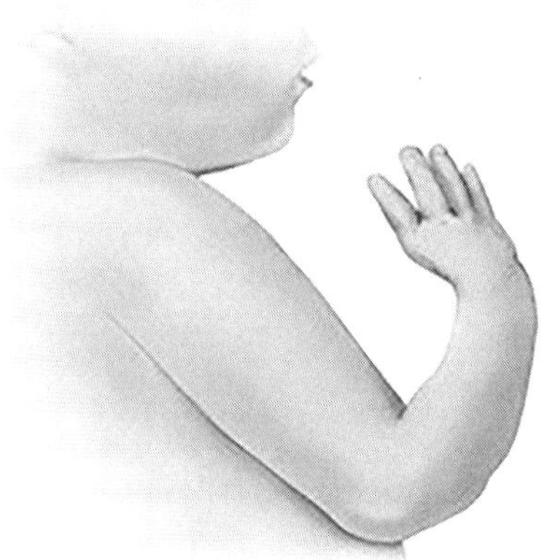

**Figure 14.3.** Longitudinal Reduction Defect of Radius

## WHAT WE STILL DO NOT KNOW ABOUT UPPER- AND LOWER-LIMB REDUCTION DEFECTS

### What Causes Limb Reduction Defects

The cause of limb reduction defects is unknown. However, research has shown that certain behaviors or exposures during pregnancy can increase the risk of having a baby with a limb reduction defect. These include:

- Exposure of the mother to certain chemicals or viruses while she is pregnant
- Exposure of the mother to certain medications
- Possible exposure of the mother to tobacco smoking (although more research is needed)

The CDC works with many researchers to study risk factors that can increase the chance of having a baby with limb reduction defects, as well as outcomes of babies with the defect. Following are examples of what this research has found:

- A woman taking multivitamins before she gets pregnant might decrease her risk for having a baby with limb reduction defects, although more research is needed.
- Certain sets of limb reduction defects might be associated with other birth defects, such as heart defects, omphalocele, and gastroschisis.

### Can Limb Reduction Defects Be Prevented?

There is no known way to prevent this type of defect, but some of the problems experienced later in life by a person born with a limb reduction defect can be prevented if the defect is treated early.

Even so, mothers can take steps before and during pregnancy to have a healthy pregnancy. Steps include taking a daily multivitamin with folic acid (400 micrograms), not smoking, and not drinking alcohol during pregnancy.

## Section 14.6 | Down Syndrome

This section contains text excerpted from the following sources: Text beginning with the heading "What Is Down Syndrome?" is excerpted from "Facts about Down Syndrome," Centers for Disease Control and Prevention (CDC), November 1, 2018; Text under the heading "Treatment of Down Syndrome" is excerpted from "What Are Common Treatments for Down Syndrome?" *Eunice Kennedy Shriver* National Institute of Child Health and Human Development (NICHD), January 31, 2017.

### WHAT IS DOWN SYNDROME?

Down syndrome (DS) is a condition in which a person has an extra chromosome. Chromosomes are small "packages" of genes in the body. They determine how a baby's body forms during pregnancy and how the baby's body functions as it grows in the womb and after birth. Typically, a baby is born with 46 chromosomes. Babies with DS have an extra copy of one of these chromosomes, chromosome 21. A medical term for having an extra copy of a chromosome is "trisomy." DS is also referred to as "Trisomy 21." This extra copy changes how the baby's body and brain develop, which can cause both mental and physical challenges for the baby.

Even though people with DS might act and look similar, each person has different abilities. People with DS usually have an IQ (a measure of intelligence) in the mildly-to-moderately low range and are slower to speak than other children.

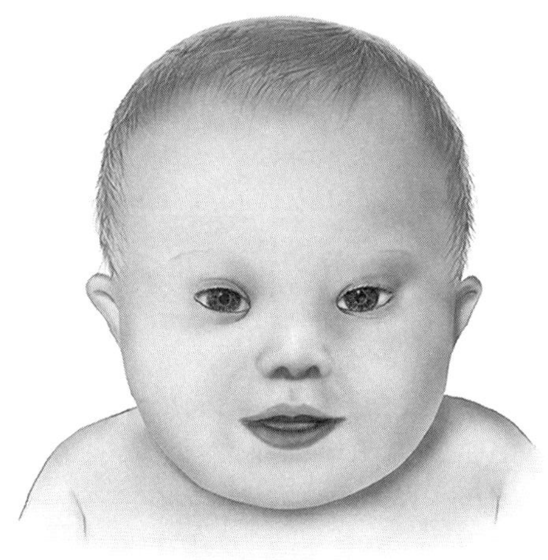

**Figure 14.4.** Birth Defects

Some common physical features of DS include:

- A flattened face, especially the bridge of the nose
- Almond-shaped eyes that slant up
- A short neck
- Small ears
- A tongue that tends to stick out of the mouth
- Tiny white spots on the iris (colored part) of the eye
- Small hands and feet
- A single line across the palm of the hand (palmar crease)
- Small pinky fingers that sometimes curve toward the thumb
- Poor muscle tone or loose joints
- Shorter in height as children and adults

### Occurrence of Down Syndrome

Down syndrome remains the most common chromosomal condition diagnosed in the United States. Each year, about 6,000 babies born in the United States have DS. This means that DS occurs in about 1 out of every 700 babies.

## TYPES OF DOWN SYNDROME

There are 3 types of DS. People often cannot tell the difference between each type without looking at the chromosomes because the physical features and behaviors are similar.

- **Trisomy 21.** About 95 percent of people with DS have Trisomy 21.2. With this type of DS, each cell in the body has 3 separate copies of chromosome 21 instead of the usual 2 copies.

- **Translocation Down syndrome.** This type accounts for a small percentage of people with DS (about 3%). This occurs when an extra part or a whole extra chromosome 21 is present, but it is attached or "trans-located" to a different chromosome rather than being a separate chromosome 21.
- **Mosaic Down syndrome.** This type affects about 2 percent of the people with DS. Mosaic means mixture or combination. For children with mosaic DS, some of their cells have 3 copies of chromosome 21, but other cells have the typical 2 copies of chromosome 21. Children with mosaic DS may have the same features as other children with DS. However, they may have fewer features of the condition due to the presence of some (or many) cells with a typical number of chromosomes.

## CAUSES AND RISK FACTORS OF DOWN SYNDROME

- The extra chromosome 21 leads to the physical features and developmental challenges that can occur among people with DS. Researchers know that DS is caused by an extra chromosome, but no one knows for sure why DS occurs or how many different factors play a role.
- One factor that increases the risk for having a baby with DS is the mother's age. Women who are 35 years or older when they become pregnant are more likely to have a pregnancy affected by DS than women who become pregnant at a younger age. However, the majority of babies with DS are born to mothers less than 35 years old, because there are many more births among younger women.

## DIAGNOSIS OF DOWN SYNDROME

There are two basic types of tests available to detect DS during pregnancy: screening tests and diagnostic tests. A screening test can tell a woman and her healthcare provider whether her pregnancy has a lower or higher chance of having DS. Screening tests do not provide an absolute diagnosis, but they are safer for the mother and the developing baby. Diagnostic tests can typically detect whether or not a baby will have DS, but they can be more risky for the mother and developing baby. Neither screening nor diagnostic tests can predict the full impact of DS on a baby; no one can predict this.

## SCREENING TESTS OF DOWN SYNDROME

Screening tests often include a combination of a blood test, which measures the amount of various substances in the mother's blood, and an ultrasound, which creates a picture of the baby. During an ultrasound, one of the things the technician looks at is the fluid behind the baby's neck. Extra fluid in this region could indicate a genetic problem. These screening tests can help determine the baby's risk of DS. Rarely, screening tests can give an abnormal result even when there is nothing wrong with the baby. Sometimes, the test results are normal and yet they miss a problem that does exist.

## DIAGNOSTIC TESTS OF DOWN SYNDROME

Diagnostic tests are usually performed after a positive screening test in order to confirm a DS diagnosis. Types of diagnostic tests include:

- **Chorionic villus sampling (CVS)**—examines material from the placenta
- **Amniocentesis**—examines the amniotic fluid (the fluid from the sac surrounding the baby)
- **Percutaneous umbilical blood sampling (PUBS)**—examines blood from the umbilical cord

These tests look for changes in the chromosomes that would indicate a DS diagnosis.

## OTHER HEALTH PROBLEMS OF DOWN SYNDROME

Many people with DS have the common facial features and no other major birth defects. However, some people with DS might have one or more major birth defects or other medical problems. Some of the more common health problems among children with DS are listed below:

- Hearing loss
- Obstructive sleep apnea, which is a condition where the person's breathing temporarily stops while asleep
- Ear infections
- Eye diseases
- Heart defects present at birth

Healthcare providers routinely monitor children with DS for these conditions.

## TREATMENT OF DOWN SYNDROME

There is no single, standard treatment for DS. Treatments are based on each individual's physical and intellectual needs as well as her or his personal strengths and limitations. People with DS can receive proper care while living at home and in the community.

A child with DS likely will receive care from a team of health professionals, including, but not limited to, physicians, special educators, speech therapists, occupational therapists, physical therapists, and social workers. All professionals who interact with children with DS should provide stimulation and encouragement.

## Pediatric Rehabilitation

People with DS are at a greater risk for a number of health problems and conditions than are those who do not have DS. Many of these associated conditions may require immediate care right after birth, occasional treatment throughout childhood and adolescence, or long-term treatments throughout life. For example, an infant with DS may need surgery a few days after birth to correct a heart defect; or a person with DS may have digestive problems that require a lifelong special diet.

Children, teens, and adults with DS also need the same regular medical care as those without the condition, from well-baby visits and routine vaccinations as infants to reproductive counseling and cardiovascular care later in life. Like other people, they also benefit from regular physical activity and social activities.

- Early intervention and educational therapy
- Treatment therapies
- Drugs and supplements
- Assistive devices

## Early Intervention and Educational Therapy

"Early intervention" refers to a range of specialized programs and resources that professionals provide to very young children with DS and their families. These professionals may include special educators, speech therapists, occupational therapists, physical therapists, and social workers.

Research indicates that early intervention improves outcomes for children with DS. This assistance can begin shortly after birth and often continues until a child reaches age 3. After that age, most children receive interventions and treatment through their local school district.

Most children with DS are eligible for free, appropriate public education under federal law. Public Law 105-17 (2004): The Individuals with Disabilities Education Act (IDEA) makes it possible for children with disabilities to get free educational services and devices to help them learn as much as they can. Each child is entitled to these services from birth through the end of high school, or until age 21, whichever comes first. Most early intervention programs fall under this legislation.

The National Early Childhood Technical Assistance Center (NECTAC), run by the U.S. Department of Education (ED), provides information and resources for parents and families looking for early intervention programs.

The law also states that each child must be taught in the least restrictive environment that is appropriate. This statement does not mean that each child will be placed in a regular classroom. Instead, educators will work to provide an environment that best fits the child's needs and skills.

The following information may be helpful for those considering educational assistance programs for a child with DS:

- The child must have certain cognitive or learning deficits to be eligible for free special education programs. Parents can contact a local school principal or special education coordinator to learn how to have a child examined to see if she or he qualifies for services under the IDEA.
- If a child qualifies for special services, a team of people will work together to design an Individualized Educational Plan (IEP) for the child. The team may include parents or caregivers, teachers, a school psychologist, and other specialists in child development or education. The IEP includes specific learning goals for that child, based on her or his needs and capabilities. The team also decides how best to carry out the IEP.
- Children with DS may attend a school for children with special needs. Parents may have a choice between a school where most of the children do not have disabilities and one for children with special needs. Educators and healthcare providers can help families with the decision about what environment is best. Integration into a regular school has become much more common in recent decades, and IDEA requires that public schools work to maximize a child's access to typical learning experiences and interactions.

The U.S. Department of Education funds the Parent Center Network, which provides resources, contacts, and assistance for parents and families trying to navigate special education programs.

## Treatment Therapies

A variety of therapies can be used in early intervention programs and throughout a person's life to promote the greatest possible development, independence, and productivity. Some of these therapies are listed below.

- **Physical therapy** includes activities and exercises that help build motor skills, increase muscle strength, and improve posture and balance.
  - Physical therapy is important, especially early in a child's life, because physical abilities lay the foundation for other skills. The ability to turn over, crawl, and reach helps infants learn about the world around them and how to interact with it.
  - A physical therapist also can help a child with DS compensate for physical challenges, such as low muscle tone, in ways that avoid long-term problems. For example, a physical therapist might help a child establish an efficient walking pattern, rather than one that might lead to foot pain.
- **Speech-language therapy** can help children with DS improve their communication skills and use language more effectively.

  - Children with DS often learn to speak later than their peers. A speech-language therapist can help them develop the early skills necessary for communication, such as imitating sounds. The therapist also may help an infant breastfeed because breastfeeding can strengthen muscles that are used for speech.
  - In many cases, children with DS understand language and want to communicate before they can speak. A speech-language therapist can help a child use alternate means of communication, such as sign language and pictures, until she or he learns to speak.
  - Learning to communicate is an ongoing process, so a person with DS also may benefit from speech and language therapy in school as well as later in life. The therapist may help with conversation skills, pronunciation skills, understanding what is read (called "comprehension"), and learning and remembering words.
- **Occupational therapy** helps find ways to adjust everyday tasks and conditions to match a person's needs and abilities.
  - This type of therapy teaches self-care skills5 such as eating, getting dressed, writing, and using a computer.
  - An occupational therapist might offer special tools that can help improve everyday functioning, such as a pencil that is easier to grip.
  - At the high school level, an occupational therapist could help teenagers identify jobs, careers, or skills that match their interests and strengths.
- **Emotional and behavioral therapies** work to find useful responses to both desirable and undesirable behaviors. Children with DS may become frustrated because of difficulty communicating, may develop compulsive behaviors, and may have attention deficit hyperactivity disorder and other mental-health issues. These types of therapists try to understand why a child is acting out, create ways and strategies for avoiding or preventing these situations from occurring, and teach better or more positive ways to respond to situations.
  - A psychologist, counselor, or other mental-health professional can help a child deal with emotions and build coping and interpersonal skills.
  - The changes in hormone levels that adolescents experience during puberty can cause them to become more aggressive. Behavioral therapists can help teenagers recognize their intense emotions and teach them healthy ways to reach a feeling of calmness.
  - Parents may also benefit from guidance on how to help a child with DS manage day-to-day challenges and reach her or his full potential.

### Drugs and Supplements

Some people with DS take amino acid supplements or drugs that affect their brain activity. However, many of the recent clinical trials of these treatments were poorly controlled and revealed adverse effects from these treatments. Since then, newer psychoactive drugs that are much more specific have been developed. No controlled clinical studies of these medications for DS have demonstrated their safety and efficacy, however.

Many studies of drugs to treat symptoms of dementia in DS have included only a few participants. The results of these studies have not shown clear benefits of these drugs, either. Similarly, studies of antioxidants for dementia in DS have shown that these supplements are safe, but not effective.

### Assistive Devices

More and more often, interventions for children with DS involve assistive devices—any type of material, equipment, tool, or technology that enhances learning or makes tasks easier to complete. Examples include amplification devices for hearing problems, bands that help with movement, special pencils to make writing easier, touchscreen computers, and computers with large-letter keyboards.

### DS-Connect®: The Down Syndrome Registry

Parents and families of children with DS can connect with other families and people with DS from around the world to learn more and share information. The NICHD-led DS-Connect® is a safe and secure registry to help families and researchers identify similarities and differences in the symptoms and treatment of people with DS and guide future research.

# Chapter 15 | Geriatric Rehabilitation

**Chapter Contents**

## Section 15.1 | **Diabetic Neuropathy**

This section includes text under the heading "Diabetic Neuropathy Information Page," National Institute of Neurological Disorders and Stroke (NINDS), March 27, 2019.

Diabetic neuropathy is a peripheral nerve disorder caused by diabetes or poor blood sugar control. The most common types of diabetic neuropathy results in problems with sensation in the feet. It can develop slowly after many years of diabetes or may occur early in the disease. The symptoms are numbness, pain, or tingling in the feet or lower legs. The pain can be intense and require treatment to relieve the discomfort. The loss of sensation in the feet may also increase the possibility that foot injuries will go unnoticed and develop into ulcers or lesions that become infected. In some cases, diabetic neuropathy can be associated with difficulty walking and some weakness in the foot muscles. There are other types of diabetic-related neuropathies that affect specific parts of the body. For example, diabetic amyotrophy causes pain, weakness and wasting of the thigh muscles, or cranial nerve infarcts that may result in double vision, a drooping eyelid, or dizziness. Diabetes can also affect the autonomic nerves that control blood pressure, the digestive tract, bladder function, and sexual organs. Challenges involving the autonomic nerves may cause lightheadedness, indigestion, diarrhea or constipation, difficulty with bladder control, and impotence.

### TREATMENT OF DIABETIC NEUROPATHY

The goal of treating diabetic neuropathy is to prevent further tissue damage and relieve discomfort. The first step is to bring blood sugar levels under control by diet and medication. Another important part of treatment involves taking special care of the feet by wearing proper-fitting shoes and routinely checking the feet for cuts and infections. Analgesics, low doses of antidepressants, and some anticonvulsant medications may be prescribed for relief of pain, burning, or tingling. Some individuals find that walking regularly, taking warm baths, or using elastic stockings may help relieve leg pain.

### PROGNOSIS OF DIABETIC NEUROPATHY

The prognosis for diabetic neuropathy depends largely on how well the underlying condition of diabetes is handled. Treating diabetes may halt the progression and improve symptoms of the neuropathy, but recovery is slow. The painful sensations of diabetic neuropathy may become severe enough to cause depression in some patients.

## Section 15.2 | **Peripheral Neuropathies**

This section includes text excerpted from "Peripheral Neuropathy Fact Sheet," National Institute of Neurological Disorders and Stroke (NINDS), August 13, 2019.

Peripheral neuropathy refers to the many conditions that involve damage to the peripheral nervous system, the vast communication network that sends signals between the central nervous system (the brain and spinal cord) and all other parts of the body. Peripheral nerves send many types of sensory information to the central nervous system (CNS), such as a message that the feet are cold. They also carry signals from the CNS to the rest of the body. Best known are the signals to the muscles that tell them to contract, which is how there is movement, but there are different types of signals that help control everything from heart and blood vessels, digestion, urination, sexual function, bones, and immune system. The peripheral nerves are such as the cables that connect the different parts of a computer or connect to the Internet. When they malfunction, complex functions can grind to a halt.

Nerve signaling in neuropathy is disrupted in three ways:

- Loss of signals normally sent (such as a broken wire)
- Inappropriate signaling when there should not be any (such as static on a telephone line)
- Errors that distort the messages being sent (such as a wavy television picture)

Symptoms can range from mild to disabling and are rarely life-threatening. The symptoms depend on the type of nerve fibers affected and the type and severity of damage. Symptoms may develop over days, weeks, or years. In some cases, the symptoms improve on their own and may not require advanced care. Unlike nerve cells in the central nervous system, peripheral nerve cells continue to grow throughout life.

Some forms of neuropathy involve damage to only one nerve (called "mononeuropathy"). Neuropathy affecting two or more nerves in different areas is called "multiple mononeuropathy" or "mononeuropathy multiplex." More often, many or most of the nerves are affected (called "polyneuropathy").

More than 20 million people in the United States have been estimated to have some form of peripheral neuropathy, but this figure may be significantly higher—not all people with symptoms of neuropathy are tested for the disease and tests currently do not look for all forms of neuropathy. Neuropathy is often misdiagnosed due to its complex array of symptoms.

## HOW ARE THE PERIPHERAL NEUROPATHIES CLASSIFIED?

More than 100 types of peripheral neuropathy have been identified, each with its own symptoms and prognosis. Symptoms vary depending on the type of nerves—motor, sensory, or autonomic—that are damaged.

- Motor nerves control movements of all muscles under conscious control, such as those used for walking, grasping things, or talking.
- Sensory nerves transmit information such as the feeling of a light touch, temperature, or the pain from a cut.
- Autonomic nerves control organs to regulate activities that people do not control consciously, such as breathing, digesting food, and heart and gland functions.

Most neuropathies affect all three types of nerve fibers to varying degrees; others primarily affect one or two types. Doctors use terms such as predominantly motor neuropathy, predominantly sensory neuropathy, sensory-motor neuropathy, or autonomic neuropathy to describe different conditions.

About three-fourths of polyneuropathies are "length-dependent," meaning the farthest nerve endings in the feet are where symptoms develop first or are worse. In severe cases, such neuropathies can spread upwards toward the central parts of the body. In nonlength dependent polyneuropathies, the symptoms can start more toward the torso, or are patchy.

## WHAT TREATMENTS ARE AVAILABLE

Treatments depend entirely on the type of nerve damage, symptoms, and location. Your doctor will explain how nerve damage is causing specific symptoms and how to minimize and manage them. With proper education, some people may be able to reduce their medication dose or manage their neuropathy without medications. Definitive treatment can permit functional recovery over time, as long as the nerve cell itself has not died.

Specific symptoms can usually be improved—

- For motor symptoms, mechanical aids such as hand or foot braces can help reduce physical disability and pain. Orthopedic shoes can improve gait disturbances and help prevent foot injuries. Splints for carpal tunnel problems can help position the wrist to reduce pressure of the compressed nerve and allow it to heal. Some people with severe weakness benefit from tendon transfers or bone fusions to hold their limbs in a better position, or to release a nerve compression.
- Autonomic symptoms require detailed management depending on what they are. For example, people with orthostatic hypotension (significant drop in blood pressure when standing quickly) can learn to

prevent drops by standing up slowly and taking medications to improve blood pressure swings. Many people use complementary methods and techniques such as acupuncture, massage, herbal medications, and cognitive-behavioral or other psychotherapy approaches to cope with neuropathic pain.

- Sensory symptoms, such as neuropathic pain or itching caused by an injury to a nerve or nerves, are more difficult to control without medication. Some people use behavioral strategies to cope with chronic pain as well as depression and anxiety that many may feel following nerve injury.

Medications recommended for chronic neuropathic pain are also used for other medical conditions. Among the most effective are a class of drugs first marketed to treat depression. Nortriptyline and newer serotonin-norepinephrine reuptake inhibitors such as duloxetine hydrochloride modulate pain by increasing the brain's ability to inhibit incoming pain signals. Another class of medications that quiets nerve cell electrical signaling is also used for epilepsy. Common drugs include gabapentin, pregabalin, and less often topiramate and lamotrigine. Carbamazepine and oxcarbazepine are particularly effective for trigeminal neuralgia, a focal neuropathy of the face.

Local anesthetics and related drugs that block nerve conduction may help when other medications are ineffective or poorly tolerated. Medications put on the skin (topically administered) are generally appealing because they stay near the skin and have fewer unwanted side effects.

Lidocaine patches or creams applied to the skin can be helpful for small painful areas, such as localized chronic pain from mononeuropathies such as shingles. Another topical cream is capsaicin, a substance found in hot peppers that can desensitize peripheral pain nerve endings. Doctor-applied patches that contain higher concentrations of capsaicin offer longer-term relief from neuropathic pain and itching, but they worsen small-fiber nerve damage. Weak over-the-counter formulations also are available. Lidocaine or longer-acting bupivacaine are sometimes given using implanted pumps that deliver tiny quantities to the fluid that bathes the spinal cord, where they can quiet excess firing of pain cells without affecting the rest of the body. Other drugs treat chronic painful neuropathies by calming excess signaling.

Narcotics (opioids) can be used for pain that does not respond to other pain-control medications and if disease-improving treatments are not fully effective. Because pain relievers that contain opioids can lead to dependence and addiction, their use must be closely monitored by a physician. One of the newest drugs approved for treating diabetic neuropathy is tapentadol, which has both opioid activity and norepinephrine-reuptake inhibition activity of an antidepressant.

Surgery is the recommended treatment for some types of neuropathies. Protruding disks ("pinched nerve") in the back or neck that compress nerve roots are commonly treated surgically to free the affected nerve root and allow it to heal. Trigeminal neuralgia on the face is also often treated with neurosurgical decompression. Injuries to a single nerve (mononeuropathy) caused by compression, entrapment, or rarely tumors or infections may require surgery to release the nerve compression. Polyneuropathies that involve more diffuse nerve damage, such as diabetic neuropathy, are not helped by surgical intervention. Surgeries or interventional procedures that attempt to reduce pain by cutting or injuring nerves are not often effective as they worsen nerve damage and the parts of the peripheral and central nervous system above the cut often continue to generate pain signals ("phantom pain"). More sophisticated and less damaging procedures such as electrically stimulating remaining peripheral nerve fibers or pain-processing areas of the spinal cord or brain have largely replaced these surgeries.

Transcutaneous electrical nerve stimulation (TENS) is a noninvasive intervention used for pain relief in a range of conditions. TENS involves attaching electrodes to the skin at the site of pain or near associated nerves and then administering a gentle electrical current. Although data from controlled clinical trials are not available to broadly establish its efficacy for peripheral neuropathies, in some studies TENS has been shown to improve neuropathic symptoms associated with diabetes.

## Section 15.3 | **Motor Neuron Diseases**

This section includes text excerpted from "Motor Neuron Diseases Fact Sheet," National Institute of Neurological Disorders and Stroke (NINDS), August 13, 2019.

### WHAT ARE MOTOR NEURON DISEASES?

The motor neuron diseases (MNDs) are a group of progressive neurological disorders that destroy motor neurons, the cells that control essential voluntary muscle activity such as speaking, walking, breathing, and swallowing. Normally, messages from nerve cells in the brain (called "upper motor neurons") are transmitted to nerve cells in the brain stem and spinal cord (called "lower motor neurons") and from them to particular muscles. Upper motor neurons direct the lower motor neurons to produce movements such as walking or chewing. Lower motor neurons control movement in the arms, legs, chest, face, throat, and tongue. Spinal motor neurons are also called "anterior horn cells." Upper motor neurons are also called "corticospinal neurons."

When there are disruptions in the signals between the lowest motor neurons and the muscle, the muscles do not work properly; the muscles gradually weaken and may begin wasting away and develop uncontrollable twitching (called "fasciculations"). When there are disruptions in the signals between the upper motor neurons and the lower motor neurons, the limb muscles develop stiffness (called "spasticity"), movements become slow and effortful, and tendon reflexes such as knee and ankle jerks become overactive. Over time, the ability to control voluntary movement can be lost.

## WHO IS AT RISK?

The motor neuron diseases occur in adults and children. In children, particularly in inherited or familial forms of the disease, symptoms can be present at birth or appear before the child learns to walk. In adults, MNDs occur more commonly in men than in women, with symptoms appearing after age 40.

## WHAT CAUSES MOTOR NEURON DISEASES

Some motor neuron diseases are inherited, but the causes of most MNDs are not known. In sporadic or noninherited MNDs, environmental, toxic, viral, or genetic factors may be implicated.

## HOW ARE MOTOR NEURON DISEASES CLASSIFIED?

The motor neuron diseases are classified according to whether they are inherited or sporadic, and to whether degeneration affects upper motor neurons, lower motor neurons, or both. In adults, the most common MND is amyotrophic lateral sclerosis (ALS), which affects both upper and lower motor neurons. It has inherited and sporadic forms and can affect the arms, legs, or facial muscles. Primary lateral sclerosis is a disease of the upper motor neurons, while progressive muscular atrophy affects only lower motor neurons in the spinal cord. In progressive bulbar palsy, the lowest motor neurons of the brain stem are most affected, causing slurred speech and difficulty chewing and swallowing. There are almost always mildly abnormal signs in the arms and legs.

If the MND is inherited, it is also classified according to the mode of inheritance. Autosomal dominant means that a person needs to inherit only one copy of the defective gene from one affected parent to be at risk of the disease. There is a 50 percent chance that each child of an affected person will be affected. Autosomal recessive means the individual must inherit a copy of the defective gene from both parents. These parents are likely to be asymptomatic (without symptoms of the disease). Autosomal recessive diseases often affect more than one person in the same generation (siblings or cousins). In X-linked inheritance, the mother carries the defective gene on one of her X chromosomes and passes the disorder along to her sons. Males inherit an X chromosome from their mother and a Y chromosome from their father, while females inherit an X chromosome from each parent. Daughters have a 50 percent chance of inheriting their mother's faulty X chromosome and a safe X chromosome from their father, which would make them asymptomatic carriers of the mutation

## WHAT ARE THE SYMPTOMS OF MOTOR NEURON DISEASES?

A brief description of the symptoms of some of the more common MNDs follows.

**Amyotrophic lateral sclerosis (ALS)**, also called "Lou Gehrig disease" or "classical motor neuron disease," is a progressive, ultimately fatal disorder that disrupts signals to all voluntary muscles. Many doctors use the terms motor neuron disease and ALS interchangeably. Both upper and lower motor neurons are affected. Symptoms are usually noticed first in the arms and hands, legs, or swallowing muscles. Approximately 75 percent of people with classic ALS will develop weakness and wasting of the bulbar muscles (muscles that control speech, swallowing, and chewing). Muscle weakness and atrophy occur on both sides of the body. Affected individuals lose strength and the ability to move their arms and legs, and to hold the body upright. Other symptoms include spasticity, spasms, muscle cramps, and fasciculations. Speech can become slurred or nasal. When muscles of the diaphragm and chest wall fail to function properly, individuals lose the ability to breathe without mechanical support. Although the disease does not usually impair a person's mind or personality, several recent studies suggest that some people with ALS may develop cognitive problems involving word fluency, decision-making, and memory. Most individuals with ALS die from respiratory failure, usually within 3 to 5 years from the onset of symptoms. However, about 10 percent of affected individuals survive for 10 or more years.

Amyotrophic lateral sclerosis most commonly strikes people between 40 and 60 years of age, but younger and older individuals also can develop the disease. Men are affected more often than women. Most cases of ALS occur sporadically, and family members of those individuals are not considered to be at increased risk for developing the disease. Familial forms of ALS account for 10 percent or less of cases of ALS, with more than 10 genes identified to date. However, most of the gene mutations discovered account for a very small number of cases. The most common familial forms of ALS in adults are caused by mutations of the superoxide dismutase gene, or *SOD1*, located on chromosome 21. There are also rare juvenile-onset forms of familial ALS.

**Progressive bulbar palsy,** also called "progressive bulbar atrophy," involves the brain stem—the bulb-shaped region containing lower motor neurons needed for swallowing, speaking, chewing, and other functions. Symptoms include pharyngeal muscle weakness (involved with swallowing), weak jaw and facial muscles, progressive loss of speech, and tongue muscle atrophy. Limb weakness with both lower and upper motor neuron signs is almost always evident but less prominent. Individuals are at increased risk of choking and aspiration pneumonia, which is caused by the passage of liquids and food through the vocal folds and into the lower airways and lungs. Affected persons have outbursts of laughing or crying (called "emotional lability"). Stroke and myasthenia gravis may have certain symptoms that are similar to those of progressive bulbar palsy and must be ruled out prior to diagnosing this disorder. In about 25 percent of individuals with ALS, early symptoms begin with bulbar involvement. Some 75 percent of individuals with classic ALS eventually show some bulbar involvement. Many clinicians believe that progressive bulbar palsy by itself, without evidence of abnormalities in the arms or legs, is extremely rare.

**Pseudobulbar palsy**, which shares many symptoms of progressive bulbar palsy, is characterized by degeneration of upper motor neurons that transmit signals to the lower motor neurons in the brain stem. Affected individuals have progressive loss of the ability to speak, chew, and swallow. Progressive weakness in facial muscles leads to an expressionless face. Individuals may develop a gravelly voice and an increased gag reflex. The tongue may become immobile and unable to protrude from the mouth. Individuals may have outbursts of laughing or crying.

**Primary lateral sclerosis (PLS)** affects the upper motor neurons of the arms, legs, and face. It occurs when specific nerve cells in the motor regions of the cerebral cortex (the thin layer of cells covering the brain which is responsible for most high-level brain functions) gradually degenerate, causing the movements to be slow and effortful. The disorder often affects the legs first, followed by the body trunk, arms and hands, and, finally, the bulbar muscles. Speech may become slowed and slurred. When affected, the legs and arms become stiff, clumsy, slow and weak, leading to an inability to walk or carry out tasks requiring fine hand coordination. Difficulty with balance may lead to falls. Speech may become slow and slurred. Affected individuals commonly experience pseudobulbar affect and an overactive startle response. PLS is more common in men than in women, with a very gradual onset that generally occurs between ages 40 and 60. The cause is unknown. The symptoms progress gradually over years, leading to progressive stiffness and clumsiness of the affected muscles. PLS is sometimes considered a variant of ALS, but the major difference is the sparing of lower motor neurons, the slow rate of disease progression, and normal lifespan. PLS may be mistaken for spastic paraplegia, a hereditary disorder of the upper motor neurons that causes spasticity in the legs and usually starts in adolescence. Most neurologists follow the affected individual's clinical course for at least 3 to 4 years before making a diagnosis of PLS. The disorder is not fatal but may affect quality of life.

**Progressive muscular atrophy** is marked by slow but progressive degeneration of only the lower motor neurons. It largely affects men, with onset earlier than in other MNDs. Weakness is typically seen first in the hands and then spreads into the lower body, where it can be severe. Other symptoms may include muscle wasting, clumsy hand movements, fasciculations, and muscle cramps. The trunk muscles and respiration may become affected. Exposure to cold can worsen symptoms. The disease develops into ALS in many instances.

**Spinal muscular atrophy (SMA)** is a hereditary disease affecting the lower motor neurons. It is an autosomal recessive disorder caused by defects in the gene SMN1, which makes a protein that is important for the survival of motor neurons (SMN protein). In SMA, insufficient levels of the SMN protein lead to degeneration of the lower motor neurons, producing weakness and wasting of the skeletal muscles. This weakness is often more severe in the trunk and upper leg and arm muscles than in muscles of the hands and feet. SMA in children is classified into three types, based on ages of onset, severity, and progression of symptoms. All three types are caused by defects in the *SMN1* gene.

SMA type I, also called "Werdnig-Hoffmann disease," is evident by the time a child is 6 months old. Symptoms may include hypotonia (severely reduced muscle tone), diminished limb movements, lack of tendon reflexes, fasciculations, tremors, swallowing and feeding difficulties, and impaired breathing. Some children also develop scoliosis (curvature of the spine) or other skeletal abnormalities. Affected children never sit or stand and the vast majority usually die of respiratory failure before the age of 2. However, the survival in individuals with SMA type I has increased in recent years, in relation to the growing trend toward more proactive clinical care.

Symptoms of SMA type II, the intermediate form, usually begin between 6 and 18 months of age. Children may be able to sit but are unable to stand or walk unaided, and may have respiratory difficulties. The progression of disease is variable. Life expectancy is reduced but some individuals live into adolescence or young adulthood.

Symptoms of SMA type III (Kugelberg-Welander disease) appear between 2 and 17 years of age and include abnormal gait; difficulty running, climbing steps, or rising from a chair; and a fine tremor of the fingers. The lower extremities are most often affected. Complications include scoliosis and joint contractures—chronic shortening of muscles or tendons around joints, caused by abnormal muscle tone and weakness, which prevents the joints from moving freely. Individuals with SMA type III may be prone to respiratory infections, but with care may have a normal lifespan.

Congenital SMA with arthrogryposis (persistent contracture of joints with fixed abnormal posture of the limb) is a rare disorder. Manifestations include severe contractures, scoliosis, chest deformity, respiratory problems, unusually small jaws, and drooping of the upper eyelids.

Kennedy disease, also known as "progressive spinobulbar muscular atrophy," is an X-linked recessive disease caused by mutations in the gene for the androgen receptor. Daughters of individuals with Kennedy disease are carriers and have a

50 percent chance of having a son affected with the disease. The onset of symptoms is variable and the disease may first be recognized between 15 and 60 years of age. Symptoms include weakness and atrophy of the facial, jaw, and tongue muscles, leading to challenges involving chewing, swallowing, and changes in speech. Early symptoms may include muscle pain and fatigue. Weakness in arm and leg muscles closest to the trunk of the body develops over time, with muscle atrophy and fasciculations. Individuals with Kennedy disease also develop sensory loss in the feet and hands. Nerve conduction studies confirm that nearly all individuals have a sensory neuropathy (pain from sensory nerve inflammation or degeneration). Affected individuals may have enlargement of the male breasts or develop noninsulin-dependent diabetes mellitus.

The course of the disorder varies but is generally slowly progressive. Individuals tend to remain ambulatory until late in the disease. The life expectancy for individuals with Kennedy disease is usually normal.

**Postpolio syndrome** is a condition that can strike polio survivors decades after their recovery from poliomyelitis. Polio is an acute viral disease that destroys motor neurons. Many people who are affected early in life recover and develop new symptoms many decades later. After acute polio, the surviving motor neurons expand the amount of muscle that each controls. Postpolio syndrome and Postpolio are thought to occur when the surviving motor neurons are lost in the aging process or through injury or illness. Many scientists believe postpolio syndrome is latent weakness among muscles previously affected by poliomyelitis and not a new MND. Symptoms include fatigue, slowly progressive muscle weakness, muscle atrophy, fasciculations, cold intolerance, and muscle and joint pain. These symptoms appear most often among muscle groups affected by the initial disease, and may consist of difficulty breathing, swallowing, or sleeping. Other symptoms of postpolio syndrome may be caused by skeletal deformities such as long-standing scoliosis that led to chronic changes in the biomechanics of the joints and spine. Symptoms are more frequent among older people and those individuals most severely affected by the earlier disease. Some individuals experience only minor symptoms, while others develop muscle atrophy that may be mistaken for ALS. Postpolio syndrome is not usually life-threatening. Doctors estimate that 25 to 50 percent of survivors of paralytic poliomyelitis usually develop postpolio syndrome.

## HOW ARE MOTOR NEURON DISEASES DIAGNOSED?

There are no specific tests to diagnose most MNDs although there are now gene tests for SMA. Symptoms may vary among individuals and, in the early stages of the disease, may be similar to those of other diseases, making diagnosis difficult. A physical exam should be followed by a thorough neurological exam. The neurological exam will assess motor and sensory skills, nerve function, hearing and speech, vision, coordination and balance, mental status, and changes in mood or behavior.

Tests to rule out other diseases or to measure muscle involvement may include the following:

Electromyography (EMG) is used to diagnose disorders of lower motor neurons, as well as disorders of muscle and peripheral nerves. In an EMG, a physician inserts a thin needle electrode, attached to a recording instrument, into a muscle to assess the electrical activity during a voluntary contraction and at rest. The electrical activity in the muscle is caused by the lower motor neurons. When motor neurons degenerate, characteristic abnormal electrical signals occur in the muscle. Testing usually lasts about an hour or more, depending on the number of muscles and nerves tested.

Electromyography is usually done in conjunction with a nerve conduction velocity study. Nerve conduction studies measure the speed and size of the impulses in the nerves from small electrodes taped to the skin. A small pulse of electricity (similar to a jolt from static electricity) is applied to the skin to stimulate the nerve that directs a particular muscle. The second set of electrodes transmits the responding electrical signal to a recording machine. Nerve conduction studies help to differentiate lower motor neuron diseases from peripheral neuropathy and can detect abnormalities in sensory nerves.

Laboratory tests of blood, urine, or other substances can rule out muscle diseases and other disorders that may have symptoms similar to those of MND. For example, analysis of the fluid that surrounds the brain and spinal cord can detect infections or inflammation that can also cause muscle stiffness. Blood tests may be ordered to measure levels of the protein creatine kinase (which is needed for the chemical reactions that produce energy for muscle contractions); high levels may help diagnose muscle diseases such as muscular dystrophy.

Magnetic resonance imaging (MRI) uses a powerful magnetic field to produce detailed images of tissues, organs, bones, nerves, and other body structures. MRI is often used to rule out diseases that affect the head, neck, and spinal cord. MRI images can help diagnose brain and spinal cord tumors, eye disease, inflammation, infection, and vascular irregularities that may lead to stroke. MRI can also detect and monitor inflammatory disorders such as multiple sclerosis and can document brain injury from trauma. Magnetic resonance spectroscopy is a type of MRI scan that measures chemicals in the brain and may be used to evaluate the integrity of the upper motor neurons.

Muscle or nerve biopsy can help confirm nerve disease and nerve regeneration. A small sample of the muscle or nerve is removed under local anesthetic and studied under a microscope. The sample may be removed either surgically, through a slit made in the skin, or by needle biopsy, in which a thin hollow needle is inserted through the skin and into the muscle. A small piece of muscle remains in the hollow needle when it is removed from the body. Although this test can provide valuable information about the degree of damage, it is an invasive procedure and many experts do not believe that a biopsy is always needed for diagnosis.

Transcranial magnetic stimulation was first developed as a diagnostic tool to study areas of the brain related to motor activity. It is also used as a treatment for certain disorders. This noninvasive procedure creates a magnetic pulse inside the brain that evokes motor activity in an area of the body. Electrodes taped to different areas of the body pick up and record the electrical activity in the muscles. Measures of the evoked activity may help in diagnosing upper motor neural dysfunction in MND or monitoring disease progression.

## HOW ARE MOTOR NEURON DISEASES TREATED?

There is no cure or standard treatment for the MNDs. Symptomatic and supportive treatment can help people be more comfortable while maintaining their quality of life. Multidisciplinary clinics, with specialists from neurology, physical therapy, respiratory therapy, and social work are particularly important in the care of individuals with MNDs.

The drug riluzole (Rilutek®) has been approved by the U.S. Food and Drug Administration (FDA) to treat ALS, prolongs life by 2 to 3 months but does not relieve symptoms. The drug reduces the body's natural production of the neurotransmitter glutamate, which carries signals to the motor neurons. Scientists believe that too much glutamate can harm motor neurons and inhibit nerve signaling. The FDA has also approved the use of edaravone (Radicava™) to slow the clinical decline seen in individuals with ALS.

The FDA has approved nusinersen (Spinraza™) as the first drug approved to treat children and adults with spinal muscular atrophy. The drug is administered by intrathecal injection into the fluid surrounding the spinal cord. It is designed to increase production of the full-length SMN protein, which is critical for the maintenance of motor neurons.

Other medicines may help with symptoms. Muscle relaxants such as baclofen, tizanidine, and the benzodiazepines may reduce spasticity. Botulinum toxin may be used to treat jaw spasms or drooling. Excessive saliva can be treated with amitriptyline, glycopyrrolate, and atropine or by botulinum injections into the salivary glands. Combinations of dextromethorphan and quinidine have been shown to reduce pseudobulbar affect. Anticonvulsants and nonsteroidal anti-inflammatory drugs may help relieve pain, and antidepressants may be helpful in treating depression. Panic attacks can be treated with benzodiazepines. Some individuals may eventually require stronger medicines such as morphine to cope with musculoskeletal abnormalities or pain, and opiates are used to provide comfort care in terminal stages of the disease.

Physical therapy, occupational therapy, and rehabilitation may help to improve posture, prevent joint immobility, and slow muscle weakness and atrophy.

### Geriatric Rehabilitation

Stretching and strengthening exercises may help reduce spasticity, increase range of motion, and keep circulation flowing. Some individuals require additional therapy for speech, chewing, and swallowing difficulties. Applying heat may relieve muscle pain. Assistive devices such as supports or braces, orthotics, speech synthesizers, and wheelchairs may help some people retain independence.

Proper nutrition and a balanced diet are essential to maintaining weight and strength. People who cannot chew or swallow may require insertion of a feeding tube. In ALS, insertion of a percutaneous gastronomy tube (to help with feeding) is frequently carried out even before it is needed, when the individual is strong enough to undergo this minor surgery. Noninvasive ventilation at night can prevent apnea in sleep, and some individuals may also require assisted ventilation due to muscle weakness in the neck, throat, and chest during daytime.

## WHAT IS THE PROGNOSIS?

Prognosis varies depending on the type of MND and the age of onset. Some MNDs, such as PLS or Kennedy disease, are not fatal and progress slowly. People with SMA may appear to be stable for long periods, but improvement should not be expected. Some MNDs, such as ALS and some forms of SMA, are fatal.

# Section 15.4 | **Preventing Osteoporosis after Immobilization**

This section includes text excerpted from "Bed Rest and Immobilization: Risk Factors for Bone Loss," NIH Osteoporosis and Related Bone Diseases—National Resource Center (NIH ORBD—NRC), November 2018.

Bone is living tissue that responds to exercise by becoming stronger. Young women and men who exercise regularly generally have greater bone mass (bone density and strength) than those who do not. For most people, bone mass peaks by the late twenties. After the age of 30, women and men can help prevent bone loss with regular exercise. The best activities for bones are weight-bearing and resistance exercises. Weight-bearing exercises force you to work against gravity. They include walking, hiking, jogging, climbing stairs, playing tennis, and dancing. Resistance exercises–such as lifting weights–can also strengthen bones. Swimming and bicycling are examples of nonweight-bearing exercises.

Although weight-bearing and resistance activities contribute to the development and maintenance of bone mass, weightlessness and immobility can result in bone loss. Space travel has provided significant research data on the subject of weightlessness and bone loss. Astronauts exposed to the microgravity of space experience significant bone loss, leaving their bones weak and less able to support the body's weight and movement upon return to Earth.

## THE IMPACT OF BED REST AND INACTIVITY

Some people cannot perform weight-bearing activity. They include, for example, people who are on prolonged bed rest because of surgery, serious illness, or complications of pregnancy; and those who are experiencing immobilization of some part of the body because of stroke, fracture, spinal cord injury, or other chronic conditions. These people often experience a significant bone loss and are at high risk for developing osteoporosis and having a fracture.

Bone loss typically occurs over several months and then gradually levels off as the bones adjust to the state of weightlessness.

## MAINTAINING BONE HEALTH

In general, healthy people who undergo prolonged periods of bed rest or immobilization can regain bone mass when they resume weight-bearing activities. Studies suggest that there is a good chance to fully recover the lost bone if the immobilization period is limited to one to two months. Additionally, even brief intervals of weight-bearing activity during periods of limited mobility or bed rest can help lessen bone loss.

The greatest concern is for people who cannot resume weight-bearing activities and, therefore, typically do not regain lost bone density. Studies suggest that taking an osteoporosis treatment medication and reducing or eliminating other risk factors for osteoporosis can help slow the rate of bone loss.

## THE BOTTOM LINE

- A lifetime of weight-bearing exercise is important for building and maintaining bone mass, improving balance and coordination, and promoting overall good health
- Weight-bearing exercise should be resumed and maintained after a prolonged period of bed rest or immobilization to help recover bone loss during disuse
- Those who cannot resume weight-bearing exercise are at significant risk for osteoporosis. In this case, it is important to reduce or eliminate other risk factors for osteoporosis, such as smoking and excessive alcohol consumption, and to eat a diet rich in calcium and vitamin D. Taking an osteoporosis medication may also be an option to minimize bone loss.

## Section 15.5 | **Preventing Future Fractures**

This section includes text excerpted from "Once Is Enough: A Guide to Preventing Future Fractures," NIH Osteoporosis and Related Bone Diseases—National Resource Center (NIH ORBD—NRC), November 2018.

Only those who have experienced a fracture can truly understand how painful and debilitating it can be. Recovering should be your first priority. However, you and your doctor will also want to determine whether this fracture is a symptom of osteoporosis. If you have this underlying disorder, it puts you at greater risk for future fractures. If you are age 50 or older, there is a very good chance your fracture is related to osteoporosis. This section will help you better understand the relationship between fracture and osteoporosis, so you can act now to strengthen and protect your bones.

Many people are unaware of the link between a broken bone and osteoporosis. Osteoporosis, or "porous bone," is a disease characterized by low bone mass. It makes bones fragile and more prone to fractures, especially the bones of the hip, spine, and wrist. Osteoporosis is called a "silent disease" because bone loss occurs without symptoms. People typically do not know that they have osteoporosis until their bones become so weak that a sudden strain, twist, or fall results in a fracture.

In the United States, more than 53 million people either already have osteoporosis or are at high risk due to low bone mass. The disease can occur in both men and women and at any age, but it is most common in older women.

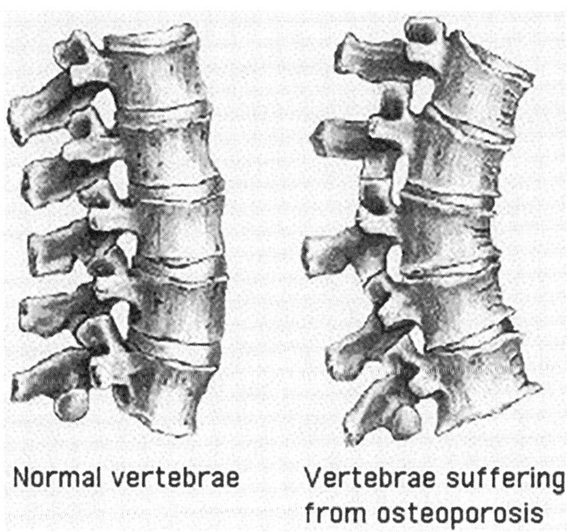


**Figure 15.1.** Normal versus Vertebrae with Osteoporosis
*(Source: National Aeronautics and Space Administration (NASA).)*

The majority of all hip and spine fractures among older white women can be attributed to underlying bone fragility. Moreover, women near or past menopause who have sustained a fracture in the past are more likely to experience another fracture. Yet, unfortunately, few patients with osteoporotic fractures are referred for an osteoporosis evaluation and medical treatment.

## THE OSTEOPOROSIS EVALUATION

If you already had a fracture. It is never too late to talk to your doctor about osteoporosis. Ideally, you should talk to your doctor during your recovery about whether you might be a candidate for an osteoporosis evaluation. But, even if your fracture has healed, you can be evaluated and begin taking steps to protect your bones now.

### What Kind of Doctor Should You See about Getting an Osteoporosis Evaluation?

Many different kinds of doctors can evaluate and treat osteoporosis. You might start with your primary care doctor or the doctor treating your fracture. She or he probably can conduct the evaluation and may then refer you to a specialist, such as an endocrinologist or rheumatologist, if you require treatment.

### What Does an Osteoporosis Evaluation Involve?

One thing your doctor will do is ask about your medical history and lifestyle to determine whether you have risk factors for osteoporosis. Some of the factors that increase the risk of developing osteoporosis include personal or family history of fractures; low levels of the hormone estrogen or testosterone; and the use of certain medications, such as glucocorticoids or antiseizure medications, that may contribute to bone fragility. Your doctor may want to test your blood or urine and may suggest that you have a bone mineral density test.

### What Is a Bone Mineral Density Test? Is It Painful?

A bone mineral density (BMD) test is the best way to determine your bone health. This test can identify osteoporosis, determine your risk for fractures (broken bones), and measure your response to osteoporosis treatment. The most widely recognized BMD test is called "a dual-energy x-ray absorptiometry," or "DXA" test. The test is painless, similar to having an x-ray, but with much less exposure to radiation. It can measure bone density at your hip and spine and takes only 15 minutes to complete. For a DXA test, you will be asked to lie on a table while a machine above you measures your bone density.

## STRATEGIES TO REDUCE YOUR RISK OF FRACTURES

### If You Are Diagnosed with Osteoporosis, What Should You Do Next?

You may feel concerned or even frightened after being diagnosed with osteoporosis. However, the good news is that, armed with information and the support of your doctor, you can significantly improve your bone health and reduce your risk of future fractures with a combination of medication, diet, exercise, and lifestyle modifications.

## Some of Your Friends Take Medication for Osteoporosis. Should You Talk to Your Doctor about This?

Yes. Several medications are available to prevent and treat osteoporosis, including: bisphosphonates; estrogen (hormone therapy); estrogen agonists/antagonists (also called "selective estrogen receptor modulators" or "SERMs"); parathyroid hormone (PTH) analog; parathyroid hormone-related protein (PTHrp) analog; RANK ligand (RANKL) inhibitor; and tissue-selective estrogen complex (TSEC). Your doctor can help you understand the benefits and risks of each of these medications and select one that is right for you, if appropriate.

In men, reduced levels of testosterone may be linked to the development of osteoporosis. Men with abnormally low levels of testosterone may be prescribed testosterone replacement therapy to help prevent or slow bone loss.

## What Else Can You Do to Protect Your Bones?

In addition to taking your medication, some of the most important things you can do are to follow a diet rich in calcium and vitamin D, maintain an adequate daily intake of protein, monitor your sodium intake, and get plenty of exercise.

- **Calcium** is needed to maintain healthy, strong bones throughout your life. Unfortunately, most Americans do not get enough calcium from their diets. Dairy products such as milk, cheese, and yogurt are excellent sources of calcium, and some nondairy foods such as broccoli, almonds, and sardines can provide smaller amounts. In addition, many foods that you may already enjoy—juices, breads, and cereals—can now be found fortified with calcium. Calcium supplements can ensure that you get enough calcium each day, especially in people with a proven milk allergy. The Institute of Medicine recommends a daily calcium intake of 1,000 mg (milligrams) for men and women up to age 50, increasing to 1,200 mg for women over age 50 and men over age 70. Calcium supplements are available without a prescription in a wide range of preparations and strengths. Many people ask which calcium supplement they should take. The "best" supplement is the one that meets your needs based on tolerance, convenience, cost, and availability. In general, you should choose calcium supplements that are well known brand names with proven reliability. Also, you will absorb calcium better if you take it several times a day in smaller amounts of 500 mg or less each time.

- **Vitamin D** plays a significant role in helping your body absorb calcium. The relationship between calcium and vitamin D is similar to that of a locked door and a key. Vitamin D is the key that unlocks the door, allowing calcium to enter your bloodstream. As age increases, bodies become less able to absorb calcium, which makes getting enough vitamin D even more important. The recommended daily intake for vitamin D is 600 IU (international units) up to age 70. Men and women over age 70 should increase their uptake to 800 IU daily. Many people get this amount by consuming vitamin D-fortified foods such as milk. In addition, many calcium supplements are fortified with vitamin D.
- **Sodium**, a main component of table salt, affects the need for calcium by increasing the amount of it excreted in urine. As a result, people with diets high in sodium, or table salt, appear to need more calcium than people with low sodium diets to ensure that, on balance, they retain enough calcium for their bones.
- **Protein** in excess amounts also increases the amount of calcium excreted in urine, but it provides benefits for bone health as well. For example, protein is needed for fracture healing. In addition, studies have shown that elderly people with a hip fracture who do not have enough protein in their diets are more likely to experience loss of independence, institutionalization, and even death after their fracture. The recommended daily intake for protein is 56 grams for men and 46 grams for women.

## You Have Always Been Active, but You Do Not Want to Risk Breaking Another Bone. Maybe You Need to Spend More Time "On the Sidelines" from Now On.

It is perfectly understandable that you want to avoid another fracture. No one who has broken a bone wants to revisit that pain and loss of independence. However, living your life "on the sidelines" is not an effective way to protect your bones. Remaining physically active reduces your risk of heart disease, colon cancer, and type 2 diabetes. It may also protect you against prostate and breast cancer, high blood pressure, obesity, and mood disorders such as depression and anxiety. If that is not enough to convince you to stay active, consider this: exercise is one of the best ways to preserve your bone density and prevent falls as you age.

## What Type of Exercise Is Best to Reduce Your Risk of Another Fracture?

Exercise can reduce your risk of fracturing in two ways—by helping you build and maintain bone density and by enhancing your balance, flexibility, and strength, all of which reduce your chance of falling.

- **Building and maintaining bone density:** Bone is a living tissue that responds to exercise by becoming stronger. Just as a muscle gets stronger and bigger with use, a bone becomes stronger and denser when it is called upon to bear weight. Two types of exercise are important for building and maintaining bone density: weight-bearing and resistance. Weight-bearing exercises are those in which your bones and muscles work against gravity. Examples include walking, climbing stairs, dancing, and playing tennis. Resistance exercises are those that use muscular strength to improve muscle mass and strengthen bone. The best example of a resistance exercise is weight training, with either free weights or weight machines.
- **Reducing the risk of falling:** You can significantly reduce your risk of falling by engaging in activities that enhance your balance, flexibility, and strength—
  - Balance is the ability to maintain your body's stability while moving or standing still. You can improve your balance with activities such as tai chi and yoga.
  - Flexibility refers to the range of motion of a muscle or group of muscles. You can improve your flexibility through tai chi, swimming, yoga, and gentle stretching exercises.
  - Strength refers to your body's ability to develop and maintain strong muscles. Lifting weights will increase your strength.

## How Can You Exercise Safely If You Have Osteoporosis?

If you have osteoporosis, it is important for you to get plenty of exercise. However, you will need to choose your activities carefully. Be sure to avoid activities with a high risk of falling, such as skiing or skating; those that have too much impact, such as jogging and jumping rope; and those that cause you to twist or bend, such as golf.

Unfortunately, some people become so afraid of breaking another bone that they become more sedentary, which leads to further loss of bone and muscle. Rest assured, however, that by practicing proper posture and learning the correct way to move, you can protect your bones while remaining physically active. Every activity can be adapted to meet your age, ability, lifestyle, and strength. Your doctor or a physical therapist can help you design a safe and effective exercise program. In the meantime, here are some general guidelines for safe movement:

Do not

- Wear shoes with slippery soles
- Slouch when standing, walking, or sitting at a desk
- Move too quickly

- Engage in sports or activities that require twisting the spine or bending forward from the waist, such as conventional sit-ups, toe touches, or swinging a golf club

Do

- Pay attention to proper posture. This includes lifting your breastbone, keeping your head erect and eyes forward, keeping your shoulders back, lightly "pinching" your shoulder blades, and tightening your abdominal muscles and buttocks.
- Make sure to use a handrail when climbing stairs
- Bend from the hips and knees and never from the waist, especially when lifting

## Fracture Happened after Tripping on a Rug at Home. How to Prevent Another Fall?

Falls are a major source of fractures. The likelihood that you will fall depends on both personal and environmental factors.

- **Personal factors**: A fall may occur because your reflexes have slowed over time, making them less able to react quickly to a sudden shift in body position. Loss of muscle mass may occur as you age, which can diminish your strength. Changes in vision and hearing can also affect your balance, as can the use of alcohol and certain medications. People with chronic illnesses that affect their circulation, sensation, mobility, or mental alertness are more likely to fall. To reduce your risk of falling, keep this personal safety checklist in mind:
- **Personal safety checklist**
    - Stay active to maintain muscle strength, balance, and flexibility.
    - Have your vision and hearing checked regularly and corrected as needed.
    - Discuss your medications with your doctor to see if one of them (or their combination) might lead to falls.
- **Environmental factors**: At any age, people can make changes in their environment to reduce their risk of falling and breaking a bone. The following safety checklists provide a few tips that should help:
- **Indoor safety checklist**
    - Use nightlights throughout your home.
    - Keep all rooms free from clutter, especially the floors.
    - Keep floor surfaces smooth but not slippery. When entering rooms, be aware of differences in floor levels and thresholds.
    - Wear supportive, low-heeled shoes even at home. Avoid walking around in socks, stockings, or floppy slippers.

- Check that all carpets and area rugs have skid-proof backing or are tacked to the floor, including carpeting on stairs.
- Keep electrical cords and telephone lines out of walkways.
- Be sure that all stairways are well lit and that stairs have handrails on both sides.
- Consider placing fluorescent tape on the edges of top and bottom steps.
- Install grab bars on bathroom walls beside tubs, showers, and toilets. If you are unstable on your feet, consider using a plastic chair with a back and nonskid leg tips in the shower.
- Use a rubber bath mat in the shower or tub.
- Keep a flashlight with extra batteries beside your bed.
- Add ceiling fixtures to rooms lit only by lamps, or install lamps that can be turned on by a switch near the entrance to the room.
- Use at least 100-watt light bulbs in your home.

- **Outdoor safety checklist**
  - In bad weather, consider using a cane or walker for extra stability.
  - In winter, wear warm boots with rubber soles for added traction.
  - Look carefully at floor surfaces in public buildings. Many floors are made of highly polished marble or tile that can be very slippery. When floors have plastic or carpet runners in place, try to stay on them whenever possible.
  - Use a shoulder bag, fanny pack, or backpack to leave hands free.
  - Stop at curbs to check height before stepping up or down. Be cautious at curbs that have been cut away to allow access for bikes or wheelchairs. The incline may lead to a fall.

## Is There Anything Else I Can Do Prevent Bone Loss and Fracture?

If you smoke, now would be a good time to quit. Tobacco is toxic to your bones, putting you at higher risk for low bone mass and osteoporosis. Excessive alcohol intake also may be damaging to your bones, and people who drink heavily tend to have more bone loss and fractures due to poor nutrition and an increased risk of falling.

# Section 15.6 | **Urinary Incontinence in Older Adults**

This section contains text excerpted from the following sources: Text in this section begins with excerpts from "Urinary Incontinence in Older Adults," National Institute of Aging (NIA), National Institutes of Health (NIH), May 16, 2017; Text under the heading "Kegel Exercises" is excerpted from "Kegel Exercises," National Kidney Disease Educational Program (NKDEP), National Institute of Diabetes and Digestive and Kidney Diseases (NIDDK), April 2014. Reviewed November 2019.

Urinary incontinence means a person leaks urine by accident. While it may happen to anyone, urinary incontinence is more common in older people, especially women. Incontinence can often be cured or controlled. Talk to your healthcare provider about what you can do.

What happens in the body to cause bladder control problems? The body stores urine in the bladder. During urination, muscles in the bladder tighten to move urine into a tube called "urethra." At the same time, the muscles around the urethra relax and let the urine pass out of the body. When the muscles in and around the bladder do not work the way they should, urine can leak. Incontinence typically occurs if the muscles relax without warning.

## CAUSES OF URINARY INCONTINENCE

Incontinence can happen for many reasons. For example, urinary tract infections, vaginal infection or irritation, constipation. Some medicines can cause bladder control problems that last a short time. When incontinence lasts longer, it may be due to:

- Weak bladder muscles
- Overactive bladder muscles

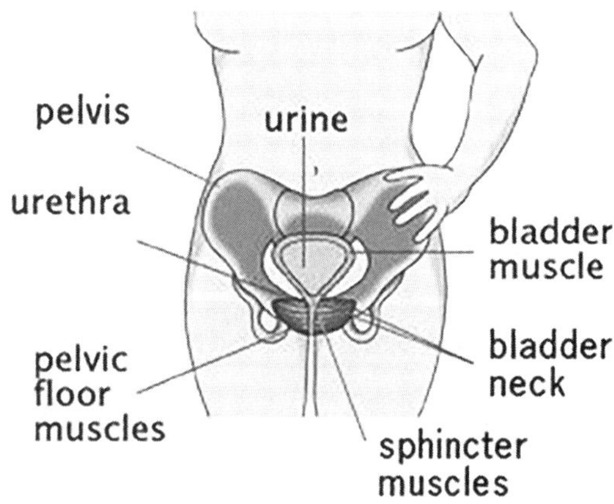


**Figure 15.2.** Bladder Control System *(Source: National Institute of Diabetes and Digestive and Kidney Diseases (NIDDK).*

- Weak pelvic floor muscles
- Damage to nerves that control the bladder from diseases such as multiple sclerosis, diabetes, or Parkinson disease
- Blockage from an enlarged prostate in men
- Diseases such as arthritis that may make it difficult to get to the bathroom in time
- Pelvic organ prolapse, which is when pelvic organs (such as the bladder, rectum, or uterus) shift out of their normal place into the vagina. When pelvic organs are out of place, the bladder and urethra are not able to work normally, which may cause urine to leak.

Most incontinence in men is related to the prostate gland. Male incontinence may be caused by:

- Prostatitis—a painful inflammation of the prostate gland
- Injury, or damage to nerves or muscles from surgery
- An enlarged prostate gland, which can lead to Benign Prostate Hyperplasia (BPH), a condition where the prostate grows as men age

## DIAGNOSIS OF URINARY INCONTINENCE

The first step in treating incontinence is to see a doctor. She or he will give you a physical exam and take your medical history. The doctor will ask about your symptoms and the medicines you use. She or he will want to know if you have been sick recently or had surgery. Your doctor also may do a number of tests. These might include:

- Urine and blood tests
- Tests that measure how well you empty your bladder

In addition, your doctor may ask you to keep a daily diary of when you urinate and when you leak urine. Your family doctor may also send you to a urologist, a doctor who specializes in urinary tract problems.

## TYPES OF URINARY INCONTINENCE

There are different types of incontinence:

- **Stress incontinence** occurs when urine leaks as pressure is put on the bladder, for example, during exercise, coughing, sneezing, laughing, or lifting heavy objects. It is the most common type of bladder control problem in younger and middle-aged women. It may begin around the time of menopause.
- **Urge incontinence** happens when people have a sudden need to urinate and cannot hold their urine long enough to get to the toilet. It may be a problem for people who have diabetes, Alzheimer disease, Parkinson disease, multiple sclerosis, or stroke.

- **Overflow incontinence** happens when small amounts of urine leak from a bladder that is always full. A person can have trouble emptying his bladder if an enlarged prostate is blocking the urethra. Diabetes and spinal cord injuries can also cause this type of incontinence.
- **Functional incontinence** occurs in many older people who have normal bladder control. They just have a problem getting to the toilet because of arthritis or other disorders that make it hard to move quickly.

## TREATMENT FOR URINARY INCONTINENCE

There are more treatments for urinary incontinence than ever before. The choice of treatment depends on the type of bladder control problem you have, how serious it is, and what best fits your lifestyle. As a general rule, the simplest and safest treatments should be tried first.

Bladder control training may help you get better control of your bladder. Your doctor may suggest you try the following:

- **Pelvic muscle exercises** (also known as "Kegel exercises") work the muscles that you use to stop urinating. Making these muscles stronger helps you hold urine in your bladder longer.
- **Biofeedback** uses sensors to make you aware of signals from your body. This may help you regain control over the muscles in your bladder and urethra. Biofeedback can be helpful when learning pelvic muscle exercises.
- **Timed voiding** may help you control your bladder. In timed voiding, you urinate on a set schedule, for example, every hour. You can slowly extend the time between bathroom trips. When timed voiding is combined with biofeedback and pelvic muscle exercises, you may find it easier to control urge and overflow incontinence.
- **Lifestyle changes** may help with incontinence. Losing weight, quitting smoking, saying "no" to alcohol, drinking less caffeine (found in coffee, tea, and many sodas), preventing constipation and avoiding lifting heavy objects may help with incontinence. Choosing water instead of other drinks and limiting drinks before bedtime may also help.

## MANAGING URINARY INCONTINENCE

Besides bladder control training, you may want to talk with your doctor about other ways to help manage incontinence:

- Medicines can help the bladder empty more fully during urination. Other drugs tighten muscles and can lessen leakage.
- Some women find that using an estrogen vaginal cream may help relieve stress or urge incontinence. A low dose of estrogen cream is applied directly to the vaginal walls and urethral tissue.

- A doctor may inject a substance that thickens the area around the urethra to help close the bladder opening. This can reduce stress incontinence in women. This treatment may need to be repeated.
- Some women may be able to use a medical device, such as a urethral insert, a small disposable device inserted into the urethra. A pessary (stiff ring) is inserted into the vagina and may help prevent leaking if you have a prolapsed bladder or vagina.
- Nerve stimulation, which sends mild electric current to the nerves around the bladder that help control urination, may be another option.
- Surgery can sometimes improve or cure incontinence if it is caused by a change in the position of the bladder or blockage due to an enlarged prostate.

Even after treatment, some people still leak urine from time to time. There are bladder control products and other solutions, including adult diapers, furniture pads, urine deodorizing pills, and special skin cleansers that may make leaking urine bother you a little less.

## KEGEL EXERCISES

### What Are Kegel Exercises?

To do Kegel exercises, you just squeeze your pelvic floor muscles. The part of your body including your hip bones is the pelvic area. At the bottom of the pelvis, several layers of muscle stretch between your legs. The muscles attach to the front, back, and sides of the pelvic bone. Kegel exercises are designed to make your pelvic floor muscles stronger. These are the muscles that hold up your bladder and help keep it from leaking. Building up your pelvic muscles with Kegel exercises can help with your bladder control.

### How Do You Exercise Your Pelvic Muscles?

Find the right muscles. Try one of the following ways to find the right muscles to squeeze.

- Imagine that you are trying to stop passing gas. Squeeze the muscles you would use. If you sense a "pulling" feeling, you are squeezing the right muscles for pelvic exercises.
- Imagine that you are sitting on a marble and want to pick up the marble with your vagina. Imagine "sucking" the marble into your vagina.
- Lie down and put your finger inside your vagina. Squeeze as if you were trying to stop urine from coming out. If you feel tightness on your finger, you are squeezing the right pelvic muscles.

Let your doctor, nurse, or therapist help you. Many people have trouble finding the right muscles. Your doctor, nurse, or therapist can check to make sure you are doing the exercises correctly. You can also exercise by using special weights or biofeedback. Ask your healthcare team about these exercise aids.

Do not squeeze other muscles at the same time. Be careful not to tighten your stomach, legs, or other muscles. Squeezing the wrong muscles can put more pressure on your bladder control muscles. Just squeeze the pelvic muscle. Do not hold your breath.

Repeat, but do not overdo it. At first, find a quiet spot to practice—your bathroom or bedroom—so you can concentrate. Lie on the floor. Pull in the pelvic muscles and hold for a count of 3. Then relax for a count of 3. Work up to 10 to 15 repeats each time you exercise.

Do your pelvic exercises at least three times a day. Every day, use three positions: lying down, sitting, and standing. You can exercise while lying on the floor, sitting at a desk, or standing in the kitchen. Using all three positions makes the muscles stronger.

Be patient. Do not give up. It is just 5 minutes, three times a day. You may not feel your bladder control improve until after 3 to 6 weeks. Still, most women do notice an improvement after a few weeks.

# Chapter 16 | Sports Injury Rehabilitation

**Chapter Contents**

## Section 16.1 | **Sports Injuries and Recovery of Function**

This section includes text excerpted from "Sports Injuries," National Institute of Arthritis and Musculoskeletal and Skin Diseases (NIAMS), February 2016. Reviewed November 2019.

### WHAT ARE SPORTS INJURIES?

The term "sports injury" refers to the kinds of injuries that most commonly occur during sports or exercise. Sports injuries can result from:

- Accidents
- Improper equipment
- Insufficient warm-up and stretching
- Lack of conditioning
- Poor training practices

The most common sports injuries include:

- Muscle sprains and strains
- Tears of the ligaments that hold joints together
- Tears of the tendons that support joints and allow them to move
- Dislocated joints
- Fractured bones, including vertebrae

Regardless of the specific structure affected, musculoskeletal sports injuries can generally be classified in one of two ways: acute or chronic.

#### Acute Injuries

Acute injuries, such as a sprained ankle, strained back, or fractured hand, occur suddenly during activity. Signs of an acute injury include:

- Sudden, severe pain
- Swelling
- Inability to place weight on a lower limb
- Extreme tenderness in an upper limb
- Inability to move a joint through its full range of motion
- Extreme limb weakness
- Visible dislocation or break of a bone

#### Chronic Injuries

Chronic injuries usually result from overusing one area of the body while playing a sport or exercising over a long period. The following are signs of a chronic injury:

- Pain when performing an activity
- A dull ache when at rest
- Swelling

## WHO GETS SPORTS INJURIES

Anyone can get a sports injury.

## TYPES OF SPORTS INJURIES

### Sprains and Strains

A sprain is a stretch or tear of a ligament, the band of connective tissue that joins the end of one bone with another. Sprains are caused by trauma such as a fall or blow to the body that knocks a joint out of position and, in the worst case, ruptures the supporting ligaments. Sprains can range from first degree (minimally stretched ligament) to third-degree (a complete tear). Areas of the body most vulnerable to sprains are ankles, knees, and wrists.

A strain is a twist, pull, or tear of a muscle or tendon, a cord of tissue connecting muscle to bone. It is an acute, noncontact injury that results from overstretching or over contraction. Although it is hard to tell the difference between mild and moderate strains, severe strains not treated professionally can cause damage and loss of function.

### Knee Injuries

The knee is a complex structure and is weight-bearing and can be a commonly injured joint. Knee injuries can range from mild to severe. Some of the less severe injuries to the knee can include:

- Runner's knee, which causes pain or tenderness close to or under the kneecap at the front or side of the knee
- Iliotibial band syndrome, which causes pain on the outer side of the knee
- Tendinitis, also called "tendinosis," which shows degeneration within a tendon, usually where it joins the bone

More severe injuries include bone bruises or damage to the cartilage or ligaments. There are two types of cartilage in the knee. One is the meniscus, a crescent-shaped disc that absorbs shock between the thigh (femur) and lower leg bones (tibia and fibula). The other is a surface-coating (or articular) cartilage. It covers the ends of the bones where they meet, allowing them to glide against one another. The four major ligaments that support the knee are the:

- Anterior cruciate ligament (ACL)
- Posterior cruciate ligament (PCL)
- Medial collateral ligament (MCL)
- Lateral collateral ligament (LCL)

Knee injuries can result from a blow to or twist of the knee; from improper landing after a jump; or from running too hard, too much, or without proper warm up.

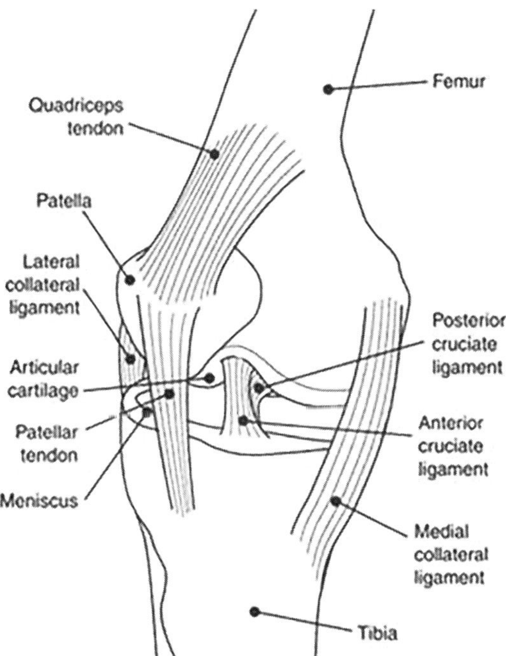


**Figure 16.1.** View of the Knee

## Compartment Syndrome

In many parts of the body, muscles, along with the nerves and blood vessels that run alongside and through them, are enclosed in a "compartment" formed of a tough membrane called "fascia." When muscles become swollen, they can fill the compartment to capacity, causing interference with nerves and blood vessels as well as damage to the muscles themselves. The resulting painful condition is referred to as "compartment syndrome."

Compartment syndrome may be caused by:

- A one-time traumatic injury, also known as "acute compartment syndrome," such as a fractured bone or a hard blow to the thigh.
- Repeated hard blows or by ongoing overuse, also known as "chronic exertional compartment syndrome." For example, long-distance running can lead to this syndrome.

## Shin Splints

Although the term "shin splints" has been widely used to describe any sort of leg pain associated with exercise, the term actually refers to pain along the tibia or shin bone, the large bone in the front of the lower leg. This pain can occur at the front of the outside part of the lower leg, including the foot and ankle (anterior shin splints) or at the inner edge of the bone where it meets the calf muscles (medial shin splints).

Shin splints are primarily seen in runners, particularly those just starting a running program. Risk factors for shin splints include:

- Overuse or incorrect use of the lower leg
- Improper stretching, warm-up, or exercise technique
- Overtraining
- Running or jumping on hard surfaces
- Running in shoes that do not have enough support

These injuries are often associated with flat (overpronated) feet.

## Achilles Tendon Injuries

An Achilles tendon injury results from a stretch, tear, or irritation to the tendon connects the calf muscle to the back of the heel. These injuries can be so sudden and agonizing that they have been known to bring down charging professional football players in shocking fashion.

The most common cause of Achilles tendon tears is a problem called "tendinitis," a degenerative condition caused by aging or overuse. When a tendon is weakened, trauma can cause it to rupture.

Achilles tendon injuries are common in middle-aged "weekend warriors" who may not exercise regularly or take time to stretch properly before an activity. Among professional athletes, most Achilles injuries seem to occur in quick-acceleration, jumping sports such as football and basketball, and almost always end the season's competition for the athlete.

## Fractures

A fracture is a break in the bone that can occur from either a quick, one-time injury to the bone, also known as "an acute fracture," or from repeated stress to the bone overtime, also known as "a stress fracture."

Acute fractures can be:

- Simple, usually a clean break with little damage to the surrounding tissue
- Compound, meaning a break in which the bone pierces the skin with little damage to the surrounding tissue

Most acute fractures are emergencies. One that breaks the skin is especially dangerous because there is a high risk of infection.

Stress fractures occur largely in the feet and legs and are common in sports that require repetitive impact, primarily running or jumping sports such as

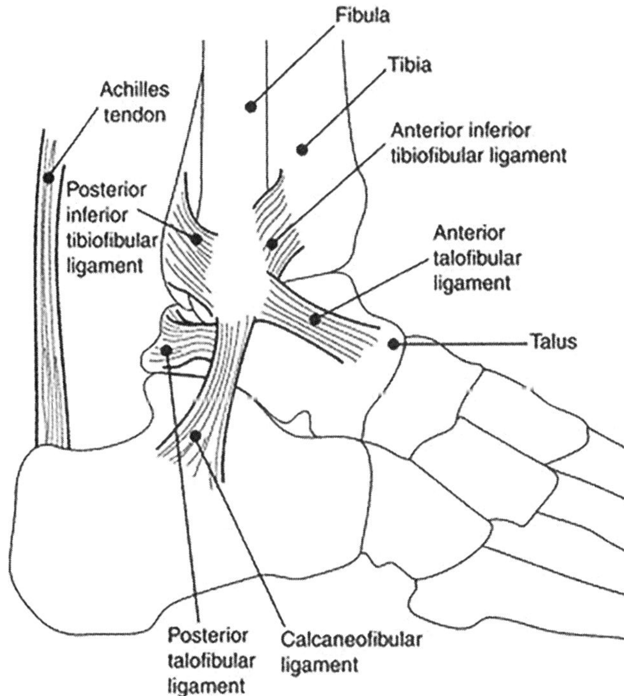


**Figure 16.2.** Lateral View of the Ankle

gymnastics or track and field. Running creates forces two to three times a person's body weight on the lower limbs.

The most common symptom of a stress fracture is pain at the site that worsens with weight-bearing activity. Tenderness and swelling often accompany the pain.

### Dislocations

When the two bones that come together to form a joint become separated, the joint is described as dislocated. Contact sports such as football and basketball, as well as high-impact sports and sports that can result in excessive stretching or falling, cause most dislocations. A dislocated joint is an emergency that requires medical treatment.

The joints most likely to be dislocated are some of the hand joints. Aside from these joints, the joint most frequently dislocated is the shoulder. Dislocations of the knees, hips, and elbows are uncommon.

## WHAT CAUSES SPORTS INJURIES

The cause of sports injuries can include:

- Accidents
- Poor training practices

- Improper gear
- Being out of condition
- Not warming up or stretching before you play or exercise

## SYMPTOMS OF SPORTS INJURIES

The symptoms of a sports injury will depend on the type of injury you have.

Symptoms of an acute injury include:

- Sudden, severe pain
- Swelling
- Not being able to place weight on a leg, knee, ankle, or foot
- An arm, elbow, wrist, hand, or finger that is very tender
- Not being able to move a joint as normal
- Extreme leg or arm weakness
- A bone or joint that is visibly out of place

In addition, signs and symptoms of strains or sprains may also include:

- Varying degrees of tenderness or pain
- Bruising
- Inflammation
- Joint looseness, laxity, or instability
- Muscle spasm
- Loss of strength

Symptoms of a chronic injury include:

- Pain when you play
- Pain when you exercise
- A dull ache when you rest
- Swelling

## DIAGNOSIS OF SPORTS INJURIES

To help diagnose your sports injury, your doctor may:

- Ask about the injury
- Examine the area of the injury
- Order an x-ray to make sure you do not have a fracture

Your doctor may order a magnetic resonance imaging (MRI) to look closely at the area of the injury or pain. An MRI is a noninvasive procedure in which a machine with a strong magnet passes a force through the body to produce a series of cross-sectional images.

## TREATMENT OF SPORTS INJURIES

Whether an injury is acute or chronic, there is never a good reason to try to "work through" the pain of an injury. When you have pain from a particular movement or activity, stop! Continuing the activity only causes further harm.

## When to Seek Medical Treatment

You should call a healthcare professional if:

- The injury causes severe pain, swelling, or numbness
- You cannot tolerate any weight on the area
- The pain or dull ache of an old injury is accompanied by increased swelling or joint abnormality or instability

## When and How to Treat at Home

If you do not have any of the above symptoms, it is probably safe to treat the injury at home at least at first. If pain or other symptoms worsen, it is best to check with your healthcare provider. Use the R-I-C-E method to relieve pain and inflammation and speed healing. Follow these four steps immediately after injury and continue for at least 48 hours.

- **Rest**. Reduce regular exercise or activities of daily living as needed. If you cannot put weight on an ankle or knee, crutches may help. If you use a cane or one crutch for an ankle injury, use it on the uninjured side to help you lean away and relieve weight on the injured ankle.
- **Ice**. Apply an ice pack to the injured area for 20 minutes at a time, four to eight times a day. A cold pack, ice bag, or plastic bag filled with crushed ice and wrapped in a towel can be used. To avoid cold injury and frostbite, do not apply the ice for more than 20 minutes. (Note: Do not use heat immediately after an injury. This tends to increase internal bleeding or swelling. Heat can be used later to relieve muscle tension and promote relaxation.)
- **Compression**. Compression of the injured area may help reduce swelling. Compression can be achieved with elastic wraps, special boots, air casts, and splints. Ask your healthcare provider for advice on which one to use.
- **Elevation**. If possible, keep the injured ankle, knee, elbow, or wrist elevated on a pillow, above the level of the heart, to help decrease swelling.

Other treatments may include:

- Nonsteroidal anti-inflammatory drugs, also known as "NSAIDs." The moment you are injured, chemicals are released from damaged tissue cells. This triggers the first stage of healing: inflammation. Inflammation causes tissues to become swollen, tender, and painful. Although inflammation is needed for healing, it can actually slow the healing process if left unchecked. To reduce inflammation and pain, healthcare providers often recommend taking an over-the-counter NSAID, such as aspirin, ibuprofen, or naproxen sodium. For severe pain and inflammation, doctors may prescribe one of several dozen NSAIDs available in prescription strength.

- Immobilization is a common treatment for musculoskeletal sports injuries that may be done immediately by a trainer or paramedic. Immobilization involves reducing movement in the area to prevent further damage. By enabling the blood supply to flow more directly to the injury (or the site of surgery to repair damage from an injury), immobilization reduces pain, swelling, and muscle spasm and helps the healing process begin. Following are some devices used for immobilization:
  - Slings, to immobilize the upper body, including the arms and shoulders.
  - Splints and casts, to support and protect injured bones and soft tissue. Cast can be made from plaster or fiberglass. Splints can be custom made or ready-made. Standard splints come in a variety of shapes and sizes and have Velcro straps that make them easy to put on and take off or adjust. Splints generally offer less support and protection than a cast and, therefore, may not always be a treatment option.
  - Leg immobilizers, to keep the knee from bending after injury or surgery. Made from foam rubber covered with fabric, leg immobilizers enclose the entire leg, fastening with Velcro straps.
- Surgery is needed in some cases to repair torn connective tissues or to realign bones with compound fractures. The vast majority of musculoskeletal sports injuries do not require surgery.

## Rehabilitation

A key part of rehabilitation from sports injuries is a graduated exercise program designed to return the injured body part to a normal level of function.

With most injuries, early mobilization—getting the part moving as soon as possible—will speed healing. Generally, early mobilization starts with gentle range-of-motion exercises and then moves on to stretching and strengthening exercises when you can without increasing pain. For example, if you have a sprained ankle, you may be able to work on range of motion for the first day or two after the sprain by gently tracing letters with your big toe. Once your range of motion is fairly good, you can start doing gentle stretching and strengthening exercises. When you are ready, weights may be added to your exercise routine to further strengthen the injured area. The key is to avoid movement that causes pain.

As damaged tissue heals, scar tissue forms, which shrinks and brings torn or separated tissues back together. As a result, the injury site becomes tight or stiff, and damaged tissues are at risk of re-injury. That is why stretching and strengthening exercises are so important. You should continue to stretch the muscles daily and as the first part of your warm up before exercising.

When planning your rehabilitation program with a healthcare professional, remember that progression is the key principle. Start with just a few exercises, do them often, and then gradually increase how much you do. A complete rehabilitation program should include exercises for flexibility, endurance, and strength; instruction in balance and proper body mechanics related to the sport; and a planned return to full participation.

Throughout the rehabilitation process, avoid painful activities and concentrate on those exercises that will improve function in the injured part. Do not resume your sport until you are sure you can stretch the injured tissues without any pain, swelling, or restricted movement, and monitor any other symptoms. When you do return to your sport, start slowly and gradually build up to full participation.

## Rest

Although it is important to get moving as soon as possible, you must also take time to rest following an injury. All injuries need time to heal; proper rest will help the process. Your healthcare professional can guide you regarding the proper balance between rest and rehabilitation.

## Other Therapies

Other therapies used in rehabilitating sports injuries include:

- **Cold/cryotherapy**. Ice packs reduce inflammation by constricting blood vessels and limiting blood flow to the injured tissues. Cryotherapy eases pain by numbing the injured area. It is generally used for only the first 48 hours after injury.
- **Heat/thermotherapy**. Heat, in the form of hot compresses, heat lamps, or heating pads, causes the blood vessels to dilate and increase blood flow to the injury site. Increased blood flow aids the healing process by removing cell debris from damaged tissues and carrying healing nutrients to the injury site. Heat also helps to reduce pain. It should not be applied within the first 48 hours after an injury.
- **Ultrasound**. High-frequency sound waves produce deep heat that is applied directly to an injured area. Ultrasound stimulates blood flow to promote healing.
- **Massage**. Manual pressing, rubbing, and manipulation soothe tense muscles and increase blood flow to the injury site.

Most of these therapies are administered or supervised by a licensed healthcare professional.

## WHO TREATS SPORTS INJURIES

Although severe injuries will need to be seen immediately in an emergency room, particularly if they occur on the weekends or after office hours, most musculoskeletal sports injuries can be evaluated and, in many cases, treated by your primary healthcare provider.

Depending on your preference and the severity of your injury or the likelihood that your injury may cause ongoing, long-term problems, you may want to see, or have your primary healthcare professionals refer you to one of the following.

- An orthopedic surgeon is a doctor specializing in the diagnosis and treatment of the musculoskeletal system, which includes bones, joints, ligaments, tendons, muscles, and nerves.
- A physical therapist/physiotherapist is a healthcare professional who can develop a rehabilitation program. Your primary care physician may refer you to a physical therapist after you begin to recover from your injury to help strengthen muscles and joints and prevent further injury.

## PREVENTION OF SPORTS INJURIES

These tips can help you avoid sports injuries:

- Do not bend your knees more than halfway when doing knee bends.
- Do not twist your knees when you stretch. Keep your feet as flat as you can.
- When jumping, land with your knees bent.
- Do warmup exercises before you play any sport.
- Always stretch before you play or exercise.
- Do not overdo it.
- Cool down after hard sports or workouts.
- Wear shoes that fit properly, are stable, and absorb shock.
- Use the softest exercise surface you can find; don't run on asphalt or concrete.
- Run-on flat surfaces.

### For Adults

- Don't be a "weekend warrior." Don't try to do a week's worth of activity in a day or two.
- Learn to do your sport right. Use proper form to reduce your risk of "overuse" injuries.
- Use safety gear.
- Know your body's limits.

- Build up your exercise level gradually.
- Strive for a total body workout of cardiovascular, strength training, and flexibility exercises.

## For Parents and Coaches

- Group children by their skill level and body size, not by their age, especially for contact sports.
- Match the child to the sport. Don't push the child too hard to play a sport that she or he may not like or be able to do.
- Try to find sports programs that have certified athletic trainers.
- See that all children get a physical exam before playing.
- Don't play a child who is injured.
- Get the child to a doctor, if needed.
- Provide a safe environment for sports.

## For Children

- Be in proper condition to play the sport.
- Get a physical exam before you start playing sports.
- Follow the rules of the game.
- Wear gear that protects, fits well, and is right for the sport.
- Know how to use athletic gear.
- Don't play when you are very tired or in pain.
- Always warm up before you play.
- Always cool down after you play.

# PROGNOSIS OF SPORTS INJURIES

From the moment a bone breaks or a ligament tears, your body goes to work to repair the damage. Here is what happens at each stage of the healing process:

- **At the moment of injury.** Chemicals are released from damaged cells, triggering a process called "inflammation." Blood vessels at the injury site become dilated; blood flow increases to carry nutrients to the site of tissue damage.
- **Within hours of injury.** White blood cells (leukocytes) travel down the bloodstream to the injury site where they begin to tear down and remove damaged tissue, allowing other specialized cells to start developing scar tissue.
- **Within days of injury.** Scar tissue is formed on the skin or inside the body. The amount of scarring may be proportional to the amount of swelling, inflammation, or bleeding within. In the next few weeks, the damaged area will regain a great deal of strength as scar tissue continues to form.

- **Within a month of injury.** Scar tissue may start to shrink, bringing damaged, torn, or separated tissues back together. However, it may be several months or more before the injury is completely healed.

## Section 16.2 | **Return to Sport**

This section includes text excerpted from "Returning to Sports and Activities," Centers for Disease Control and Prevention (CDC), February 12, 2019.

After an injury, an athlete should only return to sports practices with the approval and under the supervision of their healthcare provider. When available, be sure to also work closely with your team's certified athletic trainer.

Below are six gradual steps that you, along with a healthcare provider, should follow to help safely return an athlete to play. Remember, this is a gradual process. These steps should not be completed in one day, but instead over days, weeks, or months.

### SIX-STEP RETURN TO PLAY PROGRESSION

It is important for an athlete's parent(s) and coach(es) to watch for injury symptoms after each day's return to play progression activity. An athlete should only move to the next step if they do not have any symptoms at the existing step. If an athlete's symptoms come back or if she or he gets symptoms, this is a sign that the athlete is pushing too hard. The athlete should stop these activities and the athlete's medical provider should be contacted. After more rest and no injury symptoms, the athlete can start at the previous step.

#### Step 1: Back to Regular Activities (Such as School)

Athlete is back to their regular activities (such as school) and has the green-light from their healthcare provider to begin the return to play process. An athlete's return to regular activities involves a stepwise process. It starts with a few days of rest (2 to 3 days) and is followed by light activity (such as short walks) and moderate activity (such as riding a stationary bike) that do not worsen symptoms.

#### Step 2: Light Aerobic Activity

Begin with light aerobic exercise only to increase an athlete's heart rate. This means about 5 to 10 minutes on an exercise bike, walking, or light jogging. No weight lifting at this point.

### Step 3: Moderate Activity

Continue with activities to increase an athlete's heart rate with body or head movement. This includes moderate jogging, brief running, moderate-intensity stationary biking, moderate-intensity weightlifting (less time and/or less weight from their typical routine).

### Step 4: Heavy, Noncontact Activity

Add heavy noncontact physical activity, such as sprinting/running, high-intensity stationary biking, regular weightlifting routine, noncontact sport-specific drills (in three planes of movement).

### Step 5: Practice and Full Contact

Athlete may return to practice and full contact (if appropriate for the sport) in controlled practice.

### Step 6: Competition

Athlete may return to competition.

# Chapter 17 | **Ortho-Bionomy: Painless Self-Care**

When a physical injury disrupts the body's natural ability to heal, the body tries to adapt to the injury to the best of its ability. Yet, during this process, there is a possibility of creating even greater stress. Ortho-Bionomy® is a type of therapy that focuses on improving your posture and structural imbalances by means of gentle massage. The treatment helps ease muscle tension and pain without the use of medication or physical stressors in an effort to help the body to heal naturally. The practitioner uses gentle movements that position the body properly and manipulates specific trigger points in a manner that enables the body to self-correct its reflexes. The simplicity and gentleness of the ortho-bionomic techniques used by the practitioner re-educate the dysfunctional patterns stored in the body with the goal of restoring normal functioning. Ortho-Bionomy® therapy is based on the principle of allowing the body to heal itself.

## ORIGIN OF ORTHO-BIONOMY®

Ortho-Bionomy® was invented by Dr. Arthur Lincoln Pauls, a Canadian-born British national who was an osteopath and martial-arts instructor. He discovered the roots of Ortho-Bionomy® by observing the movements and energy flow of judo combined with his working knowledge of homeopathy. He believed that the body can regain its balance on its own when we work with it rather than against it, and avoiding using force. Ortho-Bionomy® is a combination of *ortho*, meaning "straight," *bio*, meaning "life," and *nomy*, meaning "pertaining to laws." The practitioner helps the body understand its own functioning by manipulating its physical and energetic patterns. The treatment is based on the belief that, when the structure of the body is positioned properly, one's overall well-being is enhanced due to improved circulation. Since this is a relatively new approach toward massage therapy, more research is required to validate its effectiveness for various ailments.

## ORTHO-BIONOMY® SESSION

In a typical Ortho-Bionomy® session, the patient lies fully clothed on a massage table and identifies areas of bodily discomfort for the practitioner. The practitioner then applies brief compressions and subtle contacts to unlock tension and reduce stress. These techniques help break the cycle of pain and correct structural and physical dysfunctions of the body through compression or constriction of muscles to release tension, loosen joints, and improve overall functionality. This release of stress and tension relieves the body of pain and discomfort. Ortho-Bionomy® does not incorporate deep-tissue treatments as a regular therapeutic massage does, but instead concentrates on gentle movements and slight manipulations of the limbs and joints to increase range of motion with the utmost care paid to the patient's comfort.

## EFFECTS OF ORTHO-BIONOMY®

Ortho-Bionomy® is often used as an alternative to osteopathy, which uses stress to physically manipulate bones and muscles. Ortho-Bionomy® involves a gentler approach that is particularly helpful in cases in which the patient is emotionally and physically fragile, such as in the aftermath of an injury. The therapist helps strengthen the ability of the patient's body to self-regulate and heal by releasing stress from the body and correcting its structural imbalance.

Targeted outcomes for patients undergoing Ortho-Bionomy® treatment include:

- Dissolution of knots in the body's tissue
- Softening of tissue surrounding an injury
- Experiences of comfort and relaxation
- Changes to the body's temperature

The practitioner relies on verbal responses from the patient to ensure that techniques that best enable the body to return to its natural alignment are used. The practitioner may also teach the patient specific self-care release techniques that further assist in relieving pain and restoring function.

## BENEFITS OF ORTHO-BIONOMY®

At least three Ortho-Bionomy® sessions are recommended for an improved outcome. Habitual movements or body stances may be altered after a physical injury and Ortho-Bionomy® helps to reinstate the body's natural function and performance over the course of these sessions. Sessions may also be used to improve a patient's posture in cases in which the body has been damaged by years of poor habitual movements and/or complications resulting from injuries sustained many years ago. Ortho-Bionomy® is commonly recommended when a patient has a low tolerance for pain since the technique uses no forceful movements or pressure and relies only on this noninvasive process of healing.

The benefits experienced as a result of Ortho-Bionomy® include:

- Better energy flow and relief from chronic pain
- Release of structural and muscular imbalances
- Relief from emotional tension and trauma-related symptoms
- Enhanced healing capacity
- A profound feeling of relaxation and comfort

Ortho-Bionomy® is also used to provide relief from conditions such as headaches, sports injuries, restricted movement (frozen shoulder), acute/chronic pain, and neuromuscular dysfunction (lower back pain).

It is important to find a qualified practitioner with appropriate credentials to perform Ortho-Bionomy® treatment. The patient must also communicate specific needs and level of comfort with the practitioner prior to arranging and throughout each session.

## References

1. Chrystele. "What Is Ortho-Bionomy?" Luxmama Club & ParentPrep, February 3, 2018.
2. "What Makes Ortho-Bionomy Different from All the Rest?" Zoee, February 1, 2002.
3. "OrthoBionomy® Unraveling the Mystery," Angelauriel.com, February 1, 2001.
4. "Is Orthobionomy Right for Me?" Society of Ortho-Bionomy International®, n.d.
5. "What Is Ortho-Bionomy?" Society of Ortho-Bionomy International®, n.d.

# Chapter 18 | Chronic Myofascial Pain and Treatment Options

Chronic myofascial pain (CMP), also known as "myofascial pain syndrome (MPS)," is a chronic, painful condition that affects the muscles, in particular the covering layer of the muscle, known as the "fascia." When repetitive or excessive stress is placed on a muscle, it can create sensitive areas called "myofascial trigger points (MTrPs)" that can cause pain throughout the muscle. These trigger points can also cause pain in unrelated parts of the body, a phenomena called "referred pain."

Myofascial pain is dull, aching, and deep. Along with pain, individuals may experience sleep problems as well as decreased muscle flexibility and strength. The trigger point may be active ( consistently painful) or latent (pain and tenderness only when touched).

## POSSIBLE CAUSES OF TRIGGER POINTS

Although what causes trigger points is not completely understood, potential contributing factors include:

- Poorly conditioned muscles
- Chronic overload of muscles associated with repetitive movements
- Poor ergonomics and postural stress such as sitting for prolonged duration of time
- A difference in length between the patient's legs
- Lifting or moving objects without using proper techniques
- Increased muscle tension due to anxiety or depression, Fatigue, trauma, and cold weather

## DIAGNOSING CHRONIC MYOFASCIAL PAIN

Healthcare providers diagnose CMP by completing a physical examination of the painful areas and collecting a detailed history from the patient. During the examination, the doctors may apply gentle pressure in a certain way to the trigger points to check for a referred pattern of pain or a muscle twitch. They will also feel for the texture of the muscle fibers and do tests to determine the strength and flexibility of the muscles.

Chronic myofascial pain is common in people between the ages of 30 and 60, affecting both men and women equally. Recent research has identified myofascial trigger points as a contributing factor in chronic headaches, tension type headaches, neck pain, and shoulder disorders.

## MANAGING MYOFASCIAL PAIN SYNDROME

Treatment consists of 3 main components:

1. Reducing the chronic overload of the muscles. Identify the factors and correct it.
2. Eliminate the trigger point. There are several methods used to do this.
3. Strengthen the affected group of muscles.

## TREATMENT OPTIONS FOR CHRONIC MYOFASCIAL PAIN

### Medications

- Pain relievers—Over-the-counter (OTC) pain relievers, including ibuprofen (Advil, Motrin IB, others) and naproxen sodium (Aleve), may relieve pain.
- Antidepressants—Can reduce pain and improve sleep.
- Sedatives—Can help to relax muscles; however, they should be used under a doctor's supervision since they can be addictive.

### Physical Therapy

A physical therapist may treat chronic myofascial pain using one or more of the following methods:

- Stretching exercises—loosen tight muscles and releases trigger points
- Strengthening exercises—build up muscle strength and prevents early muscle fatigue
- Massage therapy—helps muscles relax and prevents spasms or cramps.
- Hot packs or hot shower
- Ultrasound—Uses high-frequency sound waves to promote healing in the muscle tissue and helps release triggers.

### Needle Procedures

There are two types of needle procedures:

- Wet needling. Therapeutic practice in which a numbing agent or steroid is injected by needle into the trigger point to relieve the pain.
- Dry needling. Involves inserting an acupuncture needle into the trigger point. This results in a reduction of substances that interact with nearby nociceptors (the parts of nerves that sense pain) and ultimately provide pain relief.

## Self-Care Measures

Along with the treatment, patients can employ a variety of measures that can prevent recurrence and aid in better treatment outcomes:

- **Exercise:** Regular exercise and an active lifestyle can help patients cope with pain
- **Relaxation:** Various relaxation methods can help reduce tension and stress. Deep breathing exercises, listening to soothing music, meditation, and talking with friends can help.
- **Taking time for yourself:** Taking care of yourself by eating healthy and getting enough sleep will help relieve pain and the associated stress
- **Support group:** Talking to a counselor or joining a support group can help patients cope with pain

## References


1. "Chronic Myofascial Pain (CMP)," Cleveland Clinic, March 1, 2013.
2. "Dry Needling," Physiopedia, n.d.
3. "Myofascial Pain Syndrome," MayoClinic, December 9, 2014.

# Chapter 19 | Rehabilitation Engineering

## WHAT IS REHABILITATION ENGINEERING?

Rehabilitation engineering is the use of engineering science and principles to:

- Develop technological solutions and devices to assist individuals with disabilities
- Aid the recovery of physical and cognitive functions lost because of disease or injury

Rehabilitation engineers design and build devices and systems to meet a wide range of needs that can assist individuals with mobility, communication, hearing, vision, and cognition. These tools help people with day-to-day activities and tasks related to employment, independent living, and education. Rehabilitation engineering may involve relatively simple observations of how

workers perform tasks and then making accommodations to eliminate further injuries and discomfort. On the other end of the spectrum, more complex rehabilitation engineering is the design of sophisticated brain-computer interfaces that allow a severely individual with a disability to operate computers, and other assistive devices simply by thinking about the task they want to perform.

Rehabilitation engineers also develop and improve rehabilitation methods used by individuals to regain functions lost due to disease or injury, such as limb (arm and or leg) mobility following a stroke or a joint replacement.

## TYPES OF ASSISTIVE DEVICES DEVELOPED THROUGH REHABILITATION ENGINEERING

The following are examples of the many types of assistive devices.

- Wheelchairs, scooters, and prosthetic devices, such as artificial limbs that provide mobility for people with physical disabilities that affect movement

This chapter includes text excerpted from "Rehabilitation Engineering," National Institute of Biomedical Imaging and Bioengineering (NIBIB), October 2018.

- Kitchen implements with large, cushioned grips to help people with weakness or arthritis in their hands with everyday living tasks
- Automatic page-turners, book holders, and adapted pencil grips, that allow participation in educational activities in school and at home
- Medication dispensers with alarms that can help people remember to take their medicine on time
- Specially engineered computer programs that provide voice recognition to help people with sensory impairments use computer technology

## REHABILITATION ENGINEERING RESEARCH WILL IMPROVE THE QUALITY OF LIFE FOR INDIVIDUALS

Ongoing research in rehabilitation engineering involves the design and development of new, innovative assistive devices. An important research area focuses on the development of new technologies and techniques for improved therapies that help people regain physical or cognitive functions lost because of disease or injury. For example:

- **Rehabilitation robotics** that involves the use of robots as therapy aids instead of solely as assistive devices. Intelligent rehabilitation robotics aids mobility training in individuals suffering from impaired movement, such as following a stroke.
- **Virtual rehabilitation**, which uses virtual reality simulation exercises for physical and cognitive rehabilitation. Compared to conventional therapies, virtual rehabilitation can offer several advantages. It is entertaining and motivates patients. It provides objective measures such as range of motion or game scores that can be stored on the computer operating the simulation. The virtual exercises can be performed at home by a patient and monitored by a therapist over the Internet (known as "telerehabilitation"), which offers convenience as well as reduced costs.
- **Improved prosthetics**, such as smarter artificial legs. This is an area where researchers continue to make advances in design and function to better mimic natural limb movement and user intent.
- **Increasingly sophisticated use of computers** as the interface between the user and various devices to enable severely impaired individuals increased independence and integration into the community. For example, brain-computer interfaces that use the brain's electrical impulses to allow individuals to learn to move a computer cursor or a robotic arm that can reach and grab items.
- **Development of new technologies** to analyze human motion, to better understand the electrophysiology of muscle and brain activity, and to more accurately monitor human functions. These technologies will

continue to drive innovation in assistive devices and rehabilitation strategies.

## DEVELOPMENT IN THE AREA OF REHABILITATION ENGINEERING

### Artificial Hands Capable of Complex Movements and Sensation

Persons with hand amputations expect modern hand prostheses to function similar to intact hands. State-of-the-art prosthetic hands simply control two movements "open" and "close." As a result, researchers are developing new artificial hand systems that would perform complex hand motions based on measurements of the residual electrical signals from the remaining muscles of an amputee's forearm. Signals from the muscles and nerves have the potential to result in much finer control of the fingers in the artificial hand. In addition, work is on to capture the sense of touch, so in the future the users will be able to also "feel" what they are holding with their artificial hand.

### Closed-Loop Braces for Limbs, Spine*

Traditional orthosis, or braces, were purely mechanical, passive devices to provide structural, postural, and functional characteristics of the musculoskeletal system. By incorporating electronic sensors, controllers, and motors, it is possible to greatly increase functional performance for users. One approach is to build an ankle-foot brace with a hydraulically adjustable stiffness to mimic the muscles and tendons in a healthy individual. This team is developing a child-size version of the device, which adjusts to maintain a proper fit as the child grows. Another approach is to develop a hydraulic system to use forces from a user's un-impaired or less-impaired limb to support motion by the impaired limb. And yet a third approach is to build an electromechanical control system capable of supporting a complete range of motion for individuals with thoracic/lumbar vertebrae that are compressed or crushed.

**Text excerpted from "Rehabilitation Engineering," National Institute of Biomedical Imaging and Bioengineering (NIBIB), October 2018.*

### Navigation Aids*

Individuals who are visually impaired require assistance to navigate through unfamiliar locations. Researchers are developing a cane that is enhanced with computer vision and vibration feedback. The cane uses advanced image processing to map the structure of a room, identify important features (door, stairs, obstacles), and create a navigation plan to guide the user towards his destination. It provides feedback in the form of either speech or vibrations through the handle.

**Text excerpted from "Rehabilitation Engineering," National Institute of Biomedical Imaging and Bioengineering (NIBIB), October 2018.*

### Neurostimulation in Individuals with Spinal Cord Injury

Researchers are developing the next generation of high-density electrode arrays for stimulation of the spinal cord. The first patient received a current generation electrical stimulator implant in his lower back. The electrical stimulation and locomotor training resulted in the ability to stand independently for several minutes, some voluntary leg control, and regained blood pressure control, bladder, bowel, and sexual function. Three more patients have received this treatment and had similar results. This is to enhance recovery of voluntary control of standing and movement, and involuntary control of blood pressure, bladder and sexual functions.

## Prosthesis Control*

Standard-of-care prostheses for amputees, while increasing in sophistication, lack the ability to reliably detect a user's fine motor commands. Several teams are developing technologies to more accurately record and transmit the user's intent to use their hands to grasp, grip or pinch by recording the electrical signals sent by the user. By implanting electrodes in the residual arm muscles, peripheral nerves, spinal cord, and brain, it is possible to detect these electrical signals, convert them into digital commands, and drive the motors in a hand prosthesis to significantly improve function. Researchers are fine-tuning the system for each limb as well as the different needs of each amputee. By exploring all of these approaches simultaneously, it should be possible to advance the state of the art faster. Several studies have FDA approval for clinical trials, and the others are still undergoing preclinical research prior to advancing to trial.

**Text excerpted from "Rehabilitation Engineering," National Institute of Biomedical Imaging and Bioengineering (NIBIB), October 2018.*

## Restoring Muscle Control*

People with spinal cord injuries have limited or no ability to control muscle groups below the site of the injury. This often requires assistive mobility devices (crutches, wheelchairs, or powered wheelchairs) and part- or full-time caregiver support. One research team is investigating a technological approach to bypass the injury. They have built a fully-implantable system that uses a sensor to measure voluntary muscle contractions above the injury; the sensor in turn sends electrical signals to trigger muscle activity below the injury. The technology has enabled restoration of standing, stepping, cycling, and hand grasp. Another research team is using electrical stimulus in conjunction with physical therapy to more effectively train the central nervous system to enhance the function of the few remaining neurons at the site of the injury. The team uses a completely noninvasive system to train the nervous system below the injury how to walk. This approach has improved walking speed long after the therapy has ended.

Another approach uses implantable spinal cord stimulators, originally designed to reduce pain, to alter the neural activity in the spine to restore control of standing and stepping in patients.

**Text excerpted from "Rehabilitation Engineering," National Institute of Biomedical Imaging and Bioengineering (NIBIB), October 2018.*

### Smart Environment Technologies

As the population ages, increasing numbers of Americans are unable to live independently. Researchers are working on creating smart environments that aid with home health monitoring and intervention allowing individuals with health issues to remain safely at home. For example, researchers are analyzing the needs and limitations of Alzheimer disease patients to develop automated and reminder-based technologies that can be integrated into the home to help with everyday tasks.

### Wireless Tongue Drive System for Paralyzed Patients

Tongue drive system (TDS) technology exploits the fact that even individuals with severe paralysis that impairs limb movement, breathing, and speech can still move their tongue. Simple tongue movements send commands to the computer allowing users to steer their wheelchairs, operate their computers, and generally control their environment in an independent fashion.

# Part 3 | **Treatment Plans, Exercise Regimens, and Physical Modalities**

# Chapter 20 | Physical Therapy Assessments and Evaluation

Assessment done on the person served is relevant with the core values, and mission of the organization. Physical medicine and rehabilitation service (PM&R) staff perform various methods of assessments on the person served. The assessments can before and after surgical procedures; during admission to the rehabilitation unit, consult response to any program. Data are collected from patient electronic record and via personal interview and examination of the patient. Programs are established on collective interventions among the interdisciplinary team or individual procedures that include:

- Initial assessment
- Re-assessment
- Treatment plan
- Quantity and duration of care
- Treatment implementation
- Patient family education
- Discharge planning
- Interdisciplinary management
- Follow-up

## ASSESSMENT PROCESS AND DOCUMENTATION

A thorough initial assessment is performed by all members of the interdisciplinary rehabilitation team. This assessment gathers pathophysiological, functional, cognitive, communicative, behavioral and emotional, pharmacological, physical, and social data from qualified individuals regarding each veteran's

This chapter contains text excerpted from the following sources: Text in this chapter begins with excerpts from "Physical Medicine and Rehabilitation Service," U.S. Department of Veterans Affairs (VA), January 25, 2018; Text beginning with the heading "Assessment Process and Documentation" is excerpted from "Physical Medicine and Rehabilitation Service (PM&RS) Procedures," U.S. Department of Veterans Affairs (VA), May 2, 2014. Reviewed November 2019.

goals, impairments, activity limitations, participation restrictions, discharge environment, and need for care. This data is analyzed to:

- Create the information necessary to decide the approach and timeframes to meet the patient's rehabilitation care needs.
- Enable decisions establishing the patient's interdisciplinary plan of care. Evaluation and treatment are initiated according to the timeframe established.

## PHYSICAL THERAPY EVALUATION

- Evaluation in muscle strength, balance and coordination, joint flexibility, physical endurance, locomotion and transfer mobility, and pain.
- Specific assessment techniques are manual muscle tests, gait analysis, range of motion, and neurological examination.

Common interventions are therapeutic exercises, manual intervention, neuromuscular re-education, resistive muscle strengthening, gait training, and use of prostheses and orthoses; recommendations for specialized equipment; use of modalities such as transcutaneous electrical nerve stimulator (otherwise known as "TENS"), functional muscle stimulation, ultrasound; and patient, caregiver, and family education.

## INTERDISCIPLINARY PLAN OF CARE

The interdisciplinary plan of care is utilized by the rehabilitation team as a method of compiling the assessment information of the interdisciplinary team (IDT) members into a single custom plan of care for the patient. The plan of care represents the overall direction that the IDT is working towards assisting the patient to achieve improvements in independence, function, and quality of life.

**NOTE:** An interdisciplinary plan of care can be used for both inpatients and outpatients.

Each member of the IDT administers discipline-specific evaluations based on the individual medical and surgical diagnoses, impairments, and sequelae of the patient. These evaluations assist the IDT to establish the projected achievable goals and timelines for rehabilitation. The physiatrist or physician with extensive rehabilitation experience provides oversight to the interdisciplinary rehabilitation plan of care. The interdisciplinary plan and any changes to the plan, made by the IDT or the veteran are communicated in the electronic medical record to the interdisciplinary team.

The interdisciplinary plan of care is a participant centered, coordinated, and collaborative plan based on active involvement of the patient, family, and rehabilitation team members or other support system participants identified by the patient and IDT. The plan synthesizes information gathered from the patient, the patient's family, and discipline-specific evaluations, allowing for the completion of a functional impairment list, identified interventions, and expected short-term, long-term, and discharge goals. Based on input from the patient and the overall IDT assessment, the strengths, abilities, needs, and preferences of the patient are identified and noted in the plan of care. The interdisciplinary plan must include measurable goals, discharge planning, and patient education. The IDT determines the frequency of treatment and the estimated length of stay at admission, which are reviewed with the patient. Regular and frequent assessments must be performed on a discipline-specific and interdisciplinary basis, including a revision of program goals and areas of identified need, as required by the patient's condition. This includes specific and detailed information regarding the progress of the individual as determined by the re-evaluations of each consulted discipline to ensure that appropriate adjustments are made to the plan of care, and facilitate discharge planning. The results of re-evaluations are documented in the medical record and communicated to the team and the patient during the IDT meeting. Assessment and reassessment timeframes are determined within local medical facility policy.

# Chapter 21 | **Modalities Used during Physical Therapy**

**Chapter Contents**

## Section 21.1 | Thermal Agents



Heat and cold have been used for centuries to relieve pain, heal tissue, and manage joint pain. In physical rehabilitation, superficial heat may be applied to improve blood circulation, promote tissue healing, and relax stiff joints. Superficial heat helps relax the muscles and loosen the joints prior to rehabilitation exercises routines that are designed to help patients regain limb functions. Heat, along with physical therapy, is used during rehabilitation to stimulate muscles and enhance mobility.

The two major types of thermal agents available for tissue heating are:

- **Superficial-heating agents.** Surface-tissue temperature rises to varying degrees due to the use of superficial thermal agents, depending on the intensity of the heat and the medium used. The most commonly used thermal agents are hot packs and paraffin. The normal estimated amount of penetration for most superficial thermal modalities is one centimeter, or a little less than half an inch.
- **Deep-heating agents.** Deep-heat modalities consist of ultrasound, shortwave diathermy (SWD), and microwave diathermy (MWD). Heat from these modalities may penetrate as far as 3–5 centimeters, or a little over 1 to nearly 2 inches, without overheating the underlying subcutaneous tissue or skin.

### THERMOTHERAPY

The therapeutic application of heat over a targeted region of the body to induce a biological response is referred to as "thermotherapy," or "heat therapy." Thermotherapy is known to improve strength and endurance during physical rehabilitation. Aside from conductive agents such as heating pads and paraffin wax, radiation using infrared waves and convection are also used as thermal agents during rehabilitation. Convection is the transfer of heat between different areas of temperature by means of liquid or gas.

Thermotherapy is used during the healing process that follows an injury. It is used mainly to restore the structure and function of injured or diseased tissue. Heat or thermal agents are applied to the affected area to expedite healing by increasing blood flow to the injured area. Selective heating, which allows stiff muscles to stretch, uses infrared radiation to accelerate the absorption of hematomas, or a collection of blood outside a blood vessel (bruising). This enables the patient to easily exercise and strengthen mobility during the rehabilitation process. Thermotherapy has a similar effect as cryotherapy (cold therapy) with regards to nerve functions.

## CLASSIFICATION OF THERMAL AGENTS

Heat therapy can be broadly classified into two major categories based on the application of heat. They are:

- Direct contact
- Infrared radiation

### Direct Contact

This involves the application of heat directly onto a particular region of the body by using specific warming devices. Thermotherapy is known to improve vasodilation, which is the expansion of blood capillaries. This increases blood flow, enhances muscle strength, and enables the injury to heal faster.

### Infrared Radiation

Infrared radiation is the process through which infrared waves are directed at a certain wavelength to penetrate deep layers of the skin in order to enhance tissue function. The effects of infrared radiation depend on the frequency of wavelength used and the amount of energy absorbed by the tissue. Infrared radiation is beneficial for the reduction of pain and inflammation, and for muscular injuries that require a long time to heal.

## KEY ASPECTS OF THERMOTHERAPY

Heat therapy is also known to reduce inflammation and edema (fluid buildup in tissues).

The following are some of the benefits of undergoing thermotherapy:

- Enhanced flexibility of tendons and ligaments
- Reduction of muscle spasms
- Increase blood flow due to vasodilation
- Amplify overall body metabolism

Heat also may induce the release of endorphins, which are helpful in blocking pain transmission.

Thermotherapy is an important component in the rehabilitation of musculoskeletal injuries. Although there are a few contradictions to the effectiveness of heat therapy, it has been proven to relieve pain and improve muscle function.

### References

1. "Heat Therapy," Elsevier, July 7, 2017.
2. "How Does Heat Therapy Work?" Spectrum physio, July 31, 2014.
3. "Thermotherapy," Physiopedia, December 5, 2012.
4. Betsaida, Angela B. "Infrared Therapy: Health Benefits and Risks," News Medical, January 30, 2019.

5. Moroz, Alex. "Treatment of Pain and Inflammation," MSD Manual Consumer Version, September 22, 2007.

## Section 21.2 | **Ultrasound and Phonophoresis**

This section contains text excerpted from the following sources: Text in this section begins with excerpts from "Ultrasound," National Institute of Biomedical Imaging and Bioengineering (NIBIB), July 2016. Reviewed November 2019; Text under the heading "Phonophoresis" is excerpted from "The Phonophoresis of Lidocaine Gel and Its Effect on Sensory Blockage," ClinicalTrials.gov, National Institutes of Health (NIH), July 28, 2011. Reviewed November 2019.

Therapeutic ultrasound uses sound waves above the range of human hearing but does not produce images. Its purpose is to interact with tissues in the body such that they are either modified or destroyed. Among the modifications possible are:

- Moving or pushing tissue
- Heating tissues
- Dissolving blood clots
- Delivering drugs to specific locations in the body

These destructive, or ablative, functions are made possible by the use of very high-intensity beams that can destroy diseased or abnormal tissues such as tumors. The advantage of using ultrasound therapies is that, in most cases, they are noninvasive. No incisions or cuts need to be made to the skin, leaving no wounds or scars.

### HOW DOES IT WORK?

Ultrasound waves are produced by a transducer, which can both emit ultrasound waves, as well as detect the ultrasound echoes reflected back. In most cases, the active elements in ultrasound transducers are made of special ceramic crystal materials called "piezoelectrics." These materials are able to produce sound waves when an electric field is applied to them, but can also work in reverse, producing an electric field when a sound wave hits them. When used in an ultrasound scanner, the transducer sends out a beam of sound waves into the body. The sound waves are reflected back to the transducer by boundaries between tissues in the path of the beam (e.g., the boundary between fluid and soft tissue or tissue and bone). When these echoes hit the transducer, they generate electrical signals that are sent to the ultrasound scanner. Using the speed of sound and the time of each echo's return, the scanner calculates the distance from the transducer to the tissue boundary. These distances are then used to generate two-dimensional images of tissues and organs.

During an ultrasound application, the physiotherapist will apply a gel to the skin. This keeps air pockets from forming between the transducer and the skin, which can block ultrasound waves from passing into the body.

### THERAPEUTIC OR INTERVENTIONAL ULTRASOUND

Therapeutic ultrasound produces high levels of acoustic output that can be focused on specific targets for the purpose of heating, ablating, or breaking up tissue. One type of therapeutic ultrasound uses high-intensity beams of sound that are highly targeted, and is called "High-Intensity Focused Ultrasound" (HIFU). HIFU is being investigated as a method for modifying or destroying diseased or abnormal tissues inside the body (e.g., tumors) without having to open or tear the skin or cause damage to the surrounding tissue.

### PHONOPHORESIS

Phonophoresis is the use of therapeutic ultrasound to increase percutaneous drug absorption. However, few studies have compared pulsed and continuous modes of therapeutic ultrasound. Pulsed ultrasound with topical lidocaine gel induces greater anesthetic effect compared with continuous ultrasound with topical lidocaine gel and lidocaine application alone. The mechanical properties of pulsed ultrasound appear to be responsible for greater drug penetration.

Lidocaine is a common local anesthetic drug that is used topically to relieve pain, itching and burning, and also for minor surgery. However, its application through this conductive method, has been confined to surface anesthesia because it seems that it is not possible to have a deep transmission with local drug massage, without injection or systemic administration. On the other hand, the injection of lidocaine can lead to tissue injury and pain, and its use is not advised in children. Phonophoresis is one of the common procedures for reducing these problems. Therefore, the main aim of this study was to compare the two modes of therapeutic ultrasound by assessing the effect of lidocaine gel phonophoresis on percutaneous absorption and sensory blockade.

## Section 21.3 | Electrical Stimulation and Iontophoresis

This section includes text excerpted from "Decision Memo for Neuromuscular Electrical Stimulation (NMES) for Spinal Cord Injury (CAG-00153R)," Centers for Medicare & Medicaid Services (CMS), July 22, 2002. Reviewed November 2019.

One type of neuromuscular electrical stimulation (NMES) that is used to enhance functional activity of patients is commonly referred to as "functional electrical stimulation" (FES). These devices use electrical impulses to activate paralyzed or weak muscles in precise sequence and have been utilized to provide SCI patients with the ability to walk. In addition, patients require many sessions of physical therapy to learn how to use the device properly. The goal of this therapy must be to train patients on the use of FES devices to achieve walking, not to reverse or retard muscle atrophy.

NMES/FES used for walking, in the setting of physical therapy or home use, will be limited to patients with all of the following characteristics:

- Persons with intact lower motor units
- Persons with muscle and joint stability for weight-bearing at upper and lower extremities that can demonstrate balance and control to maintain an upright support posture independently
- Persons that demonstrate brisk muscle contraction to NMES and have sensory perception of electrical stimulation sufficient for muscle contraction
- Persons that possess high motivation, commitment and cognitive ability to use such devices for walking
- Persons that can transfer independently and can demonstrate standing tolerance for at least three minutes
- Persons that can demonstrate hand and finger function to manipulate controls
- Persons with at least six-month postrecovery spinal cord injury and restorative surgery
- Persons without hip and knee degenerative disease and no history of long bone fracture secondary to osteoporosis

NMES/FES for walking will not be used for patients with any of the following:

- Persons with cardiac pacemakers
- Severe scoliosis or severe osteoporosis
- Skin disease or cancer at area of stimulation
- Irreversible contracture
- Autonomic dysreflexia

There are two broad categories of NMES. One type stimulates the muscle when the patient is in a resting state to treat patients with muscle atrophy. A second type is used to enhance functional activity in neurologically impaired patients. These devices use electrical impulses to activate paralyzed or weak muscles in precise sequence and have been utilized to provide patients with the ability to walk. This technology is utilized for both upper extremity (e.g., improved hand grasp function) and lower extremity rehabilitation. NMES used for this indication is also commonly called "functional electrical stimulation" (or FES). NMES is used to assist standing and ambulation in paraplegics or quadriplegics who have adequate use of their upper extremities to allow balancing with a walker (or with elbow-support crutches), assuming satisfactory pulmonary and cardiovascular functioning. However, this technology is not intended to replace the wheelchair, which still remains the main source of transportation.

The first use of NMES to enhance lower extremity functions in paraplegics began with work on the correction of foot-drop. The use of surface stimulation to assist standing and walking for persons with complete and incomplete spinal cord injury began in the 1970s. Two surface electrodes per leg were used to stimulate standing and reciprocal walking by direct activation of the quadriceps muscles.

There are three types of NMES:

- Transcutaneous (surface)
- Percutaneous
- Subcutaneous (fully implanted) systems

One such transcutaneous device is the Parastep system which is noninvasive and uses a microcomputer microchip that synchronizes stimulation at various sites. Surface or transcutaneous devices send an electric current through the skin. Generally, four electrodes are placed on the skin and current crosses through the skin to stimulate the appropriate muscles. This system generates trains of pulses to trigger action potentials of selected nerves at the quadriceps for knee extension, at the common peroneal nerve for the hip flexion withdrawal reflex and the paraspinal muscles/gluteus maximus muscle for enhancing trunk stability. Most patients use a walker for balancing support. This device has received FDA approval to enable standing and walking.

Another surface system is the hybrid body-brace system, which is a body brace/NMES combination. This system combines an orthosis with NMES. These systems are designed for standing and ambulation of SCI patients who have full use of their upper extremities so they can balance themselves by using a walker or crutches. The NMES components consist of a four-channel surface stimulator and surface electrodes placed over the rectus femoris and hamstrings. Benefits of a surface system are that they are noninvasive with relative ease in placing and removing electrodes.

- The inability to maintain isolated muscle selectivity
- Difficulty in stimulating deeper muscles
- Poor reproducibility of contraction due to variability in electrode placement
- Inconvenience in placing multiple electrodes
- Pain from stimulation

- Skin irritation from adhesives on surface electrodes
- Breakage of the wire electrodes
- Relatively greater risk of infection at the electrode site
- Early patient fatigue due to high energy demand from use of the device

The second type of device is the percutaneous system, which is implanted into the body with leads and parts of the system remaining outside the body. In this case, only electrical impulses cross the skin. Percutaneous leads require surgery and have been designed as either intramuscular electrodes that are embedded into the fibers of the muscle or epimysial electrodes that lay on the surface of the muscle. This type of system can use an 8-channel implantable receiver/stimulator and an external control unit, which powers and instructs the radio frequency signals. Percutaneous interfaces require continuous attention from the user, and the electrode site must be cleaned, dressed, and properly maintained to avoid infection and possible breakage. Although these leads can remain functional for years without infection and complication, they are generally not considered preferable for long-term clinical use. The implantable system does offer an advantage by placing the stimulating electrode close to neural structures, thus greatly increasing selectivity and efficiency of activation while simultaneously reducing required current. Furthermore, the time required for donning and doffing of this system is relatively short, as it only requires connecting electrode leads to the stimulator/controller cables and the control sensors.

The third type of system is a subcutaneous, fully implantable system, which includes both the stimulator and leads. These leads assume larger dimensions than percutaneous leads because they need to be more robust and resistant to failure. Some of the designs isolate the system subcomponents through high reliability, implantable connectors. These designs reduce the risk of infection and minimize the likelihood of damage to other implanted components.

## Section 21.4 | Transcutaneous Electrical Nerve Stimulation

This section contains text excerpted from the following sources: Text in this section begins with excerpts from "Pain: Hope through Research," National Institute of Neurological Disorders and Stroke (NINDS), August 13, 2019; Text under the heading "How Is Back Pain Treated?" is excerpted from "Low Back Pain Fact Sheet," National Institute of Neurological Disorders and Stroke (NINDS), August 13, 2019.

Electrical stimulation, including transcutaneous electrical stimulation (TENS), implanted electrical nerve stimulation, and deep brain or spinal cord stimulation, is the modern-day extension of age-old practices in which the nerves or muscles are subjected to a variety of stimuli, including heat or massage. The following techniques each require specialized equipment and personnel trained in the specific procedure being used:

Transcutaneous electrical stimulation uses tiny electrical pulses, delivered through the skin to nerve fibers, to cause changes in muscles, such as numbness or contractions. This, in turn, produces temporary pain relief. There is also evidence that TENS can activate subsets of peripheral nerve fibers that can block pain transmission at the spinal cord level, in much the same way that shaking your hand can reduce pain.

Peripheral nerve stimulation uses electrodes placed surgically or percutaneously (through the skin using a needle) on a peripheral nerve. The individual is then able to deliver an electrical current as needed to the affected nerve, using a controllable electrical generator.

Spinal cord stimulation (SCS) uses electrodes surgically or percutaneously inserted within the epidural space of the spinal cord. The individual is able to deliver a pulse of electricity to the spinal cord using an implanted electrical pulse generator that resembles a cardiac pacemaker.

Deep brain stimulation (DBS) is considered a more extreme treatment and involves surgical stimulation of the brain, usually the thalamus or motor cortex. It is used to treat chronic pain in cases that do not respond to less invasive or conservative treatments.

## HOW IS BACK PAIN TREATED?

Transcutaneous electrical stimulation involves wearing a battery-powered device consisting of electrodes placed on the skin over the painful area that generate electrical impulses designed to block incoming pain signals from the peripheral nerves. The theory is that stimulating the nervous system can modify the perception of pain. Early studies of TENS suggested that it elevated levels of endorphins, the body's natural pain-numbing chemicals.

## Section 21.5 | **Hydrotherapy**

This section contains text excerpted from the following sources: Text in this section begins with excerpts from "Water Use in Hydrotherapy Tanks," Centers for Disease Control and Prevention (CDC), October 11, 2016. Reviewed November 2019; Text beginning with the heading "Health Benefits of Water-Based Exercise" is excerpted from "Health Benefits of Water-Based Exercise," Centers for Disease Control and Prevention (CDC), May 4, 2016. Reviewed November 2019; Text under the heading "Aquatic Fitness" is excerpted from "Recreation Therapy—Aquatic Fitness," U.S. Department of Veterans Affairs (VA), November 13, 2017.

Hydrotherapy involves the use of water for soothing pains and treating certain medical conditions. Hydrotherapy equipment includes pools, whirlpools, whirlpool spas, hot tubs, and physiotherapy tanks. Patients with medical conditions, such as burns, septic ulcers, lesions, amputations, and arthritis, can benefit from the effects of sitting in warm water. For the health and safety of patients, it is vital to ensure that the water that is used in hydrotherapy is safe and clean. Many of these patients have compromised immune systems due to current infections, and are highly susceptible to infections from contaminated water in hydrotherapy pools. Potential routes of infection caused by contaminated water include accidental ingestion of the water, breathing sprays and aerosols from the water, and allowing wounds to come in direct contact with the water.

Infection control for hydrotherapy tanks, pools, or birthing tanks presents unique challenges because naturally-occurring microbes, that may not be dangerous for a healthy individual, are always present in the water during treatments. According to the Centers for Disease Control and Prevention's (CDC) Division of Healthcare Quality Promotion (DHQP) and the Healthcare Infection Control Practices Advisory Committee (HICPAC), the use of hydrotherapy for patients with wounds, burns, or other types of nonintact skin conditions should be considered on a case-by-case basis. Healthcare providers should always consider the availability of alternative aseptic techniques for wound management, as well as a risk-benefit analysis of using traditional hydrotherapy. If hydrotherapy is used, facilities should maintain strict cleaning and disinfection practices in accordance with the manufacturer's instructions.

### HEALTH BENEFITS OF WATER-BASED EXERCISE

Swimming is the fourth most popular sports activity in the United States and a good way to get regular aerobic physical activity. Just two and a half hours per week of aerobic physical activity, such as swimming, bicycling, or running can decrease the risk of chronic illnesses. This can also lead to improved health for people with diabetes and heart disease. Swimmers have about half the risk of death compared with inactive people. People enjoy water-based exercise more than exercising on land. They can also exercise longer in water than on land without increased effort or joint or muscle pain.

### WATER-BASED EXERCISE AND CHRONIC ILLNESS

Water-based exercise can help people with chronic diseases. For people with arthritis, it improves use of affected joints without worsening symptoms. People with rheumatoid arthritis have more health improvements after participating in hydrotherapy than with other activities. Water-based exercise also improves the use of affected joints and decreases pain from osteoarthritis.

### AQUATIC FITNESS

The benefits of hydrotherapy are numerous, especially for individuals who cannot bear weight and/or have difficulty engaging in a land-based program. Hydrotherapy can be useful for pain management, relaxation, reducing edema, increasing circulation and cardio capacity, reducing weight, increasing flexibility, strength, endurance, and motivation to work on goals. Engaging in aquatic exercise enables opportunities for independent movement, social interaction, and success in reaching fitness and wellness goals.

## Section 21.6 | **Aquatic Therapy**



Aquatic therapy, also called "aquatic physical therapy," has been in use for centuries and is based on the application of skilled physical practice in an aquatic environment. Although predominantly used in clinical settings for the management and rehabilitation of chronic conditions, the practice is gaining acceptance in athletic settings, particularly in areas such as recovery and rehabilitation from orthopedic dysfunction and sports injuries. The zero-gravity environment that water provides is used to intervene in a variety of conditions—including sensory integration and motor control deficits, fine motor deficits, poor social participation skills, and poor strength/endurance—to accomplish the activities of daily living.

The therapy is provided by a trained therapist and features exercise-based treatment in an aquatic environment. The buoyancy of water provides a controlled environment in which increased range of motion by all major muscle groups is possible at all angles. Water also provides a low-impact environment for exercising muscles with less strain than is for similar muscular activity on land. Treatment, which may include total or partial immersion, and helps patients maintain or improve muscular coordination, strength, flexibility, and endurance.

## HOW WATER WORKS

The physical properties of water make it a conducive therapeutic medium for a variety of chronic conditions. The natural buoyancy and drag resistance of the water makes it possible for patients to remain afloat and while experiencing a decreased effect of gravity on painful joints and muscles. The hydrostatic pressure of water stabilizes the patient and prevents falls while exercising—an important aspect of ensuring patient compliance with exercise regimens. Waves and turbulence can be simulated in pools to provide varying degrees of resistance or manipulation; this allows therapists and patients set specific exercise goals and achieve desired outcomes.

Warm water can also alleviate pain, elevate mood, improve sleep, and lower stress levels in people with depression or chronic illness, and in those seeking quick rehabilitation. Studies have also shown improved pulmonary and cardiovascular functions with aquatic therapy, particularly in patients who cannot participate in traditional land-based rehabilitation as a result of orthopedic constraints.

## INDICATIONS FOR AQUATIC THERAPY

Rehabilitation through aquatic therapy generally focuses on improving motor functions associated with disability, illness, or injury. Aquatic therapy may also be recommended for treating musculoskeletal pain and pressure ulcers. In pediatric populations, it is widely used as an intervention to improve motor skills in children with developmental disorders such as cerebral palsy or autism spectrum disorders. It may also be indicated in respiratory and circulatory disorders and is regarded as an ideal nonweight-bearing exercise during pregnancy. Prenatal aquatic therapy helps to maintain a moderate or greater intensity of exercise throughout the third trimester. Aquatic interventions are used for a wide variety of conditions, including impaired sensory and motor functions, spasticity, balance deficits, trauma, and to address motor learning and processing disorders. Special populations that require rehabilitation in neurodegenerative disorders also benefit from aquatic intervention; these populations include Parkinson disease, multiple sclerosis, amyotrophic lateral sclerosis, and Huntington disease.

## MODES OF AQUATIC THERAPY

Modes of aquatic therapy differ, but the four main modes are deepwater running, shallow-water running, water calisthenics, and underwater treadmill exercise. Each mode has its own biomechanical requirements and induces its own distinct physiological and functional responses. Physiological responses include factors such as oxygen consumption and degree of exertion, while biomechanical factors include the length or frequency of underwater strides as compared with land-based therapeutic exercise. For instance, deepwater running that does not include ground contact elicits a lower oxygen consumption than other modes of aquatic therapy.

Deepwater jogging or running mimics running on land and is popularly used to maintain fitness levels after an injury. Deepwater running is usually practiced using a flotation device (buoyancy vest or belt), which keeps the body afloat and without ground contact while executing underwater running biomechanics. Shallow-water running, on the other hand, typically includes contact with the ground and is done in shallow water below mid-chest level without the aid of buoyancy aids. Patients walk or run and propel themselves through the water. Water calisthenics includes a variety of aerobic conditioning and resistance-training exercises and is usually executed in the shallow end of a pool. Walking and running are not included in water calisthenics. Underwater treadmill exercise uses a submerged treadmill belt and may include adjustable water depth and treadmill speed in order to control exercise intensity.

## SOME POPULAR TECHNIQUES OF AQUATIC THERAPY

While dozens of techniques are used in aquatic therapy, some are more popular than others. These include:

- **Tai chi:** A therapy based on qi gong (a holistic system of traditional Chinese medicine that combines the elements of coordinated breathing, body posture, movements, and meditation) and tai chi chuan (a Chinese system of internal martial arts based on spiritual and mental aspects).
- **Bad Ragaz Ring Method:** Developed by Swiss physiotherapists, this form of aquatic therapy is based on proprioceptive neuromuscular facilitation that involves targeting specific muscle groups for improving strength and flexibility through a series of contraction and stretching movements. This is a therapist-assisted regime performed with patients lying supine on the water surface supported by rings or floats around their necks, arms, knees, and pelvis. This type of aquatic therapy finds use in the treatment of arthritic conditions, soft tissue injury, and cerebrovascular accident. It is also recommended for postfracture or postsurgery rehabilitation.
- **Halliwick aquatic therapy:** Developed in the 1940s by James McMillan, a hydromechanics engineer, this patient-specific aquatic therapy is based on the use of a ten-point structured-learning program that helps people with no experience in swimming progress toward complete independence in the water. Also referred to as water specific therapy, the ten-point program is used to address specific limitations resulting from disability or injury. The water provides a medium for

developing specific areas, including a range of movements, strength, stamina, and respiratory function. Water can also serve as a medium for sensory-integration to enhance functional independence and motor learning. Working in groups can also enhance psychological well-being and self-esteem by helping to develop social skills.

- **Watsu:** A form of passive aquatic therapy, this form of aquatic therapy is a one-to-one routine performed in chest-deep water that takes the patient into a state of deep meditation and relaxation. Watsu focuses on the application of manual pressure for manipulation and mobilization of joints and is believed to have physical and emotional benefits for a variety of orthopedic and neurological disorders. During a typical session, the therapist supports the back-floating receiver and performs a routine comprising breath coordination, gentle massage, muscle stretches, and Shiatsu, a type of Japanese bodywork based on traditional Chinese medicine.

## AQUATIC THERAPIST

An aquatic therapist works on the principle of specificity and chooses the most advantageous mode of therapy for a particular patient. Ideally, the therapist chooses a mode that is associated with minimal pain and impact, ease of mobility, and maximum relaxation while eliciting the same biomechanical and physiological responses as a parallel land-based exercise therapy.

Although aquatic therapy interventions are typically held in a fairly shallow pool, this therapy is not entirely risk-free and safety standards must be maintained in order to provide a safe environment for the patient. Toward this end, aquatic therapy practitioners should be trained in first aid, cardiopulmonary resuscitation (CPR), oxygen administration, automated external defibrillation, and risk awareness related to blood-borne pathogens.

## THE LOWDOWN ON AQUATIC THERAPY

Aquatic therapy has been shown to be an effective intervention for improving joint flexibility and functional ability, and also for decreasing pain in certain rheumatic diseases and orthopedic conditions. Its popularity as an alternative therapy notwithstanding, aquatic therapy and some of its aspects, including its role in rehabilitation medicine, still require high-quality research. While most studies to date have focused on the physiological aspects of aquatic therapy, there is a dearth of research on the biomechanical implications of this therapy. Methodologies differ as well. The absence of standardized protocols for evaluating the impact of various modes of aquatic therapy on rehabilitation creates challenges and questions regarding the veracity of published findings in this field.

## References

1. "Aquatherapy for Neurodegenerative Disorders," U.S. National Library of Medicine (NLM), 2014.
2. "The Effects of Aquatic Exercise on Pulmonary Function in Patients with Spinal Cord Injury," U.S. National Library of Medicine (NLM), 2014.
3. "What Is Aquatic Therapy?" National Rehabilitation Information Center (NARIC), June 2016.

## Section 21.7 | **Taping Techniques**



Bracing and taping are methods of wrapping that provide support to muscles, tendons, and ligaments and prevent injuries such as sprains, strains, and fractures. Bracing and taping also helps reduce the risk of re-injury when a player goes back out on the field. Ankle sprains account for 2 million sports injuries annually. Most athletes and coaches are familiar with ankle bracing and taping and routinely apply it before every game.

### WHAT IS BRACING?

Braces are suitable for athletes who require additional support following an injury. They have solid pieces of polymer or metal and can be adjusted during practice and competition. Braces are designed to enhance mobility rather than immobilize the affected area. A safe degree of movement allows bones and ligaments to heal better. Braces can also help athletes extend physical therapy by allowing them to perform strengthening exercises on their own.

### WHAT IS TAPING?

Athletic tape is self-adhesive and is used to maintain muscle and bone alignment by limiting excessive movement of the ligaments and joints. Tapes are available in various strengths and colors, with different properties including levels of flexibility and moisture-wicking ability. For optimum effect, taping should be done by a professional doctor, trainer, or physical therapist since incorrectly taping will only worsen the injury. The most significant issue with taping is that it is a temporary fix. The binding power of tape lessens due to sweat and movement. The endurance of tape will last for not more than 30 minutes with continuous sports activity.

## WHAT ARE THE DIFFERENCES BETWEEN BRACING AND TAPING?

Braces have a significant advantage over tape because they can be applied, used, and adjusted by athletes without the need for professional help.

Many studies have been conducted on the effectiveness of taping and bracing. Among the findings:

- It has been definitively established that bracing and taping offers significant benefits as compared to not using either.
- Tapes last only for three to four days before becoming ineffective while braces can help keep your active lifestyle.
- While compression can help with injury management, excessive compression can cause problems.
- Braces are more cost-effective than tapes in the long run. In a competitive season, taping is three times more expensive than bracing.
- Athletes feel less comfortable and stable wearing braces than tapes.
- Sweating when exercising and playing sports affects the position of tapes and causes tapes to slip. Braces, on the other hand, cover a larger area and can be adjusted manually. Braces are made of breathable material and allow perspiration without affecting its position.
- Applying taping incorrectly can render it ineffective or may even lead to blistering. Braces can be applied easily and effectively without much reason for concern.
- The choice of tapes or braces depends on preference and experience.

## HOW DOES BRACING AND TAPING DECREASE THE SEVERITY OF INJURIES IN ATHLETES?

Various studies have been conducted on how bracing and taping helps prevent injury and the incidence of reinjury. One theory suggests that bracing and taping increases proprioception, which is the body's unconscious ability to sense affected body part, in athletes. The traction or pressure on skin due to bracing and taping improves sensory input and proprioception where it is in space and in what direction and how fast it is moving. However, recent research also seems to indicate that wrapping actually reduces proprioceptive feedback.

Another study indicated that wearing high top shoes with taping resulted in 50 percent less injuries as compared to wearing low top shoes along with taping.

### References

1. Reeves, Douglas A. "Ankle Taping and Bracing," WebMD LLC., June 12, 2017.

2. Hamel, Andrea. "Sports Taping vs. Bracing—Which Is Right for Your Injury?" Mueller Sports Medicine, Inc., June 2, 2016.
3. "To Tape or To Brace... Is That the Question?" Nationwide Children's Hospital, n.d.
4. "Ankle Injuries: To Tape or Not to Tape?" Minnesota Sports Medicine (MSM), n.d.

# Chapter 22 | Therapeutic Exercises for Improving Motor Function

**Chapter Contents**

## Section 22.1 | **Flexibility and Stretches**

This section contains text excerpted from the following sources: Text in this section begins with excerpts from "Ways to Stretch," girlshealth.gov, Office on Women's Health (OWH), June 28, 2015. Reviewed November 2019; Text under the heading "Muscle Strengthening Exercises" is excerpted from "Parkinson Disease: Hope through Research," National Institute of Neurological Disorders and Stroke (NINDS), August 28, 2019; Text under the heading "Musculoskeletal Exercises" is excerpted from "Exercises and Stretches," Division of Occupational Health and Safety (DOHS), National Institutes of Health (NIH), September 2, 2016. Reviewed November 2019.

Stretching can help make you more flexible, so you can do activities more easily. It also lengthens and loosens tight muscles.

It is a good idea to stretch any time you work out but try for at least two or three days each week. To stretch well, try these tips:

- **Warm up before you stretch**. Stretching is more helpful when your muscles are warmed up. You can do some light exercises like walking or jogging in place for 5 to 10 minutes to warm up.
- **Stretch for around 10 minutes**. You can stretch right after you warm-up or at the end of your workout—or do both!
- **Go easy on yourself**. You will feel a gentle pull, but if it hurts, stop. And do not forget to breathe.
- **Do not bounce**. A stretch works well if you just hold it. If you are just starting out, try holding a stretch for around 15 seconds. If you are more flexible, you can hold it for a minute.
- **Make sure to repeat each stretch on both sides**. Do each stretch 2 to 4 times on each side

### MUSCLE STRENGTHENING EXERCISES

Exercise can help people improve their mobility and flexibility. Some doctors prescribe physical therapy or muscle-strengthening exercises to tone muscles and to put underused and rigid muscles through a full range of motion. The effects of exercise on disease progression are not known, but it may improve body strength so that the person is less disabled. Exercises also improve balance, helping people minimize gait problems, and can strengthen certain muscles so that people can speak and swallow better. Exercise can improve emotional well-being and general physical activity, such as walking, gardening, swimming, calisthenics, and using exercise machines, can have other benefits. A National Institute of Neurological Disorders and Stroke (NINDS)-funded clinical trial demonstrated the benefit of tai chi exercise compared to resistance or stretching exercises. People should always check with their doctors before beginning an exercise program.

## MUSCULOSKELETAL EXERCISES

### Deep Breathing

- While standing, or in an otherwise relaxed position
- Place one hand on the abdomen and one on the chest
- Inhale slowly through the nose
- Hold for 4 seconds
- Exhale slowly through the mouth
- Repeat

### Cable Stretch

- While sitting with chin in, stomach in, shoulders relaxed, hands relaxed in lap, and feet flat on the floor, imagine a cable pulling your head upward
- Hold for 3 seconds and relax
- Repeat 3 times

### Side Bend: Neck Stretch

- Tilt head to one side (ear towards shoulder)
- Hold for 15 seconds
- Relax
- Repeat 3 times on each side

### Diagonal Neck Stretch

- Turn head slightly and then look down as if looking in your pocket
- Hold for 15 seconds
- Relax
- Repeat 3 times on each side
- Shoulder Shrug
- Slowly bring shoulders up to the ears and hold for approximately 3 seconds
- Rotate shoulders back and down
- Repeat 10 times

### Executive Stretch

- While sitting, lock hands behind head
- Bring elbows back as far as possible
- Inhale deeply while leaning back and stretching
- Hold for 20 seconds
- Exhale and relax
- Repeat 1 time

### Foot Rotation

- While sitting, slowly rotate each foot from the ankle
- Rotate 3 times in one direction, then 3 times in the opposite direction
- Relax
- Repeat 1 time

### Hand Shake

- While sitting, drop arms to the side
- Shake hands downward gently
- Repeat frequently

### Hand Massage

- Massage the inside and outside of the hand using the thumb and fingers
- Repeat frequently (including before beginning work)

### Finger Massage

- Massage fingers of each hand individually, slowly, and gently
- Move toward nail gently
- Massage space between fingers
- Perform daily

### Wrist Stretch

- Hold arm straight out in front of you
- Pull the hand backward with the other hand, then pull downward
- Hold for 20 seconds
- Relax
- Repeat 3 times each

## Section 22.2 | Posture, Balance, and Coordination Exercises

This section contains text excerpted from the following sources: Text in this section begins with excerpts from "Guide to Good Posture," MedlinePlus, National Institutes of Health (NIH), January 28, 2019; Text beginning with the heading "Balance Exercises" is excerpted from "Balance," *Go4Life*®, National Institutes of Health (NIH), December 13, 2012. Reviewed November 2019.

Good posture is about more than standing up straight so you can look your best. It is an important part of your long-term health. Making sure that you hold your body the right way, whether you are moving or still, can prevent pain, injuries, and other health problems.

## WHAT IS POSTURE?

Posture is how you hold your body. There are two types:

- Dynamic posture is how you hold yourself when you are moving, like when you are walking, running, or bending over to pick up something.
- Static posture is how you hold yourself when you are not moving, like when you are sitting, standing, or sleeping.

It is important to make sure that you have a good dynamic and static posture.

The key to good posture is the position of your spine. Your spine has three natural curves—at your neck, mid-back, and low back. Correct posture should maintain these curves, but not increase them. Your head should be above your shoulders, and the top of your shoulder should be over the hips.

## HOW CAN POSTURE AFFECT YOUR HEALTH?

Poor posture can be bad for your health. Slouching or slumping over can

- Misalign your musculoskeletal system
- Wear away at your spine, making it more fragile and prone to injury
- Cause neck, shoulder, and back pain
- Decrease your flexibility
- Affect how well your joints move
- Affect your balance and increase your risk of falling
- Make it harder to digest your food
- Make it harder to breathe

## HOW CAN YOU IMPROVE YOUR POSTURE IN GENERAL?

- Be mindful of your posture during everyday activities. Activities such as watching television, washing dishes, or walking.
- Stay active. Any kind of exercise may help improve your posture, but certain types of exercises can be especially helpful. They include yoga, tai chi, and other classes that focuses on body awareness. It is also a good idea to do exercises that strengthen your core (muscles around your back, abdomen, and pelvis).
- Maintain a healthy weight. Extra weight can weaken your abdominal muscles, cause problems for your pelvis and spine, and contribute to low back pain. All of these can hurt your posture.
- Wear comfortable, low-heeled shoes. High heels, for example, can throw off your balance and force you to walk differently. This puts more stress on your muscles and harms your posture.
- Make sure work surfaces are at a comfortable height for you. Whether you are sitting in front of a computer, making dinner, or eating a meal.

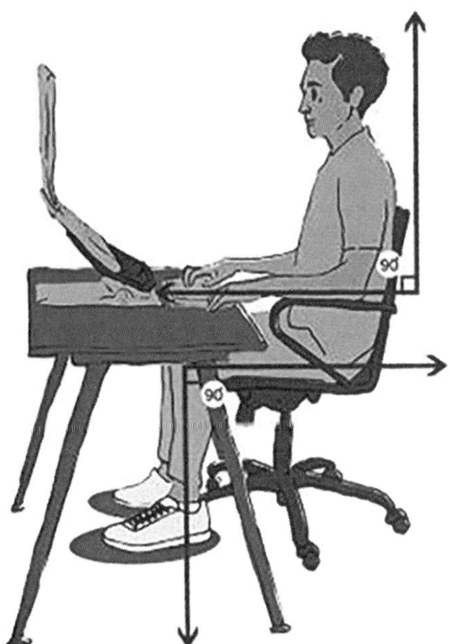


**Figure 22.1.** Man Sitting

## HOW CAN YOU IMPROVE YOUR POSTURE WHEN SITTING?

Many Americans spend a lot of their time sitting—either at work, at school, or at home. It is important to sit properly, and to take frequent breaks.

- Switch sitting positions often.
- Take brief walks around your office or home.
- Gently stretch your muscles every so often to help relieve muscle tension.
- Do not cross your legs; keep your feet on the floor, with your ankles in front of your knees.
- Make sure that your feet touch the floor, or if that is not possible, use a footrest.
- Relax your shoulders; they should not be rounded or pulled backward.
- Keep your elbows close to your body. They should be bent between 90 and 120 degrees.
- Make sure that your back is fully supported. Use a back pillow or other back support if your chair does not have a backrest that can support your lower back's curve.
- Make sure that your thighs and hips are supported. You should have a well-padded seat, and your thighs and hips should be parallel to the floor.

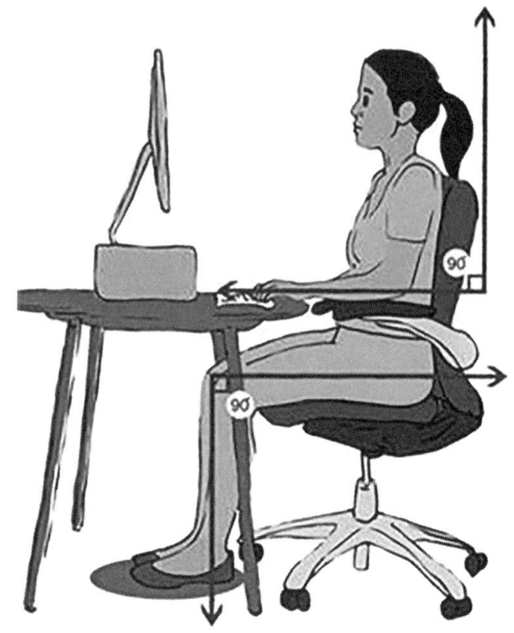


**Figure 22.2.** Woman Sitting

## HOW CAN YOU IMPROVE YOUR POSTURE WHEN STANDING?

- Stand up straight and tall.
- Keep your shoulders back.
- Pull your stomach in.
- Put your weight mostly on the balls of your feet.
- Keep your head level.
- Let your arms hang down naturally at your sides.
- Keep your feet about shoulder-width apart.

With practice, you can improve your posture; you will look and feel better.

## BALANCE EXERCISES

You can do balance exercises almost anytime, anywhere, and as often as you like. Having good balance is important for many everyday activities, such as going up and down the stairs. It also helps you walk safely and avoid tripping and falling over objects in your way.

## TAI CHI

Balance is important to help you perform many of your daily activities and prevent falls. Research has shown that tai chi can significantly reduce the risk of falls

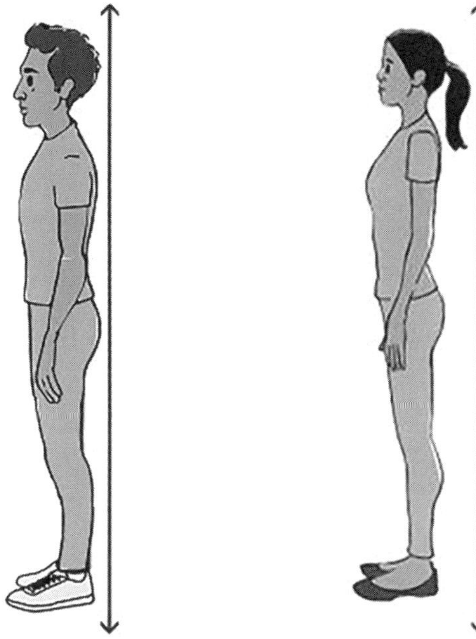

**Figure 22.3.** Man Standing **Figure 22.4.** Woman Standing

among older people. In tai chi, which is sometimes called "moving meditation," you work to improve your balance by moving your body slowly, gently, and precisely, while breathing deeply. Other benefits from practicing tai chi include:

- Improvements in bone and heart health
- Easing of pain and stiffness from osteoarthritis
- Better sleep
- Improvements in overall wellness

Try to put aside distracting thoughts and focus on being aware of your movements.

## BALANCE WALK EXERCISE

Good balance helps you walk safely and avoid tripping and falling over objects in your way.

- Raise arms to sides, shoulder height.
- Choose a spot ahead of you and focus on it to keep you steady as you walk.
- Walk-in a straight line with one foot in front of the other.
- As you walk, lift your back leg. Pause for 1 second before stepping forward.
- Repeat for 20 steps, alternating legs.

As you progress, try looking from side to side as you walk, but skip this step if you have inner ear problems.

## HEEL TO TOE WALK EXERCISE

Having good balance is important for many everyday activities, such as going up and downstairs.

- Position the heel of one foot in front of the toes of the other foot. Your heel and toes should touch or almost touch.
- Choose a spot ahead of you and focus on it to keep you steady as you walk.
- Take a step. Put your heel just in front of the toe of your other foot.
- Repeat for 20 steps.

If you are unsteady on your feet, try doing this exercise near a wall so you can steady yourself if you need to.

## STAND ON ONE FOOT EXERCISE

You can do this exercise while waiting for the bus or standing in line at the grocery. For an added challenge, you can modify the exercise to improve your balance.

- Stand on one foot behind a sturdy chair, holding on for balance.
- Hold position for up to 10 seconds.
- Repeat 10 to 15 times.
- Repeat 10 to 15 times with other leg.
- Repeat 10 to 15 more times with each leg.

As you progress in your exercise routine, try adding the following challenges to help your balance even more.

- Start by holding on to a sturdy chair with both hands for support.
- When you are able, try holding on to the chair with only one hand.
- With time, hold on with only one finger, then with no hands at all.
- If you are really steady on your feet, try doing the balance exercises with your eyes closed.

## Section 22.3 | **Aerobic Activities**

This section contains text excerpted from the following sources: Text in this section begins with excerpts from "Exercise and HIV: Entire Lesson," U.S. Department of Veterans Affairs (VA), May 10, 2019; Text under the heading "How It Works?" is excerpted from "Physical Activity Guidelines for Americans, 2nd Edition," Office of Disease Prevention and Health Promotion (ODPHP), U.S. Department of Health and Human Services (HHS), November 12, 2018; Text under the heading "Total Amount of Physical Activity," is excerpted from "Increasing Physical Activity among Adults with Disabilities," Centers for Disease Control and Prevention (CDC), September 4, 2019.

Aerobic exercise strengthens your lungs and heart. Walking, jogging, running, swimming, hiking, and cycling are forms of this exercise.

This movement increases your heart rate and the rate and depth of your breathing, which in turn increases how much blood and oxygen your heart pumps to your muscles. To achieve the maximum benefit of this kind of exercise, most experts recommend that your heart rate should reach the target rate for at least 20 minutes. It may take you weeks to reach this level if you have not been exercising much.

### HOW IT WORKS

In this kind of physical activity (also called an "endurance activity" or "cardio activity"), the body's large muscles move in a rhythmic manner for a sustained period of time. Brisk walking, running, bicycling, jumping rope, and swimming are all examples. Aerobic activity causes a person's heart to beat faster, and they will breathe harder than normal.

#### Aerobic Physical Activity Has Three Components

- Intensity, or how hard a person works to do the activity. The intensities most often studied are moderate (equivalent in effort to brisk walking) and vigorous (equivalent in effort to running or jogging).
- Frequency, or how often a person does the aerobic activity
- Duration, or how long a person does an activity in any one session

Although these components make up an aerobic physical activity profile, research has shown that the total amount of physical activity (minutes of moderate-intensity physical activity in a week, for example) is more important for achieving health benefits than is any one component (frequency, intensity, or duration). All time spent in moderate or vigorous-intensity physical activity counts toward meeting the key guidelines.

### TOTAL AMOUNT OF PHYSICAL ACTIVITY

For aerobic:

- At least 2 hours and 30 minutes (150 minutes) a week of moderate-intensity aerobic physical activity (i.e., brisk walking; wheeling oneself in a wheelchair); or

- 1 hour and 15 minutes (75 minutes) a week of vigorous-intensity aerobic physical activity (i.e., jogging, wheelchair basketball); or
- A mix of both moderate and vigorous-intensity aerobic physical activities each week. A rule of thumb is that 1 minute of vigorous-intensity activity is about the same as 2 minutes of moderate-intensity activity.

## Section 22.4 | Gait and Motion Analysis

This section includes text excerpted from "Motion Analysis and Biomechanics," Rehabilitation Research & Development Service (RR&D), U.S. Department of Veteran Affairs (VA), February 1, 2001. Reviewed November 2019.

The applications of biodynamics to the medical field are increasing as research in this area is expanded and equipment becomes available. The overall purpose of biodynamics is to provide a quantitative measurement of the function/dysfunction of the neuromuscular skeletal system. It is the responsibility of the biomechanist in cooperation with the clinician to provide information that cannot be obtained by other methods and, more importantly, to establish the clinical relevance of this information.

The most common application of motion analysis and biomechanics is gait analysis; for this reason, most clinical and research laboratories are called "gait laboratories." However, to limit the application of this equipment and the analytical tools to gait analysis would be a failure to understand the full range of medical applications. One common application is the assessment of postural balance. Although balance is understood in a lay sense as the ability to maintain physical equilibrium, it is necessary to define it in a mathematical sense if biomechanical measurements are being made. When standing quietly, an individual is said to be in perfect balance when the center of gravity (c.g.) of the body is directly over the center of pressure (COP) of the ground reaction force (GRF). The COP is measured with the force plate and can be accurately determined at any instant of time. The difficulty in obtaining rapid balance assessments is due to the inability to define the location of the center of mass in real-time. An 11-segment model of the body may be made comprising the head, trunk, two upper arms, two forearms, pelvis, two thighs, and two lower legs. Data are available for the proportion of the mass of each segment and the location of the center of mass of each segment for men and women of different sizes. However, accurate establishment of the position of each of these segments requires three markers per segment, totaling 33 markers.

The mean radius of the stabilogram can be computed and the velocity of the movement of the COP determined. These have been used as measures of postural stability. The COP must remain within the area of the base of support (the area underneath and between the feet), which decreases as the stance width decreases and increases as the feet are moved farther apart to a more stable position. Data have been collected for individuals standing with feet together, feet apart, feet tandem, or standing on one leg. In addition, eyes open and eyes closed data give the influence of vision on postural stability. Some laboratories have had the individual stand on soft mats to obtain information on proprioceptor influence on balance.

The major difficulty in using only the COP as a measure of balance is that the subject can move the position of the COP anteriorly, posteriorly, or laterally and still remain in a controlled balance position. Therefore, the data are dependent upon the individual trying to maintain balance and not deliberately perturbing the stabilogram. This is not the case when the difference between the c.g. and the COP is used as a measure of balance. Simpler models to determine the c.g. of the body are being introduced to obtain better measurement of postural balance and still maintain a workable laboratory protocol.

The ultimate goal of biodynamics is the development of predictive computer models for the neuromuscular skeletal system. This would allow the evaluation of an individual using the techniques of the indirect s model to determine joint motion and muscular activity. A computer model would then be created that could be driven using the muscle moments at the joints. Using electromyography (EMG), the temporal activity of these muscles may be determined.

# Chapter 23 | Manual Therapy—Hands On

**Chapter Contents**

## Section 23.1 | Manipulative Therapy

This section includes text excerpted from "Spinal Manipulation: What You Need to Know," National Center for Complementary and Integrative Health (NCCIH), July 2019.

### WHAT IS SPINAL MANIPULATION?

Spinal manipulation is also called "spinal manipulative therapy." It is a technique where practitioners use their hands or a device to apply a controlled thrust (i.e., a force of a specific magnitude or degree in a specific direction) to a joint of your spine. The amount of force can vary, but the thrust moves the joint more than it would on its own. Spinal manipulation is different from spinal mobilization, which does not involve a thrust (and is performed within a joint's natural range of motion and can be controlled by the patient).

Most spinal manipulations are done by chiropractors (chiropractic treatment often involves spinal manipulation), although other licensed professionals including osteopathic physicians and physical therapists also do spinal manipulations.

Spinal manipulation is one of the most common complementary health approaches used by adults and children in the United States, the 2012 National Health Interview Survey (NHIS) showed.

### WHY DO PEOPLE USE SPINAL MANIPULATION?

Among U.S. adults who used chiropractic or osteopathic manipulation, about 67 percent used it to treat a specific health condition, and 53 percent used it for wellness, the NHIS found. Specifically:

- 43 percent used it for general wellness or disease prevention
- 25 percent used it because it focuses on the whole person—their mind, body, and spirit
- 16 percent used it for improved energy
- 11 percent used it for better immune function
- 5 percent used it to improve memory or concentration.

Previous research found that people report positive experiences and reduced pain as a result of receiving spinal manipulation.

### WHO USES SPINAL MANIPULATION, AND HAS USAGE CHANGED?

Between 2012 and 2017, U.S. adults' use of chiropractic care (which usually involves spinal manipulation) during the past year increased slightly, from 9.1 percent to 10.3 percent, a comparison of NHIS data from the 2 years showed. The data also show that women were more likely than men to see a chiropractor, and that adults between the ages of 45 and 64 were more likely than people aged

18 to 44 or 65 and over to have visited one during the past year. According to the same national survey (by the Centers for Disease Control and Prevention's (CDC) National Center for Health Statistics (NCHS), non-Hispanic White adults were much more likely to visit a chiropractor (12.7%) than Hispanic (6.6%) or non-Hispanic black (5.5%) adults.

Among children, there was no significant difference in the use of chiropractic care between 2012 and 2017 (3.5% versus 3.4%). Older children (ages 12 to 17) were more likely than younger ones (ages 4 to 11) to have seen a chiropractor, but there was no significant difference in the use of chiropractic care between girls and boys. Non-Hispanic White children were more likely than non-Hispanic black or Hispanic children to have seen a chiropractor.

## WHAT ARE SOME OF THE PAIN CONDITIONS FOR WHICH SPINAL MANIPULATION HAS BEEN USED?

### For Sciatica

- Sciatica is pain associated with the sciatic nerve, which controls the muscles in the back of the knee and the lower leg; it also provides feeling to the back of the thigh, part of the lower leg, and the sole of the foot.
- Manipulation is not widely used to treat sciatica but it may help, a 2015 research review of a variety of sciatica treatments suggests. However, the studies had many limitations, the authors noted.
- In a 2014 study of 192 people with leg pain associated with back pain, participants who received spinal manipulation, personal instruction, and exercises had less pain after 12 weeks and used less medication a year later than participants who received only personal instruction and exercises. However, leg pain was the same for both groups after 1 year.

### For Low-Back Pain

Many noninvasive treatments are available for low-back pain, and these include drugs and nondrug options. In its 2017 clinical guidelines, the American College of Physicians (ACP) suggests that spinal manipulation is one of a number of therapeutic options that may help people with acute or chronic low-back pain (although the ACP says the quality of the evidence is low).

- Spinal manipulation was better than placebo for immediate, short-term relief from acute or subacute low-back and neck pain, a 2010 research review concluded. Manipulation was also better than acupuncture for chronic low-back pain. However, the results of studies comparing spinal manipulation to massage, medication, or physical therapy were mixed.
- A 2011 review of 26 studies concluded that for chronic low-back pain, spinal manipulation works as well as other commonly recommended

approaches, including exercise or physical therapy. However, the effect on pain was minimal.

- Twelve sessions of spinal manipulation may be the best "dose," according to a 2014 National Center for Complementary and Integrative Health (NCCIH) funded study of 400 people with chronic low-back pain.
- In a 2014 study of 110 participants with chronic low-back pain, those who received spinal manipulation had less sensitivity to painful stimuli right after getting spinal manipulation, compared to people who got sham spinal manipulation. But, after a couple of weeks the two groups had similar amounts of pain and disability, the study showed. The study was supported by NCCIH.
- The Agency for Healthcare Research and Quality (AHRQ) systematic review of noninvasive nonpharmacologic treatment for chronic pain reported that spinal manipulation was associated with slightly greater effects than sham manipulation, usual care, an attention control, or a placebo intervention in the short-term (i.e., 1 to 6 months following treatment) and intermediate term (i.e., 6 to 12 months). It is concluded that the strength of the evidence was low. In addition, it is concluded that there was no evidence of differences between spinal manipulation versus sham manipulation, usual care, an attention control, or a placebo intervention in short-term pain, but manipulation was associated with slightly greater effects than controls on intermediate-term pain. The standard of evidence was considered low for short-term effects and moderate for intermediate-term effects.
- The research on spinal manipulation for acute low-back pain is generally mixed and has many limitations.
- Spinal manipulation is no more effective for acute low-back pain than sham (fake) spinal manipulation, or when added to another treatment such as standard medical care, a 2012 research review of 20 studies found. Spinal manipulation appeared to be safe when compared to other treatment options.
- In a 2015 study of 220 people with acute low-back pain, participants who received physical therapy, which included spinal manipulation, fared no better than those who received standard care.
- However, a 2015 NCCIH funded study of 107 adults with onset acute and subacute low-back pain found that those receiving spinal manipulation got greater short-term relief, compared to participants getting standard medical care. Furthermore, the study compared two different techniques—manual thrust manipulation (MTM) and mechanical-assisted manipulation (MAM)—and found MTM led to

greater short-term reductions in self-reported pain and disability than MAM or usual care.

- A 2017 analysis examined data from 15 randomized controlled trials with almost 1,700 participants. The researchers concluded that spinal manipulative therapy can modestly improve pain and function in people with acute low-back pain.
- Results of a 2018 study with 750 active-duty U.S. military personnel with low-back pain found that those who received chiropractic care in addition to usual care had better short-term improvements in low-back pain intensity and pain-related disability than those who only received usual medical care.

## For Neck Pain

- For patients with acute neck pain, either spinal manipulation or home exercises appeared to be more effective than medication in the short and long term, an NCCIH-funded study of 272 patients showed in 2012. A 2015 research review that looked at results from 51 trials with 2,920 participants also reported that there is weak evidence that spinal manipulation may provide short-term relief from acute or chronic neck pain.

## For Headache

- For preventing migraines, spinal manipulation may be one of several complementary health approaches (including massage therapy) that is as helpful as medications used for migraine prevention, but the research is not conclusive.
- The AHRQ systematic review of noninvasive nonpharmacologic treatment for chronic pain reported spinal manipulation therapy was associated with slight to moderate improvements in function compared to usual care on the Headache Impact Test and the Headache Disability Inventory (scale 0 to 100) and in pain over the short term (i.e., 1 to 6 months) in one trial. The standard of evidence was rated as low.

## For Other Conditions

- Researchers have studied spinal manipulation for many other conditions, including fibromyalgia, children's ear infections, chronic obstructive pulmonary disease (COPD), infant colic, and bedwetting, but there is too little evidence to know if it helps with these problems.
- Spinal manipulation does not help with asthma, hypertension, or menstrual pain, studies show.

## IS SPINAL MANIPULATION SAFE?

Spinal manipulation is relatively safe when performed by a trained and licensed practitioner. The most common side effects of spinal manipulation are temporary muscle soreness, stiffness, or a temporary increase in pain.

Serious complications, deaths, and delays in diagnosis of serious illnesses have been associated with spinal manipulation, including in children, but are very rare.

### Strokes and Artery Tears

- A type of spinal manipulation that focuses on the neck has been linked to small, potentially dangerous tears in the artery walls in the neck, called the "cervical artery dissections" (CAD). These tears are rare but can lead to a stroke. Any kind of sudden neck movement, such as playing sports, getting whiplash, and violent vomiting or coughing may also increase the risk of tears. The available evidence suggests that the incidence of CAD in people getting spinal manipulation is low, but patients need to be informed of this potential risk.

### Spinal Manipulation and Pregnancy

- There are few spinal manipulation causing problems during pregnancy or in the period after childbirth. The problems ranged from mild, temporary pain to life-threatening injuries. Serious adverse events occurred only after cervical spinal manipulation.

## Section 23.2 | Joint Mobilization Techniques



Joints are areas in the body where two bones meet. They are surrounded by soft tissue, which is prone to physical injury or damage. Joint mobilization is a form of physical therapy in which skilled passive movements are applied at varying speeds and magnitude to the joints to restore optimal motion, function, and reduce pain. When a joint's mobility is restricted, the structure and function of the joint undergoes changes. There arises a reduction of cartilage nutrition within the joint, and the adjacent joints begin to move too much to make up for the stiff joint. These adjacent joints begin to deteriorate caused by overuse. Muscles supporting the stiff joint lose their capacity to contract and relax and become tense. Eventually, the entire area surrounding the stiff joint becomes dysfunctional. Joint mobility is difficult to assess and the quantity is graded in degrees, whereas the quality is graded by "end feel." Joint mobility can be best gauged by comparison to the uninvolved side. Joint mobilization, unlike joint manipulation, does not depend on the use of forceful techniques for strengthening joints.

## EFFECTS OF JOINT MOBILIZATION

Joint mobilization improves the range of motion and mobility of a joint by enhancing the client's awareness of the correct position and movement of a joint by simulating smooth joint function. A physical therapist manually moves a joint using small, passive movements, gently working it through a natural level of resistance. These motions stretch the tissue around the bone, which in turn helps reduce pain and increase range of motion. Joint-mobilization exercises include flexion, extension, tibiofemoral glides, patellar glides, long-axis distraction, and lateral movements and rotations. Joint-mobilization exercises can also be used to treat reversible joint hypomobility of the capsular origin.

The therapeutic effects of joint mobilization include:

- Stimulation of the synovial fluid movement to nourish cartilage
- Maintenance or promotion of periarticular extensibility
- Sensory input to the joint

Joint mobilization is generally used for the rehabilitation of the neck, upper, middle and lower back, and sacroiliac joints. It is also used for the joints of the extremities, such as the shoulder, wrist, hand, hip, knee, foot, and ankle.

## BENEFITS OF JOINT MOBILIZATION

Joint mobilization by a physical therapist does not involve the adjustment and manipulation of hard tissues, as the chiropractic technique does. Joint mobilization is a hands-on treatment, designed to provide relief from pain and muscle spasms, and to release tension and improve flexibility in a joint. The benefits that can be gained from joint mobilization are:

- Improved joint mobility
- Reduction in muscle spasms and tension
- Increased freedom of movement
- Pain relief

Joint mobilization is provided at a moderate speed, with or without oscillations or a stretch. This technique is generally graded and varies based on two factors: The patient's pain tolerance and the acuity of the patient's condition.

## THE MAITLAND JOINT MOBILIZATION GRADING SCALE

Joint mobilization is broadly classified by the Australian physiotherapist Geoffrey Douglas Maitland into five grades, each of which deals with a specific range of motion. These mobilizations help to decrease pain and increase mobility.

- **Grade I**—This involves small-amplitude rhythmic oscillating mobilization in early range-of-movement therapy
- **Grade II**—This stage makes use of relatively large-amplitude rhythmic oscillating mobilization in during the mid-range stages of movement
- **Grade III**—Utilizes large-amplitude, rhythmic oscillating mobilization to the point of limiting range of movement. It is designed to physically stretch the joints.
- **Grade IV**—Uses small-amplitude rhythmic oscillations up to the limit of the available motion and stress to address tissue resistance
- **Grade V (Thrust manipulation)**—This grade refers to the use of a single high-velocity, low-amplitude thrust performed at the end of the available joint movement therapy

Grades I and II are used primarily to reduce pain and stiffness. They provide pain relief through neuromodulation of the sensory innervation of the joint mechanoreceptors (sensory receptors that respond to mechanical pressure or distortion) and pain receptors. They also neutralize joint pressure and prevent grinding. Grades III through V are used particularly to increase mobility and joint play. They are used to treat stiffness or hypomobility. Hypomobility is when your ligaments are too tense or tight, which restricts your ability to stretch normally and results in a decreased range of motion. They help with swelling or stretching of shortened tissue.

### References

1. "Joint Mobilization," Alliant Physical Therapy, August 24, 2015.
2. "Joint Mobilization for Physical Therapy," Advance Physical & Aquatic Therapy, January 8, 2013.
3. "Joint Mobilization," ScienceDirect, July 9, 2017.
4. "Principles of Joint Mobilization," Physiopedia, February 8, 2007.

# Chapter 24 | Occupational Therapy Assessments and Evaluation

Occupational therapists provide therapeutic services designed to optimize the disabled or injured patient's ability to perform everyday activities and tasks. These therapeutic services help patients develop, recover, improve, maintain, or acquire the skills needed for daily living and working.

An occupational therapy treatment plan is based on the patient's history, ailments, and physical restrictions. Occupational therapists develop individualized therapy treatment plans based on the outcome of specific assessments and evaluations they use to determine optimal treatment methods. Assessments help occupational therapists determine a patient's current occupational performance skills and measure the extent of existing impairments. Evaluations are more complex and include interviews, observation, and assessment results, all of which allow the therapist to thoroughly determine impairments and measure function. Both elements are essential parts of occupational therapy treatment planning.

## EVALUATION TOOLS IN OCCUPATIONAL THERAPY

Evaluations take many forms. Some evaluations are designed specifically for certain patient populations or diagnoses. Specialized materials, or kits, are used to execute these tests and assessments. Occupational therapy (OT) treatment begins with these evaluations, which the therapist uses to plans the flow of the entire OT evaluation process. They also allow therapists to determine what a patient wants to get out of the therapy process, and allow the therapist to communicate to patients and patient advocates what they can expect during the therapy process. Common evaluation tools used in OT include:

- **The Comprehensive Occupational Therapy Evaluation (COTE)** is used by the therapists for patients with mental-health conditions. This scale distinguishes among 25 various behavior types that are relevant to OT practice. This scale helps the therapist determine the patient's progress.

- **The Routine Task Inventory (RTI)** concentrates on the evaluation of patients with cognitive disabilities, including but not limited to schizophrenia and depression. This inventory estimates the extent to which the patient's cognitive impairments obstruct their ability to perform occupational tasks. The therapist must observe the patient in order to complete this evaluation.
- **Activity Configuration Logs** are diaries in either physical or electronic form. Patients enter each activity in these diaries, which allows the therapist to measure the amount of time spent performing healthy or unhealthy behaviors. These logs use the designations "activity health" or "activity ill health" to classify patient behaviors. Activity-ill behaviors include the patient performing an activity out of sequence, which can lead to confusion in patients with certain ailments. These logs help occupational therapists narrow their focus for treatment and enhance the facilitation of particular tasks and activities.
- **The Barth Time Construction Tool (BTC)** requires patients to place colored papers on a chart to show the amount of time spent on work, self-care, and leisure activities in a week. This tool, often used with patients with psychosocial dysfunctions, allows occupational therapists to assess the patient's roles in various parts of their life.
- **The Milwaukee Evaluation of Daily Living Skills (MEDLS)** evaluates the ability of patients with long-term mental illness to perform various activities of daily living (ADLs). The evaluation is designed to measure ADL skills in lower-functioning patients with a mental illness. It provides the occupational therapist with a baseline for each patient that is then used to measure progress and the effectiveness of treatment. The evaluation also helps healthcare providers determine the level of assistance required for patients to perform ADLs.

Evaluations are performed by occupational therapists and certified occupational therapy assistants following established guidelines. The length of an OT evaluation ranges from 20 minutes (in a hospital) to several hours (at an outpatient facility).

The field of occupational therapy is extremely diverse, and OT evaluations performed in, for example, a newborn intensive-care unit (NICU) differ significantly from those used to evaluate an adult patient's ability to perform specific task needed for a job. Nevertheless, all OT evaluations follow a general structure.

## PATIENT INTERVIEW AND INFORMATION GATHERING

If a medical record is available, the occupational therapist will review it before the evaluation begins in order to obtain basic information about the patient's medical profile. The therapist will then interview the patient to fill in any gaps. Specific information that the therapist will be looking for includes the patient's age, referring physician, past medical history, the reason for the OT referral, the patient's diagnosis, and any needed precautions. The occupational therapist will also seek to determine what the patient's day-to-day life looked like before the incident that caused an injury or disability. This information helps the occupational therapist identify the goal-setting process and terms of a safe discharge since the objective of OT is to return the patient to the prior level of function (PLOF).

## OBJECTIVE ASSESSMENTS

After the interview, the therapist will perform assessments to obtain tactile data about the patient's general health and how the patient's diagnosis influences the potential to perform everyday activities. The therapist will assess the following:

- Pain
- Vital signs
- Mental status
- Skin health
- Joint range of motion
- Manual muscle function
- Level of assistance needed with ADLs (if any)
- Sensation
- Tone
- Coordination
- Proprioception, also referred to as "kinaesthesia," or the patient's sense of their own body movements and positions

There are other standardized assessments, ranging from sensory processing to driving safely, that the therapist may choose to perform. Whether these assessments are needed will depend on the patient's surroundings and individual needs.

## COMMONLY USED ASSESSMENT MEASURES

The following are some common types of assessment measures used by occupational therapists:

- **Occupation-focused.** Here, the patient's occupation is the primary focus of discussions and interviews, and the assessments help determine needed intervention and how to best measure outcomes.

- **Participation-focused.** Here, the chief focus is on the level of engagement and involvement that a patient has in their life.
- **Environment-focused.** Here, the main objective is to identify the effect that the environment has on the patient's occupational performance and contributions.

The therapist may also use assessment tools to determine:

- Body function
- Cognition and perception
- Development
- Eating disorders
- General health and well-being
- Mental health
- Pain

Therapists further use assessment tools to determine the level of risk in a patient's community, and educational, home, and work environments.

## GOAL SETTING

The occupational therapist will work with the patient to set short- and long-term goals for the OT treatment. The referring doctor will then approve or make adjustments to these goals, and then a customized plan is formulated for achieving them. At a minimum, the plan will include the benefits a patient can gain from the OT treatment and outline the strategies that will be used to achieve these stated goals.

### References

1. "Occupational Therapists," U.S. Bureau of Labor Statistics (BLS), September 4, 2019.
2. Lyon, Sarah. "What to Expect during an OT Evaluation," Verywell Health, June 23, 2019.
3. "Assessment Process in Occupational Therapy: Methods, Tools and Examples," Study.com, March 12, 2018.
4. "Occupational Therapy Terminology Supporting Occupation-Centred Practice," Royal College of Occupational Therapists, October 9, 2016.

# Chapter 25 | **Occupational Therapy Interventions**

**Chapter Contents**

## Section 25.1 | Functional and Adaptive Training in Daily Living

"Functional and Adaptive Training in Daily Living," © 2020 Omnigraphics. Reviewed November 2019.

Functional training has its origins in rehabilitation. It is a form of exercise that involves training the body for the activities performed in daily life. Physical and occupational therapists and chiropractors often make use of this method to retrain patients with movement disorders. The main objective in physical rehabilitation is to restore and enhance function within the patient's environment and to execute specific activities of daily living. The entire rehabilitation process must be concentrated on improving the functional aspect of the patient.

The principles of functional training include level-dependent generalized-movement literacy (learning-to-move basics, depending on skill level and previous training), strength, conditioning (energy- or skill-based), and sports-specific movements, if appropriate.

The general goal of a functional exercise program is to return patients to their preinjury level as quickly and as safely as possible by reducing the amount of measurable dysfunction within basic and functional movement patterns. Specific training activities are allocated to restore both dynamic joint stability and functional skills. The functional rehabilitation program not only involves strength, flexibility, and agility training, but also teaching the patient how to move effectively from a supine to a sitting position.

### COMPONENTS OF A FUNCTIONAL EXERCISE PROGRAM

Functional rehabilitation is typically applied to sports medicine; however, this approach is also useful for individuals returning to work or basic activities of daily living after traumatic injuries, neurological injuries, or strokes. Functional rehabilitation can be modified to suit an individual's requisite or goals by being specific to the individual's state of health, including the presence or history of injury. An evaluation must be completed to assist the therapist with exercise selection and training load.

A functional exercise program should cover a number of different elements to be effective:

- Training based on functional tasks directed toward everyday life activities
- Integrated training, involving a variety of exercises that work on flexibility, core, balance, strength and power, and focus on multiple movement planes
- Progressive and periodic training by steadily increasing the difficulty and variation of tasks with distributed practice

- Making use of real-life object manipulation
- Repetitive training performed in context-specific environments
- Self-feedback as well as trainer/therapist feedback, following a performance

## ADVANTAGES OF FUNCTIONAL TRAINING

Functional rehabilitation combines various techniques in an attempt to return an injured person to an optimal level of performance. Functional training may improve impairments. However, during instances when the impairment cannot be changed, the therapist finds alternatives that allow the patient to compensate for and use intact systems to perform the desired function, giving the individual increased control and opportunities to participate in everyday life.

Functional training is also beneficial for improved neuromuscular coordination. Beyond improving general balance and reflex time, we can actually train our muscles and joints to perform complex movements almost automatically. Since functional training exercise utilizes many different muscles, it can make everyday activities such as grocery shopping, cleaning, and moderate lifting a lot easier.

## ADAPTIVE SKILLS TRAINING

Adaptive skills are defined as the entire range of abilities necessary to complete essentially all activities that people engage in, and the term encompasses a broad set of skills that are necessary in order to live independently. Adaptive skills involve a wide range of skills, such as maintaining health and hygiene, obtaining and maintaining one's job and place of residence, displaying the social and communication abilities required for being employed and sustaining relationships, managing money, and maintaining a household.

Adaptive behavior was first defined by the American Association on Mental Deficiency as "the effectiveness with which the individual copes with the natural and social demands of his environment." This definition includes two major facets:

1. The level to which the individual is able to function and maintain themselves independently
2. The degree to which the individual sufficiently meets the socially acceptable demands of personal and social responsibility

Adaptive behavior is also defined by The American Association on Intellectual and Developmental Disabilities (AAIDD) as the collection of conceptual, social, and practical skills that people learn and perform in their everyday lives.

## COMPONENTS OF ADAPTIVE TRAINING

Adaptive skills-training services involve the following aspects:

- They are based on a developmental perspective and target areas in which a patient is developmentally delayed.

### Occupational Therapy Interventions

- They utilize principles of applied behavior analysis, including breaking down skills into more manageable tasks or steps, and reinforcing or reward systems.
- They involve parents and caregivers, where appropriate, in order to aid in the patient's learning of new skills.

Adaptive skills training aims to increase the patient's life skills so they can have a greater level of independence both at home and in the community.

## BENEFITS OF ADAPTIVE TRAINING

The development of adaptive skills involves, but is not restricted to, the following:

- Purchasing and monetary (banking) skills
- Communication (oral or adapted)
- Self-advocacy/acceptance
- Using public transportation
- Attending community events
- Safety awareness
- Independent living skills
- Engaging in leisure and recreational skills

Adaptive training is a program designed to enhance the individual's overall quality of life. It is used to target the following skill areas: functional academics, self-help skills, safety skills, community access, communication, social skills, job prerequisites, and self-management. Therapists perform an assessment, which provides an overview of the individual's skill deficits, targeted goals, and the behavior-change procedures that will aid in the development of a suitable training program.

### References


1. "Functional Rehabilitation," American Academy of Physical Medicine and Rehabilitation (AAPMR), March 2, 2016.
2. "Adaptive Skills Training," Assessment, Consultation & Treatment, February 10, 2014.
3. "Functional Training and Advanced Rehabilitation," North American Sports Medicine Institute (NASMI) and Advances in Clinical Education, October 21, 2013.
4. "Adaptive Behavior, Life Skills, and Leisure Skills Training," Neupsy Key, November 27, 2016.
5. "Adaptive Skills Training," TOTAL Programs, March 17, 2013.

## Section 25.2 | Eating and Swallowing Performance

This section includes text excerpted from documents published by three public domain sources. Text under the headings marked 1 are excerpted from "Eating Disorders: About More than Food," National Institute of Mental Health (NIMH), 2018. Reviewed November 2019; Text under the headings marked 2 are excerpted from "Swallowing Disorders Information Page," National Institute of Neurological Disorders and Stroke (NINDS), March 27, 2019; Text under the headings marked 3 are excerpted from "Dysphagia," National Institute on Deafness and Other Communication Disorders (NIDCD), March 6, 2017.

### WHAT ARE EATING DISORDERS?[1]

Eating disorders are serious medical illnesses marked by severe disturbances to a person's eating behaviors. Obsessions with food, body weight, and shape may be signs of an eating disorder. These disorders can affect a person's physical and mental health; in some cases, they can be life-threatening. But, eating disorders can be treated.

### WHO IS AT RISK FOR EATING DISORDERS?[1]

Eating disorders can affect people of all ages, racial/ethnic backgrounds, body weights, and genders. Although eating disorders often appear during the teen years or young adulthood, they may also develop during childhood or later in life (40 years and older).

The exact cause of eating disorders is not fully understood, but research suggests a combination of genetic, biological, behavioral, psychological, and social factors can raise a person's risk.

### WHAT ARE THE COMMON TYPES OF EATING DISORDERS?[1]

Common eating disorders include anorexia nervosa, bulimia nervosa, and binge-eating disorder. If you or someone you know experiences the symptoms listed below, it could be a sign of an eating disorder—call a health provider right away for help.

### WHAT IS DYSPHAGIA?[2]

Having trouble swallowing (dysphagia) is a symptom that accompanies a number of neurological disorders. The problem can occur at any stage of the normal swallowing process as food and liquid move from the mouth, down the back of the throat, through the esophagus and into the stomach. Difficulties can range from a total inability to swallow, to coughing or choking because the food or liquid is entering the windpipe, which is referred to as aspiration. When aspiration is frequent a person can be at risk of developing pneumonia. Food may get "stuck" in the throat or individuals may drool because they cannot swallow their saliva. Neurological conditions that can cause swallowing difficulties are: stroke (the most common cause of dysphagia); traumatic brain injury; cerebral

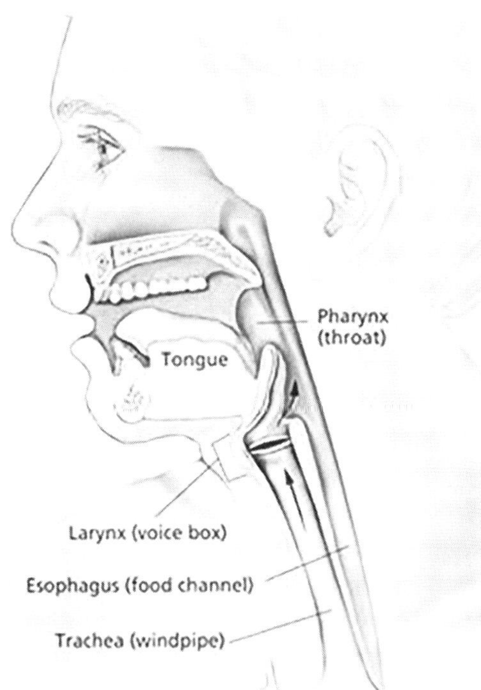


**Figure 25.1.** Parts of the Mouth and Neck Involved in Swallowing

palsy; Parkinson disease and other degenerative neurological disorders such as amyotrophic lateral sclerosis (ALS, also known as "Lou Gehrig disease"), multiple sclerosis (MS), progressive supranuclear palsy, Huntington disease, and myasthenia gravis. Muscular dystrophy (MD) and myotonic dystrophy are accompanied by dysphagia, which is also the cardinal symptom of oculopharyngeal muscular dystrophy, a rare, progressive genetic disorder.

## HOW DO WE SWALLOW?[3]

Swallowing is a complex process. Some 50 pairs of muscles and many nerves work to receive food into the mouth, prepare it, and move it from the mouth to the stomach. This happens in three stages. During the first stage, called the "oral phase," the tongue collects the food or liquid, making it ready for swallowing. The tongue and jaw move solid food around in the mouth so it can be chewed. Chewing makes solid food the right size and texture to swallow by mixing the food with saliva. Saliva softens and moistens the food to make swallowing easier. Normally, the only solid we swallow without chewing is in the form of a pill or caplet. Everything else that we swallow is in the form of a liquid, a puree, or a chewed solid.

The second stage begins when the tongue pushes the food or liquid to the back of the mouth. This triggers a swallowing response that passes the food through the pharynx, or throat. During this phase, called the "pharyngeal phase," the larynx (voice box) closes tightly and breathing stops to prevent food or liquid from entering the airway and lungs.

The third stage begins when food or liquid enters the esophagus, the tube that carries food and liquid to the stomach. The passage through the esophagus, called the "esophageal phase," usually occurs in about three seconds, depending on the texture or consistency of the food, but can take slightly longer in some cases, such as when swallowing a pill.

## HOW DOES DYSPHAGIA OCCUR?[3]

Dysphagia occurs when there is a problem with the neural control or the structures involved in any part of the swallowing process. Weak tongue or cheek muscles may make it hard to move food around in the mouth for chewing. A stroke or other nervous system disorder may make it difficult to start the swallowing response, a stimulus that allows food and liquids to move safely through the throat. Another difficulty can occur when weak throat muscles, such as after cancer surgery, cannot move all of the food toward the stomach. Dysphagia may also result from disorders of the esophagus.

## TREATMENT[2]

Changing a person's diet by adding thickeners helps many people, as does learning different ways to eat and chew that reduce the risk for aspiration. Occasionally drug therapy that helps the neurological disorder can also help dysphagia. In a few persons, botulinum toxin injections can help when food or liquid cannot enter the esophagus to get to the stomach. More severely individuals with a disability may require surgery or the insertion of feeding tubes.

## PROGNOSIS[2]

The prognosis depends upon the type of swallowing problem and the course of the neurological disorder that produces it. In some cases, dysphagia can be partially or completely corrected using diet manipulation or noninvasive methods. In others, especially when the dysphagia is causing aspiration and preventing adequate nutrition and causing weight loss, it may require aggressive intervention such as a feeding tube. For those with progressive degenerative neurological disorders, dysphagia will be only one in a cluster of symptoms and disabilities that have to be treated.

## Section 25.3 | Cognitive-Behavioral Therapy

This section includes text excerpted from "A Therapist's Guide to Brief Cognitive-Behavioral Therapy," Mental Illness Research, Education and Clinical Centers (MIRECC), U.S. Department of Veterans Affairs (VA), January 30, 2010. Reviewed November 2019.

Cognitive-behavioral therapy (CBT) combines cognitive and behavioral therapies and has strong empirical support for treating mood and anxiety disorders. The basic premise of CBT is that emotions are difficult to change directly, so CBT targets emotions by changing thoughts and behaviors that are contributing to the distressing emotions.

Cognitive-behavioral therapy builds a set of skills that enables an individual to be aware of thoughts and emotions; identify how situations, thoughts, and behaviors influence emotions; and improve feelings by changing dysfunctional thoughts and behaviors. The process of CBT skill acquisition is collaborative. Skill acquisition and homework assignments are what sets CBT apart from "talk therapies." Therapists use session time to teach skills to address the presenting problem and not simply to discuss the issue with the patient or offer advice.

Brief CBT is the compression of CBT material and the reduction of the average 12 to 20 sessions into 4 to 8 sessions. In Brief CBT, the concentration is on specific treatments for a limited number of the patient's problems. Specificity of the treatment is required because of the limited number of sessions and because the patient is required to be diligent in using extra reading materials and homework to assist in her or his therapeutic growth.

Brief CBT can range in duration from patient to patient and provider to provider. Although variability exists, therapists are encouraged to think flexibly in determining the length of treatment. Time-limited therapy may offer additional incentive for patients and therapists to work efficiently and effectively. However, the exact length of treatment will likely be determined by a host of factors involving the therapist, patient, and treatment setting. Therapists are not expected to rigidly adhere to a "set schedule" of progress or topics but rather should be flexible and adaptive in approaching all Brief CBT applications. For example, it is often helpful to work within a "session limited framework" where the patient receives four to six sessions of "active" treatment, followed by one or more follow-up sessions that occur at increasing intervals after the active treatment phase (e.g., two weeks posttreatment with an additional booster four weeks after that).

Certain problems are more appropriate for Brief CBT than others. Problems amenable to Brief CBT include, but are not limited to, adjustment, anxiety, and depressive disorders. Therapy also may be useful for problems that target specific symptoms (e.g., depressive thinking) or lifestyle changes (e.g., problem-solving, relaxation), whether or not these issues are part of a formal psychiatric diagnosis.

Brief CBT is particularly useful in a primary-care setting for patients with anxiety and depression associated with a medical condition. Because these individuals often face acute rather than chronic mental-health issues and have many coping strategies already in place, Brief CBT can be used to enhance adjustment. Issues that may be addressed in primary care with Brief CBT include, but are not limited to, diet, exercise, medication compliance, mental-health issues associated with a medical condition, and coping with a chronic illness or diagnosis.

Other problems may not be suitable for the use of Brief CBT or may complicate a straightforward application of Brief CBT. Axis II disorders such as borderline personality disorder or antisocial personality disorder typically are not appropriate for a shortened therapeutic experience because of the pervasive social, psychological, and relational problems individuals with these disorders experience. Patients exhibiting comorbid conditions or problems also may not be appropriate because the presence of a second issue may impede progress in therapy. For example, an individual with substance dependence comorbid with major depression may not be appropriate because the substance use requires a higher level of care and more comprehensive treatment than is available in a brief format. However, Brief CBT could be used with axis II and comorbid patients in dealing with specific negative behaviors or in conjunction with more intensive treatment.

## THERAPIST CONSIDERATIONS

It is important to be adequately skilled to evoke change in a patient's life in a short amount of time. Therapists should periodically assess and seek supervision/consultation regarding their capabilities in the process and content of Brief CBT.

The following are general therapist skills and abilities required for Brief CBT:

- Capability to establish a strong working relationship quickly
- Thorough knowledge of the treatments used
- Skill in structuring sessions and homework material to address all problems
- Skill in presenting material clearly and concisely with specific examples for each of the patient's issues
- Therapist interpersonal/personality variables: ability to be assertive, directive, nonjudgmental, and collaborative

## ASSESSING THE PATIENT

It is necessary to choose patients who are appropriate for Brief CBT versus traditional CBT or other types of therapy.

# Chapter 26 | Functional Mobility

An individual's ability to move around independently is known as "functional mobility." The ability of a person to move about independently can decrease as a result of a physical injury, which weakens the muscles and impairs balance. Physical performance and functional ability are determined by the presence of many physical and nonphysical aspects of independent living, including cognition, flexibility, social support, strength, and one's home surroundings. Physical impairments, such as the loss of range of motion and strength, can be attributed to a decrease in functional mobility, which can be enhanced and sometimes completed restored with proper therapeutic intervention and exercising.

Physical and occupational therapists help restore the functional capacity of a patient to the patient's previous level of functionality or help the patient adapt to new ways of optimal functioning. The ability of a patient to move around effortlessly after an injury may be limited following an extended period of immobilization. The patient might then require assistance getting into and out of bed or walking or sitting down. To help maintain balance, assistive devices such as canes or walkers may be recommended for use. Therapeutic exercises are commonly used with such assistive devices to improve functional mobility and achieve better results. In the United States, physical therapy involving functional mobility is commonly administered to patients recovering from critical injuries or illnesses.

The three major components of functional mobility are:

1. **Bed mobility.** The ability to move around in bed, including lying down, sitting up, turning to both sides, and rolling around.
2. **Transfers.** The process of moving from one surface to another, such as moving from a bed to a chair and vice versa.
3. **Ambulation.** The ability to walk independently or with the support of assistive devices such as walkers and crutches.

## FUNCTIONAL MOBILITY REHABILITATION

The process of working with the goal of enabling a person to return to their maximum level of independence in performing their day-to-day activities is called "functional mobility rehabilitation." This level of independence can be achieved with the help of a physical and/or occupational therapist. These medical professionals break down the tasks to be accomplished to enhance individual motions. Physical exercises are also prescribed to improve the patient's functional mobility. The therapists focus on improving the following areas:

- Strengthening muscles and bones
- Increasing flexibility
- Increasing range of motion
- Improving balance

Managing pain during physical therapy or leisure activity is another important part of recovering full strength and mobility as quickly as possible.

Therapists use specially designed routines to maximize joint and soft-tissue mobilization. Professionally developed interactive games have also proven to be helpful in improving balance and coordination in adults. The training routines established by these therapists depend on the type of ailment affecting the functional mobility of the patient. Rehabilitation is a combination of the training provided by the therapist and completion of the home exercise programs prescribed by the therapists. These programs are based on the following essential principles:

- The exercises are to be performed in a calm and relaxed manner.
- The therapist customizes the exercises as required based on the patient's medical impairments.
- The therapist adjusts the progress of the exercises when necessary.
- The patient performs the exercises by incorporating them into their daily home-exercise routine as assigned by the therapist.

## LEVELS OF ASSISTANCE

Different levels of assistance are provided to the patient based on the intensity of the injury. The various levels of assistance include the following:

- **Dependent.** During this stage, the therapist or helper performs all of the work, assists the patient in moving around, and performs most tasks due to the patient's inability to move on their own.
- **Maximum, moderate, and minimal assist.** These levels of assistance are applied based on how much the patient can move independently. The patient performs about 25 percent, 50 percent, and 75 percent of the work in minimal, moderate, and maximum assist, respectively.

- **Contact guard assist.** At this level of assistance, the therapist helps only in maintaining the patient's balance using either one or both hands as the patient performs their tasks independently.
- **Stand-by assist.** During this phase of assistance, the therapist merely stands by, in case the patient loses balance. There is no physical contact with the patient otherwise.
- **Independent.** This is the final objective of a functional rehabilitation therapist. A patient reaches this level when they are able to perform functional tasks without the need for any assistance.

Physical and occupational therapists complete their work in consultation with the doctors involved in the patient's recovery. The therapists outline a treatment plan that ensures optimal recovery with consideration given to the patient's medical history and in a manner designed to avoid setbacks or complications and then the patient's doctors vet treatment plans.

## ON THE HORIZON

Gaming and virtual reality-based rehabilitation methods are now being used in addition to physical therapy. Virtual reality-based rehabilitation training integrates action, observation, and execution. This provides strenuous, repetitive, and motivating training scenarios that lead to improvements in lower-limb motor function which, in turn, further enhance the patient's walking speed and stability. This form of rehabilitation also helps to significantly improve balance and functional mobility. This method of rehabilitation may also provide added benefits by reducing the patient's transportation costs and the effort required to monitor the patient's activity outside the clinic. Further research is needed to ascertain the advantages between clinic- and home-based virtual-reality training.

### References

1. Sears, Brett. "Assistance with Mobility in Physical Therapy," Verywell, July 5, 2019.
2. "Functional Mobility," Park Physical Therapy, May 17, 2017.
3. "Functional Rehabilitation," The OT Practice, March 30, 2017.
4. "Home-Based Virtual Reality-Augmented Training Improves Lower Limb Muscle Strength, Balance, and Functional Mobility following Chronic Incomplete Spinal Cord Injury," National Center for Biotechnology Information (NCBI), November 28, 2017.

# Chapter 27 | Speech and Language Assessments and Therapeutic Intervention

**Chapter Contents**

## Section 27.1 | **Dysphagia Therapy**

This section includes text excerpted from "Dysphagia," National Institute of Deafness and Other Communication Disorders (NIDCD), March 6, 2017.

### WHAT IS DYSPHAGIA?

People with dysphagia have difficulty swallowing and may even experience pain while swallowing (odynophagia). Some people may be completely unable to swallow or may have trouble safely swallowing liquids, foods, or saliva. When that happens, eating becomes a challenge. Often, dysphagia makes it difficult to take in enough calories and fluids to nourish the body and can lead to additional serious medical problems.

### HOW IS DYSPHAGIA TREATED?

There are different treatments for various types of dysphagia. Medical doctors and speech-language pathologists who evaluate and treat swallowing disorders use a variety of tests that allow them to look at the stages of the swallowing process. One test, the Flexible Endoscopic Evaluation of Swallowing with Sensory Testing (FEESST), uses a lighted fiber optic tube, or endoscope, to view the mouth and throat while examining how the swallowing mechanism responds to such stimuli as a puff of air, food, or liquids.

A videofluoroscopic swallow study (VFSS) is a test in which a clinician takes a videotaped x-ray of the entire swallowing process by having you consume several foods or liquids along with the mineral barium to improve visibility of the digestive tract. Such images help identify where in the swallowing process you are experiencing problems. Speech-language pathologists use this method to explore what changes can be made to offer a safe strategy when swallowing. The changes may be in food texture, size, head and neck posture, or behavioral maneuvers, such as "chin tuck," a strategy in which you tuck your chin so that food and other substances do not enter the trachea when swallowing. If you are unable to swallow safely despite rehabilitation strategies, then medical or surgical intervention may be necessary for the short-term as you recover. In progressive conditions such as amyotrophic lateral sclerosis (ALS, or Lou Gehrig disease), a feeding tube in the stomach may be necessary for the long term.

For some people, treatment may involve muscle exercises to strengthen weak facial muscles or to improve coordination. For others, treatment may involve learning to eat in a special way. For example, some people may have to eat with their head turned to one side or looking straight ahead. Preparing food in a certain way or avoiding certain foods may help in some situations. For instance, people who cannot swallow thin liquids may need to add special thickeners to their drinks. Other people may have to avoid hot or cold foods or drinks.

For some, however, consuming enough foods and liquids by mouth may no longer be possible. These individuals must use other methods to nourish their bodies. Usually, this involves a feeding system, such as a feeding tube, that bypasses or supplements the part of the swallowing mechanism that is not working normally.

## Section 27.2 | **Auditory Training**

This section contains text excerpted from the following sources: Text in this section begins with excerpts from "Listening/Auditory Training," Centers for Disease Control and Prevention (CDC), March 21, 2019; Text under the heading "Music Is Effective for Auditory Training" is excerpted from "Fine-Tuned Brains," National Science Foundation (NSF), April 10, 2009. Reviewed November 2019.

Most children who have a communication disability have some hearing. This is called "residual hearing." Some parents of a child with residual hearing may choose to use a building block called "listening" (auditory training). This building block is often used in combination with other building blocks (such as hearing aids, cochlear implants, and other assistive devices)

Listening might seem easy to a person with hearing. But for a child with hearing loss, listening is often hard without proper training. As with all other building blocks, the skill of listening must be learned. Often a speech-language pathologist will work with the child and family.

### MUSIC IS EFFECTIVE FOR AUDITORY TRAINING

Musicians exhibit greater sensitivity to the nuances of emotion in speech with their fine-tuning abilities. This ability to detect emotion is a fundamental skill that is needed for social and professional interactions. Enhanced sensitivity in musicians is not surprising given that musicians must attend to the detailed acoustic properties of sound on a daily basis

What links emotion in both language and music is their common acoustic and neural processing. Research has shown that extensive experience in one area may provide benefits in the other. Scientists know that emotion is carried less by the linguistic meanings of words than by the way the sound is communicated.

In a typically functioning brainstem, inputs like music and language shape early auditory cortical processing. A disrupted auditory brainstem pathway is exhibited through language and reading disorders. Music acts as a reinforcement of the pathway and may provide preventive or rehabilitative benefits. By measuring the responses of the auditory portion of the brainstem of musicians, researchers gain better insight into how they could treat deficiencies.

Due to its spectral complexity, wide frequency range and large variations in tone duration, music serves as an extremely effective vehicle for auditory training.

## Section 27.3 | Early Intervention and Speech-Language Pathology

This section contains text excerpted from the following sources: Text under the heading "About Early Intervention" is excerpted from "Language and Speech Disorders in Children," Centers for Disease Control and Prevention (CDC), February 6, 2019; Text under the heading "About Speech-Language Pathology" is excerpted from "Speech-Language Pathologists," U.S. Bureau of Labor Statistics (BLS), U.S. Department of Labor (DOL), September 4, 2019.

### ABOUT EARLY INTERVENTION

Children with language difficulties often need extra help and special instruction. Speech-language pathologists can work directly with children and their parents, caregivers, and teachers.

Having a language or speech delay or disorder can qualify a child for early intervention (for children up to 3 years of age) and special education services (for children aged 3 years and older). Schools can do their own testing for language or speech disorders to see if a child needs intervention. An evaluation by a healthcare professional is needed if there are other concerns about the child's hearing, behavior, or emotions. Parents, healthcare providers, and the school can work together to find the right referrals and treatment.

Children with specific learning disabilities, including language or speech disorders, are eligible for special education services or accommodations at school under the Individuals with Disabilities in Education Act (IDEA) and Section 504, an antidiscrimination law.

Healthcare providers can play an important part in collaborating with schools to help a child with speech or language disorders and delays or other disabilities get the special services they need. The American Academy of Pediatrics (AAP) has created a report that describes the roles that healthcare providers can have in helping children with disabilities, including language or speech disorders.

### ABOUT SPEECH-LANGUAGE PATHOLOGY

#### What Speech-Language Pathologists Do

Speech-language pathologists typically do the following:

- Evaluate levels of speech, language, or swallowing difficulty
- Identify treatment options

- Create and carry out an individualized treatment plan that addresses specific functional needs
- Teach children and adults how to make sounds and improve their voices and maintain fluency
- Help individuals improve vocabulary and sentence structure used in oral and written language
- Work with children and adults to develop and strengthen the muscles used to swallow
- Counsel individuals and families on how to cope with communication and swallowing disorders

Speech-language pathologists work with children and adults who have problems with speech and language, including related cognitive or social communication problems. They may be unable to speak at all, or they may speak with difficulty or have rhythm and fluency problems, such as stuttering. Speech-language pathologists may work with people who are unable to understand language or with those who have voice disorders, such as inappropriate pitch or harsh voice.

Speech-language pathologists also must complete administrative tasks, including keeping accurate records and documenting billing information. They record their initial evaluations and diagnoses, track treatment progress, and note any changes in an individual's condition or treatment plan.

Some speech-language pathologists specialize in working with specific age groups, such as children or the elderly. Others focus on treatment programs for specific communication or swallowing problems, such as those resulting from strokes, trauma, or a cleft palate.

In medical facilities, speech-language pathologists work with physicians and surgeons, social workers, psychologists, occupational therapists, physical therapists, and other healthcare workers. In schools, they evaluate students for speech and language disorders and work with teachers, other school personnel, and parents to develop and carry out individual or group programs, provide counseling, and support classroom activities.

# Chapter 28 | **Upper-Limb Prostheses**

The major role of the human arm is to place the hand where it can function and to transport objects held in the hand. The energy for operation of the hand substitute in upper-extremity prostheses is derived from relative motion between two parts of the body. Energy for operation of the elbow joint, when necessary, can be obtained in the same way. The stump, of course, is also a source of energy for control of the prosthesis in all except the shoulder disarticulation and forequarter cases. Force and motion can be obtained through a cable connected between the device to be operated and a harness across the chest or shoulders.

## HAND SUBSTITUTES TERMINAL DEVICES

All upper-extremity prostheses for amputation at the wrist level and above have in common the problem of selection of the "terminal device," a term applied to artificial hands and substitute devices such as hooks. In some areas of the world there is a tendency to supply the arm amputee with a number of devices, each designed for specific tasks such as eating, shaving, hair grooming, etc. In the United States, such an approach has been considered too clumsy, and opinion has been that the terminal device should be designed so that most upper-extremity amputees can perform the activities of daily living with a single device, or at most with two devices.

The so-called split hooks are much more functional than any artificial hand devised to date. The arm amputee must rely heavily upon visual cues in handling objects and the hook offers more visibility. The hook also offers more prehension facility, and can be more easily introduced into and withdrawn from pockets than a device in the form of a hand. Therefore, the hook is used in manual occupations and those avocations requiring manual dexterity. When extensive contact with the public is necessary and for social occasions, the hand is of course generally preferred. Many amputees have both types of devices, using each as the occasion

This chapter includes text excerpted from "Limb Prosthetics Services and Devices," National Institute of Standards and Technology (NIST), April 28, 2017.

warrants. Two basic types of mechanism have been developed for terminal device operation; voluntary opening and voluntary closing. In the former, tension on the control cable opens the fingers against an elastic force; in the latter, tension in the control cable closes the fingers against an elastic force. Each type of mechanism has its advantages and disadvantages, neither being superior to the other when used in a wide range of activities. Both hands and hooks are available with either type of mechanism.

## PROSTHESES FOR THE WRIST DISARTICULATION CASE

One of the problems in fitting the wrist disarticulation in the past has been to keep the overall length of the prosthesis commensurate with the unaffected arm. The development of very short wrist units, especially for wrist disarticulation cases, has materially reduced this problem. However, these units are available in only the screw, or thread, type, and cannot be obtained in the bayonet type which lends itself to quick interchange of terminal devices.

The socket for the wrist disarticulation case need not extend the full length of the forearm and is fitted somewhat loosely at the upper, or proximal, end to permit the wrist to rotate. A simple figure-eight harness and Bowden cable are used to operate the terminal device.

## PROSTHESES FOR THE LONG BELOW-ELBOW CASE

The prosthesis for the long below-elbow case is essentially the same as that for the wrist disarticulation patient except that the quick disconnect wrist unit can be used when desired.

## PROSTHESES FOR THE SHORT BELOW-ELBOW CASE

The socket for the short below-elbow stump, where there is no residual rotation of the forearm, is usually fitted snugly to the entire slump, and often rigid hinges connecting the socket to a cuff about the upper arm are used to provide additional stability. Either the figure-eight harness or the chest-strap harness may be used, the latter being preferred when heavy-duty work is required since it tends to spread the loads involved in lifting over a broader area than is the case with the figure-eight design. A wrist flexion unit, which permits the terminal device to be tilted in toward the body for effective use, can be provided in the short below-elbow prosthesis but is seldom prescribed for unilateral cases.

## PROSTHESES FOR THE VERY SHORT BELOW-ELBOW CASE

Often the very short below-elbow case cannot control the prosthesis of the short below-elbow type through the full range of motion, either because of a muscle contracture or because the stump is too short to provide the necessary leverage.

When a contracture is present that limits the range of motion of the stump, a "split socket" and "step up" hinge may be used. With this arrangement of levers and gears, movement of the stump through one degree causes the prosthetic forearm to move through two degrees; thus, a stump that has only about half the normal range of motion can drive the forearm through the desired 135 degrees. However, when the step-up hinge is used, twice the normal force is required. When the stump is incapable of supplying the force required, it can be assisted by employing the "dual control" harness wherein force in the terminal device control cable is diverted to help lift the forearm. When the elbow stump is very short or has a very limited range of motion, an elbow lock operated by stump motion is employed to obtain elbow function.

A number of prosthetists have reported success in fitting very short below-elbow cases with an arm that is bent to give a certain amount of preflexion. This type of fitting, which was developed in Munster, West Germany, eliminates the necessity for using the rather clumsy step up hinges and split socket, thus providing improved prosthetic control without disadvantageous force feedback. Furthermore, the harness is not necessary for suspension of the prosthesis. The maximum forearm flexion may be limited to about 100 deg, but this does not appear to be a significant disadvantage to unilateral amputees.

## PROSTHESES FOR THE ELBOW-DISARTICULATION CASE

Because of the length of the elbow-disarticulation stump, the elbow locking mechanism is installed on the outside of the socket. Otherwise, the prosthesis and harnessing methods are identical to those applied to the above-elbow case.

## PROSTHESES FOR THE ABOVE-ELBOW CASE

For the above-elbow prosthesis to operate efficiently, it is necessary that a lock be provided in the elbow joint, and it is, of course, preferable that the lock is engaged and disengaged without resorting to the use of the other hand or pressing the locking actuator against an external object such as a table or chair.

Several elbow units that can be locked and unlocked alternately by the same motion are available. This action is usually accomplished by the relative motion between the prosthesis and the body when the shoulder is depressed slightly and the arm is extended somewhat. The motion required is so slight that with practice the amputee can accomplish the action without being noticed. These elbow units contain a turntable above the elbow axis that permits the forearm to be positioned with respect to the humerus, supplementing the normal rotation remaining in the upper arm and thus allowing the prosthesis to be used more easily close to the midline of the body.

The elbow units described above are available with an adjustable coil spring to assist in flexing the elbow when this is desired. The flexion-assist device may be added or removed without affecting the other operating characteristics.

The plastic socket of the above-elbow prosthesis covers the entire surface of the stump. The most popular harness used is the figure-eight dual control design wherein the terminal device control cable is also attached to a lever on the forearm so that, when the elbow is unlocked, tension in the control cable produces elbow flexion, and, when the elbow is locked, the control force is diverted to the terminal device. The chest-strap harness may also be used in the dual control configuration.

## PROSTHESES FOR THE SHOULDER-DISARTICULATION AND FOREQUARTER CASES

Because of the loss of the upper-arm motion as a source of energy for control and operation of the prosthesis, restoration of the most vital functions in the shoulder-disarticulation case presents a formidable problem; for many years a prosthesis was provided for this type of amputation only for the sake of appearance. However, it has been possible to make available prostheses which provide a limited amount of function. To date, it has not been possible to devise a shoulder joint that can be activated from a harness, but a number of manually operated joints are available. Various harness designs have been employed but, because of the wide variation in the individual cases and the marginal amount of energy available, no standard pattern has developed, each design being made to take full advantage of the remaining potential of the particular patient.

## PROSTHESIS FOR BILATERAL UPPER-EXTREMITY AMPUTEES

Except for the bilateral shoulder-disarticulation case, fitting the bilateral case offers few problems not encountered with the unilateral case. The prostheses provided are generally the same as those prescribed for corresponding levels in unilateral cases. Artificial hands are rarely used by bilateral amputees because hooks afford so much more function. Many bilateral cases find that the wrist flexion unit, at least on one side, is of value. The harness for each prosthesis may be separated, but it is the general practice to combine the two. In addition to being neater, this arrangement makes the harness easier for the patient to don unassisted.

Some prosthetists have claimed success in fitting bilateral shoulder-disarticulation cases with two prostheses. Because of the lack of sufficient sources of energy for control, most cases of this type are provided with a single, functional prosthesis and a plastic cap over the opposite shoulder which provides an anchor for the harness and also fills this area to present a better appearance.

## NEUROPROSTHETICS

Prosthetic limbs are far less than optimal. All prosthetics must deal with the issues of function, control and fit. In other words, how does the prosthesis function? Can the prostheses be controlled? How does it fit? Each of these issues present significant hurdles that can only be addressed by a paradigm of neuro-implantable prostheses. Neuroprosthetics (also called "neural prosthetics") is a discipline related to neuroscience and bioengineering concerned with developing artificial prosthetic devices to replace or improve the function of an impaired nervous system. Neural prostheses are a series of devices that can substitute a motor, sensory, or cognitive modality that might have been damaged as a result of an injury or a disease. The goal of the neuroprosthetic limb is to restore an optimal degree of natural function for the missing or damaged limb.

Neuroprosthetic limbs are just now moving from beta devices to commercially available prosthetics. The integration and application of emerging technologies is moving laboratory research into commercial applications for the limb amputee. The limb amputee is beginning to see the dream become a reality. However, at this point in time, a true neuroprosthetic limb may cost up to nearly $100,000.

Here are three examples of neuroprosthetic limbs that are on the market or close to being commercialized:

## i-LIMB Hand Touch Bionics

Touch Bionics is a leading developer of advanced upper-limb prosthetics to become the world's first fully articulating and commercially available bionic hand. One of the Touch Bionics products now commercially available from the company, the i-LIMB Hand, is a first-to-market prosthetic device with five individually powered digits. This replacement hand looks and acts like a real human hand and represents a generational advance in bionics and patient care. The Touch Bionics i-LIMB Hand was developed using leading-edge mechanical engineering techniques and is manufactured using high strength plastics. The result is a next-generation prosthetic device that is lightweight, robust, and highly appealing to both patients and healthcare professionals.

The i-LIMB Hand is controlled by a unique, highly intuitive control system that uses a traditional two-input myoelectric (muscle) signal to open and close the hand's lifelike fingers. Myoelectric controls utilize the electrical signal generated by the muscles in the remaining portion of the patient's limb. This signal is picked up by electrodes that sit on the surface of the skin. Existing users of basic myoelectric prosthetic hands are able to quickly adapt to the system and can master the device's functionality within minutes. For patients, the i-LIMB Hand offers a prosthetic solution that has never before been available.

The modular construction of the i-LIMB Hand means that each individually powered finger can be quickly removed by simply removing one screw. This means that a prosthetist can easily swap out fingers that require servicing and patients can return to their everyday lives after a short clinic visit. Traditional devices would have to be returned to the manufacturer, often leaving the patient without a hand for many weeks.

## The Utah Arm Three–Motion Control

Since 1981, the Utah Arm has been the premier myoelectric arm for above-elbow amputees. It was originally developed at the University of Utah by the Center for Engineering Design, led by Dr. Steve Jacobsen. In 1987, Motion Control released the Utah Arm Two, with entirely re-engineered electronics that made the Utah Arm the most durable and dependable myoelectric arm available.

In 2004, Motion Control introduced microprocessor technology into the Utah Arm Three (U3), with a Computer Interface that allows the prosthetist or wearer to fine-tune the adjustments to achieve maximum performance. A variety of inputs may be used, so more options are available to more wearers. Meanwhile, the U3 still delivers the same sensitive, proportional control of elbow, hand, and wrist (optional), letting the wearer move the arm and hand slowly or quickly in any position. This provides a more natural response with less effort than the traditional on/off movement.

## DEKA Arm

The DEKA arm is modular and usable by anyone with any level of amputation. The arm works as though it had a very complicated set of vacuum-cleaner attachments; the hand contains separate electronics, as does the forearm. The elbow is powered, and the electronics that power it are contained in the upper arm. The shoulder is also powered and can accomplish the never-before-seen feat of reaching up as if to pick an apple off a tree.

DEKA worked closely with the Rehabilitation Institute of Chicago, where neuroscientist Todd Kuiken has had successes in surgically rerouting amputees' residual nerves—which connect the upper spinal cord to the 70,000 nerve fibers in the arm—to impart the ability to "feel" the stimulation of a phantom limb. Normally, the nerves travel from the upper spinal cord across the shoulder, down into the armpit, and into the arm. Kuiken pulled them away from the armpit and under the clavicle to connect to the pectoral muscles. The patient thinks about moving the arm, and signals travel down nerves that were formerly connected to the native arm but are now connected to the chest. The chest muscles then contract in response to the nerve signals. The contractions are sensed by electrodes on the chest, the electrodes send signals to the motors of the prosthetic arm—and the arm moves. With Kuiken's surgery, a user can control the DEKA arm with her or his own muscles, as if the arm were an extension of the person's flesh. However, the DEKA arm also provides feedback to the user without surgery.

# Chapter 29 | Lower-Limb Prostheses

## WHAT IS SYME AMPUTATION?

Developed about 1842 by James Syme, a leading Scottish surgeon, the Syme amputation leaves the long bones of the shank (the tibia and fibula) virtually intact, with only a small portion at the very end being removed. The tissues of the heel, which are ideally suited to withstand high pressures, are preserved, and this, in combination with the long bones, usually permits the patient to bear the full weight of the body on the end of the stump. Because the amputation stump is nearly as long as the unaffected limb, a person with Syme's amputation can usually get about the house without a prosthesis even though normal foot and ankle action has been lost. Atrophy of the severed muscles that were formerly attached to bones in the foot to provide ankle action results in a stump with a bulbous end which, though not of the most pleasing appearance, is quite an advantage in holding the prosthesis in place. Since its introduction, Syme's operation has been looked upon with both favor and disfavor among surgeons. It seems to be the consensus now that "the Syme" should be performed in preference to amputation at a higher level if possible. In the case of most women, though, "the Syme" is undesirable because of the difficulty of providing a prosthesis that matches the shape of the other leg.

## PROSTHESIS FOR SYME AMPUTATION

The major reason Syme amputation was held in such disfavor in some quarters was the difficulty in providing a comfortable, sufficiently strong prosthesis with a neat appearance. The short distance between the end of the stump and the floor made it extremely difficult to provide needed ankle motion. Most prostheses were of leather reinforced with steel sidebars resulting in an ungainly appearance. Research workers at the prosthetic services center at the Department of

This chapter includes text excerpted from "Limb Prosthetics Services and Devices," National Institute of Standards and Technology (NIST), April 28, 2017.

Veterans Affairs of Canada were quick to realize that the use of the proper plastic laminate might solve many of the problems long associated with the Syme prosthesis. After a good deal of experimentation, the Canadians developed a model in 1955 which, with a few variations, is used almost universally in both Canada and the United States.

Necessary ankle action is provided by making the heel of the foot of sponge rubber. The socket is made entirely of a plastic laminate. A full-length cutout in the rear permits entry of the bulbous stump. When the cutout is replaced and held in place by straps, the bulbous stump holds the prosthesis in place. In the American version, a window-type cutout is used on the side because calculations show that smaller stress concentrations are present with such an arrangement.

In those cases where, for poor surgery or other reasons, full-body weight cannot be tolerated on the end of the stump, provisions can be made to transfer all or part of the load to the area just below the kneecap. When this procedure is necessary, it can be accomplished easily by the use of the window-type cutout.

## PROSTHESIS FOR BELOW-KNEE AMPUTATIONS

Most below-knee amputees were fitted with wooden prostheses carved out by hand. A good portion of the body weight was carried on a leather thigh corset, or lacer, attached to the shank and socket by means of steel hinges. The shape of the corset and upper hinges also held the prosthesis to the stump. The distal, or lower, end of the socket was invariably left open. Other versions of this prosthesis used aluminum, fibre or molded leather, as the materials for construction of the shank and socket, but the basic principle was the same. Many thousands of below-knee amputees have gotten along well with this type of prosthesis, but there are many disadvantages. Because the human knee joint is not a simple, single axis hinge joint, relative motion is bound to occur between the prosthesis and the stump and thigh during knee motion when single jointed side hinges are used, resulting in some chafing and irritation. To date, it has not been possible to devise a hinge to overcome this difficulty. Edema, or accumulation of body fluids, was often present at the lower end of the stump. Most of these prostheses were exceedingly heavy, especially those made of wood.

In an attempt to overcome these difficulties, the biomechanics laboratory of the University of California (UC), in 1958, designed what is known as the "patellar tendon bearing (PTB)" below-knee prosthesis. In the PTB prosthesis, no lacer and side hinges are used, all of the weight being taken through the stump by making the socket high enough to cover all the tendons below the patella, or kneecap. The patellar tendon is an unusually inelastic tissue which is not unduly affected by pressure. The sides of the socket are also made much higher than had usually been the practice in the past in order to give stability against side loads. The socket is made of molded plastic laminate that provides an intimate fit over the entire area of the socket, and is lined with a thin layer of sponge rubber and leather. Because it is rare for a below-knee stump to bear much pressure on its lower end, care is taken to see that only a very slight amount is present in that area. This feature has been a big factor in eliminating the edema problem in many instances. The PTB prosthesis is generally suspended by means of a simple cuff, or strap, around the thighs just above the kneecap, but sometimes a strap from the prosthesis to a belt around the waist is used.

After the socket has been made, it is installed on a special adjustable leg so that the prosthetist can try various alignment combinations with ease. When both prosthetists and patient are satisfied, the leg is completed utilizing the alignment determined with the adjustable unit.

The shank recommended is of plastic laminate and the foot prescribed is usually the solid ankle cushion heel (SACH) design but other types can be used.

It is now general practice in many areas to prescribe the PTB prosthesis in most cases and in many old ones, and if side hinges and a corset are indicated later, these can be added.

Stumps as short as two and a half inches have been fitted successfully with the PTB prosthesis. In special cases, such as extreme flexion contracture, the so-called kneeling knee, or bent knee, prosthesis may be indicated. The prosthesis used is similar to that used for the knee-disarticulation case.

## PROSTHESES FOR THE KNEE-DISARTICULATION AND OTHER KNEE-BEARING CASES

Because of the bulbous shape of the true knee-disarticulation stump, it is not possible to use a wooden socket of the type used on the tapered above-knee stump. To allow entry of the bulbous end, a socket is molded of leather to conform to the stump and is provided with a lengthwise anterior cutout that can be laced to hold the socket in position. Because of the length of the knee-disarticulation and supracondylar stump, it is not possible to install any of the present knee units designed for above-knee prostheses and, therefore, heavy-duty below-knee joints are generally used. Most prosthetists try to provide some control of the shank during the swing phase of walking by inserting nylon washers between the mating surfaces of the joint to provide friction and by using check straps. Better devices for control of the knee joint are being developed and should be available in the near future.

## PROSTHESIS FOR ABOVE-KNEE CASES

The articulated above-knee leg is in effect a compound pendulum actuated by the thigh stump. If the knee joint is perfectly free to rotate when force is applied, the effects of inertia and gravity tend to make the shank rotates too far backward and slam into extension as it rotates forward, except at a very slow rate of walking. The method most used to permit an increase in walking speed is the introduction of some restraint in the form of mechanical friction about the knee joint. The limitation imposed by constant mechanical friction is that for each setting there is only one speed that produces a natural appearing gait. When restraint is provided in the form of hydraulic resistance, a much wider range of cadence can be obtained without introducing into the gait pattern awkward and unnatural motions.

Throughout the past century, much time and effort have been spent in providing an automatic brake, or lock, at the knee in order to provide stability during the stance phase and to reduce the possibility of stumbling. Stability during the stance phase can be obtained by aligning the leg so that the axis of the knee is behind the hip and ankle axes. For most above-knee amputees in good health, such an arrangement has been quite satisfactory, but an automatic knee brake is indicated for the weaker or infirm patients.

The prosthesis prescribed most commonly for the above-knee amputee consists of a carved wooden socket, a single axis knee unit with constant but adjustable friction, a wooden shank, and a SACH foot. The shank and socket are reinforced with an outer layer of plastic laminate to reduce the amount of wood required and thus keep weight to an optimum.

When an automatic brake is indicated, the Bock, the "Vari Gait" 100, and the Mortensen knee units are the ones most generally used. All are actuated upon contact of the heel with the ground. The Bock and "Vari-Gait" units can be used with almost any type of foot, while a foot of special design is necessary when the Mortensen mechanism is used.

The "hydra cadence" above-knee leg was the only unit available that provided hydraulic friction to control the shank during the swing phase of walking. In addition to this feature, incorporated in the hydra-cadence design is provision for coordinated motion between the ankle and the knee action. After the knee is flexed 20 degrees, the toe of the foot is lifted as the knee is flexed further, thus giving more clearance between the foot and the ground as the leg swings through. Other hydraulic units made available are the Regnell (a Swedish design) and the DuPaCo. Still, others are in advanced stages of development.

A number of methods for suspending the above-knee leg are available. For younger, healthy patients, the suction socket is generally the method of choice. In this design the socket is simply fitted tightly enough to retain sufficient negative pressure, or suction, between the stump and the bottom of the socket when the leg is off the ground. Special valves are used to control the amount of negative pressure created so as not to cause discomfort. No stump sock is worn with the suction socket. A major advantage of this type of suspension is the freedom of motion permitted the wearer, thus allowing the use of all the remaining musculature of the stump. Another important advantage is the decreased amount of piston action between stump and socket. Additional comfort is also obtained by elimination of all straps and belts.

In some cases additional suspension is provided by adding a "silesian bandage," a light belt attached to the socket in such a way that there is very little restriction to motion of the various parts of the body.

Patients with weak stumps and most of those with very short stumps will require a pelvic belt connected to the socket by means of a "hip" joint. Because the connecting joint cannot be placed to coincide with the typical joint, certain motions are restricted. Pelvic-belt suspension is generally indicated for the older patient because of the problems encountered in donning the suction socket, especially that of bending over to remove the donning socks.

Shoulder straps, at one time the standard method of suspending above knee prostheses, are still sometimes indicated for the elderly patient.

Prior to the introduction of the suction socket into the United States soon after the close of World War II, virtually all above-knee sockets had a conical shaped interior and were known as "plug fits," with most of the weight being borne along the sides of the stump. Such a design does not permit the remaining musculature to perform to its full capabilities. In the development of the suction socket, a design known as the "quadrilateral socket" evolved, and now is virtually the standard for above-knee sockets regardless of the type of suspension used. When the pelvic belt or suspender straps are used, the socket is fitted somewhat looser than in the case of the suction socket, and the stump sock is generally worn to reduce skin irritation from the pumping action of the loose socket. Most of the body weight is taken on the ischium of the pelvis, that part which assumes the load when an individual is sitting.

The quadrilateral socket, because of the method employed to permit full use of the remaining muscles, does not resemble the shape of the stump but, as the name implies, is rectangular in shape. The standard method of fitting a quadrilateral socket called for no contact over the lower end of the stump, a hollow space being left in this area. Although this method was quite successful there remained a sufficient number of cases that persistently developed ulcers or edema over the end of the stump. Experiments involving the use of slight pressure over the stump end led to the development of what is known as the "plastic total contact socket." As the name implies, the socket is in contact with the entire surface of the stump. The total contact socket has helped to cure most of the problem cases and is now being used routinely in many areas.

In fitting the above-knee prosthesis, the prosthetist carves the interior of the socket using measurements of the stump as a guide. When a satisfactory fit has been achieved the socket is usually mounted on an adjustable leg for alignment trial, after which the wooden shank and the knee are substituted for the adjustable unit and the leg is finished by applying a thin layer of plastic laminate over the shank and thigh piece.

In the case of the total contact socket, the prosthetist obtains a plaster cast of the stump, usually with the aid of a special casting jig, and thus obtains a model of the stump over which the plastic socket can be formed.

## PROSTHESIS FOR HIP-DISARTICULATION AND HEMI-PELVECLOMY CASES

A prosthesis developed by the Canadian Department of Veterans Affairs in 1954 and modified slightly through the years has become accepted as standard practice. In the Canadian design a plastic-laminate socket is used, and the "hip" joint is placed on the front surface in such a position that, when used with an elastic strap connecting the rear end of the socket to a point on the shank ahead of the femur, stability during standing and walking can be achieved without the use of a lock at the hip joint. The location of the hip joint in the Canadian design also facilitates sitting, a real problem in earlier designs.

A constant friction knee unit is most often used with the hip-disarticulation prosthesis, but some prosthetists have reported successful use of hydraulic knee units.

The hemipelvectomy patient is provided with the same type of prosthesis but the socket design is altered to allow for the loss of part of the pelvis.

# Chapter 30 | **Bionic Movements**

When you lose the use of a limb, even the simplest of daily tasks can turn into a challenge. High-tech devices can help restore independence. New technologies are even making it possible to connect the mind to an artificial limb. These artificial limbs are called "bionic prosthetic devices."

"To get back some of that lost function, you need some sort of assistive tool or technology to either enhance recovery or restore the capability of the anatomy that's missing now," says Dr. Nick Langhals, who oversees National Institutes of Health (NIH)-supported prosthetic engineering research.

This fast-moving research aims to improve people's lives by restoring both movement and feeling.

## PROSTHETIC CONTROL

Traditional prosthetic devices use a body-powered harness to control a hand device. These are easy to use. With a shrug of your shoulder, the prosthetic hand or hook opens. With the release of your shoulder, the prosthesis closes. Through the feel of the cable tension across your shoulders, you know whether the prosthesis is open or closed without looking at it.

Newer, motorized hands are not as easy to learn how to use. To close the device, you contract the remaining muscles in your arm. An electrical sensor placed over those muscles detects the contraction and tells the hand to close. Since the original muscles that controlled the hand are gone, the remaining muscles must be retrained. Learning how to open and close a prosthetic hand in this way takes some time. And you still need to watch the device to know what it is doing.

To make motorized hands more intuitive to use, researchers are developing ways to detect the electrical signals in your brain and nerves to help control advanced bionic prosthetics. This can be done in many ways, such as by

This chapter includes text excerpted from "Bionic Movements," *NIH News in Health*, National Institutes of Health (NIH), August 2018.

implanting tiny sensors in the parts of the brain that control movement or by attaching small electrodes to the amputated nerves. Either way, the patients simply think about moving their hand and computers translate it into the movements of a bionic prosthetic hand.

## TWO-WAY COMMUNICATION

To regain a sense of wholeness, a person with a bionic limb needs to do more than controlling the device. They also need to "feel" what it is doing. New bionic devices can send sensation from the device back to the brain. This allows a person with a bionic device to feel like they are using their own limb

"The most important thing about the research that we're doing is this sense of wholeness," says Dr. Paul Marasco, a biomedical engineering researcher at Cleveland Clinic.

One way to help a person feel their prosthetic hand is to move the remaining sensory nerves from the amputated hand to the skin of the upper arm. You can then use small robots to press on the skin of the upper arm when the hand is touching something.

Marasco's team devised a similar system to restore the feeling of movement, too. The bionic hand sends signals to a computerized control system outside of the body. The computer then tells a small robot worn on the arm to send vibrations to the arm muscle. These vibrations deep in the muscle create an illusion of movement that tells the brain when the hand is closing or opening.

Marasco's team tested this feedback system with several people who had a hand prosthesis. The study participants were able to operate the bionic hand and know what position it was in just as well as with their natural hand. With this feedback system, they didn't have to look at the bionic hand to know when it was open or closed, or when it was reaching for an object.

"We fool their brains into believing that the prosthesis is actually part of their body," Marasco says. This advancement directly taps into the way that the brain senses movement, which helps improve the two-way communication between prosthetic device and mind.

## WEARABLE ROBOTS

Research teams are also trying to help people who have lost the use of their legs. By wearing a robotic device called an "exoskeleton," some people with leg paralysis have been able to regain the ability to walk.

A group led by Dr. Thomas Bulea, a biomedical engineer at the NIH Clinical Center, created a wearable exoskeleton for children with cerebral palsy (CP). CP is a brain disorder that makes it hard to stand up straight, balance, and walk. The motorized, robotic exoskeleton changes the way the children walk by helping them straighten their knees at key points during the walking cycle. While the exoskeleton can make walking easier, children must be able to navigate at least small distances on their own to use it.

"The ultimate goal really is to have a person wear this outside of NIH Clinical Center lab, or even outside of the clinical setting," Bulea explains. "To do that you have to have a really robust control system that makes sure that the robot is behaving properly in all different kinds of environments."

# Chapter 31 | Community-Based Rehabilitation

The goal of community-based rehabilitation (CBR) is to provide primary rehabilitation therapy to people with disabilities within their communities. The core concept of CBR is that community-based medical rehabilitation using an integrated design will help equalize vocational and financial opportunities for people with disabilities. The combined efforts of both government and nongovernmental organizations (NGOs) are designed to provide health, vocational, and other social services at the community level.

## INITIATION AND EARLY DAYS

The CBR model was initiated by the World Health Organization (WHO) in an effort to meet the basic needs of people with disabilities and their families and to improve their quality of life. This initiative was established primarily for low-income countries in an effort to ensure that people with disabilities have access to the services necessary for the best possible healthcare. The favorable outcomes of these programs led to CBR being adopted throughout the African, Asian, and South American continents. In the 1990s, other United Nations (UN) agencies, including the United Nations Educational, Scientific and Cultural Organization (UNESCO) and the United Nations Children's Fund (UNICEF), became involved. These combined efforts led to the evolution of a multidisciplinary approach to CBR.

## SECTORS AND ROLES FOR DEVELOPMENT AND IMPLEMENTATION

The following are the most relevant resources required to sustain CBR:

### People with Disabilities

People with disabilities play a significant role in CBR. Because people with disabilities have a better understanding of what their peers with disabilities are going through. They are especially effective role models and counselors.

### Families of People with Disabilities

Families of people with disabilities typically provide primary care, support, and assistance to family members with disabilities. Hence, members of these families often initiate CBR programs. They are also some of the most effective contributors in these programs.

### Communities

Community members are also an essential part of CBR, since they are knowledgeable about particular environmental, economic, and political situations in the local area. This knowledge enables them to more easily establish accessible rehabilitation centers and provide training skills through the microeconomic, or individual, activities of people and organizations in the community.

## GOVERNMENTS AND NONGOVERNMENTAL ORGANIZATIONS

Governments—and this category includes local, regional, national, and international governments, as well as NGOs—have the most significant role to play in developing and sustaining CBR programs. Governments provide CBR infrastructure and pass legislation that guarantees the rights and protections extended to people with disabilities. And, NGOs are often best enabled to provide long-term care to people with disabilities who have no families to care for them.

## MEDICAL PROFESSIONALS, EDUCATORS, AND OTHER PROFESSIONALS

People with disabilities are guaranteed equal access to healthcare and other areas in which they seek opportunities that allow them to live better lives. "Professionals" refers to people who are in a position that enables them to share their knowledge and use their skills to help people with disabilities. These professionals may include therapists, trainers, and social scientists, all of whom can help develop new and effective CBR programming that benefits people with disabilities. In local environments where qualified healthcare professionals are unavailable, CBR workers must be trained to make sure they can provide such basic levels of service.

## THE PRIVATE SECTOR (BUSINESS AND INDUSTRY)

Supporting CBR programs includes fulfilling a community needs through charity work/donations or by providing resources and otherwise assisting in CBR activities. Providing this support is an efficient way for those in the private sector to guarantee support for people with disabilities while, in return, receiving social credit for their involvement. Private-sector businesses and industries can also help by making sure that private healthcare facilities are made accessible for the CBR program.

The above-mentioned resources are vital to the continued maintenance and development of the CBR. The continued collaboration, coordination, and involvement of all of these factors are deemed necessary for the CBR program to be effective.

## FUNCTIONS OF COMMUNITY-BASED REHABILITATION

The main functions of the CBR include the following:

- Provide education and training opportunities to people with disabilities.
- Provide training to the community and family members of people with disabilities in an effort to create a positive climate while helping them to better understand disability. The WHO-CBR training manual provides guidelines for this effort.
- Refer specialist services and provide rehabilitation and assistive devices (e.g., crutches, wheelchairs, and hearing aids, etc.).
- Provide programs that involve physiotherapy, and medical and surgical interventions.
- Provide financial assistance and promote the creation of income-generating opportunities for people with disabilities.
- Support social activities such as sports and recreation.

## COMMUNITY-BASED REHABILITATION NETWORKS

At present, there are three major CBR networks. These are identified based on the countries in which they are established. They are:

- CBR Africa Network (CAN)
- CBR America Network (RED de RBC de las Américas y el Caribe)
- CBR Asia–Pacific Network

These CBRs were created to promote the sharing of resources and training.

## BENEFITS OF COMMUNITY-BASED REHABILITATION

Community-based rehabilitation programming has proven to be highly advantageous, especially in developing countries. It has greatly increased the independence and mobility of people with disabilities. People undergoing brain-injury rehabilitation, in particular, have experienced a higher psychosocial outcome, including increased self-esteem and a greater degree of social inclusion, through CBR. CBR-related educational and vocational training also has been immensely beneficial in helping people with disabilities find employment. CBR has proven to be the only decentralized system that can extend long-term support to people with disabilities by meeting their basic needs. It has excelled in creating positive attitudes and providing functional rehabilitation with a potential for reaching people with disabilities across multiple regions. CBR is highly cost-effective when compared to institution-based rehabilitation. CBR is also highly effective at removing barriers that prevent people with disabilities from taking part in community activities while promoting the education, empowerment, healthcare, livelihoods, and welfare of people with disabilities at the community level.

## References

1. "Understanding Community-based Rehabilitation," Disability INFormation Resources (DINF), February 1, 2001.
2. "Community-Based Rehabilitation: CBR Guidelines," National Center for Biotechnology Information (NCBI), August 19, 2015.
3. "Community-Based Rehabilitation (CBR)," World Health Organization (WHO), February 13, 2016.

# Chapter 32 | Using Virtual Reality to Improve Health

Virtual reality (VR)—used to be science fiction. Nowadays, it is everywhere. All you need is a smartphone and a headset to immerse yourself in 3-D virtual worlds or games. This booming technology may also be useful for healthcare and research.

"In the last few years, there's been a huge expansion in the number of exciting clinical applications of virtual reality," says Dr. Andrew Huberman, a VR researcher at Stanford University.

The National Institutes of Health (NIH)-funded researchers are finding that VR may help with many areas of medicine. These include tailoring rehabilitation exercises, improving mental health, and reducing pain.

## RESTORING MOVEMENT

Scientists have been testing VR to treat movement problems. These can be caused by a stroke, a brain injury, Parkinson disease, or other conditions. Rehabilitation exercises can sometimes help people train their muscles to improve their movement. But, these exercises can be boring—especially for kids.

Dr. Amy Bastian, a movement specialist at the Kennedy Krieger Institute (KKI), is using VR to make rehabilitation exercises more engaging for kids. It also lets her team tailor the exercises to individual children's needs.

"With VR, we can do things that are really hard to do in real-world therapy," Bastian says. "If we want you to learn to reach and control your balance in one direction, we can make all the game components move things in that direction."

Virtual reality can also help kids who have trouble following directions, she explains. "We can say something like, 'just punch the red things.' This can get them to do all kinds of complex tasks."

This chapter includes text excerpted from "Beyond Games," *NIH News in Health*, National Institutes of Health (NIH), July 2019.

Bastian is also developing VR exercises for adults who have damage to the cerebellum, the part of the brain that coordinates movement. This type of brain injury makes people's movements jerky and uncoordinated.

The team is testing whether other parts of the brain can be taught to coordinate movements instead. But, this cannot happen if the eyes can see the body, because the damaged cerebellum tries to take over.

That is why her team is putting people into a VR scene where their bodies do not exist. They must reach for targets with now-invisible limbs. Because people cannot see their arms, other brain areas must take over to complete the task.

Coins fall from the virtual sky when the person makes a smooth movement to grab an object. This instant feedback for a successful movement is vital for the brain to forge new learning pathways, Bastian explains. "In VR, we can manipulate the environment in real-time to help them learn to use another brain system."

## FIGHTING FEAR

Huberman is using VR to test techniques to help people cope with fear and anxiety. VR is ideal for studying such mental states, he explains.

"Vision, more than any other sense, is the sense that humans use to navigate the world and survive. And, more than any other sense, it drives phobias and anxiety."

What you see can be easily manipulated using a virtual environment. His team is using this aspect of VR to help people learn to manage their fears.

"We can create experiences that are very realistic," Huberman explains. "We can create an experience that's a little bit threatening, or one that's very threatening."

Virtual reality can show people scenes of sharks or spiders, put them high on top of a building, or have them standing in front of a crowd to speak.

After their participants have one of these VR experiences, the team teaches them ways to manage their stress and discomfort. These include focused breathing exercises and other techniques.

The researchers then put people back into the stressful VR environment to see if the techniques can help them reduce their anxiety at the moment.

A unique advantage of VR, Huberman explains, is that researchers can directly measure signs of anxiety. These include changes in eye movements and pupil size.

## DISTRACTING FROM PAIN

In addition to helping people process uncomfortable mental experiences, VR may help people cope with physical discomfort. Researchers are testing how VR can help reduce the pain from certain medical procedures.

Dr. Sam Sharar, a pain expert at the University of Washington (UW), uses VR to distract children and adults who are recovering from burns.

"Burn pain can be really, really bad. It is hard to tolerate," Sharar says. For burns to heal, the wounds must be washed and covered again every day. These procedures are very painful. Drugs that reduce pain often provide only partial relief for people with burn injuries.

Sharar believes VR can relieve pain by distracting the brain. "People have a fixed amount of conscious attention," he says. "If you divert some of that from experiencing a painful procedure to another task, the brain experiences less pain. This happens even though the same pain signal is coming through the skin."

His team and others developed a VR program that places people in a freezing cold virtual world. It engages their eyes and ears to block out what is happening to their skin. It also has a game where people hit a target to distract more of their attention.

The team's studies have shown that the immersive program reduced people's pain during burn care by half compared with playing a regular video game.

Sharar and other researchers continue looking for ways to use virtual environments to provide more effective pain relief. For people with chronic pain, which lasts for more than three months, using VR distraction has not been found to be helpful. His team and others are now using VR to expand access to techniques that have proven to help people manage chronic pain, like cognitive-behavioral therapy (CBT).

"If VR could be used to deliver this type of therapy in an immersive, virtual environment," Sharar says, "I think that would have tremendous potential to improve self-management of pain."

Virtual reality continues to drop in cost and grow in popularity, Huberman adds. He thinks the feedback it can provide to the senses will also continue to improve. Such improvements could potentially open doors to its use in more areas of healthcare.

# Chapter 33 | **Latest Trends in Fitness and Exercise**

Physical fitness and exercise are two areas of modern life that are particularly subject to fluctuations in consumer interest. New fitness equipment and exercise programs catch the attention of those looking for the greatest results, replacing older approaches that have fallen out of favor. Some popular exercise programs quickly become fads, fading away after a brief period of widespread success in the fitness industry. Other fitness practices develop into trends, resulting in a more lasting change in the way people approach physical fitness. Some of the more popular current trends in fitness and exercise are described below.

## NEWER TRENDS

Wearable fitness trackers have become extremely popular among those with an interest in overall health and well-being. These portable devices use sensors and other technology to records various biometric data such as heart rate, and physical activities such as walking, running, stair climbing, and so on. Wearable fitness trackers often work in conjunction with smartphone apps or other web-enabled technology.

Functional fitness is a relatively new trend among fitness enthusiasts. Functional fitness refers to exercise that is performed to enhance one's ability to carry out tasks of daily living. Those who practice functional fitness generally seek to increase their strength, balance, coordination, and endurance in order to increase overall quality of life.

As the population of the U.S. ages, the popularity of fitness programs tailored specifically for older adults continues to grow. With the increase among senior citizens and retirees who are interested in continuing an active lifestyle, demand is increasing for fitness programs to serve this demographic.

High-intensity interval training (HIIT) is another popular fitness trend. This style of workout involves short periods of intense activity followed by short periods of rest. A high-intensity interval workout generally lasts about 30 minutes, although some sessions can run longer.

The use of special flexibility/mobility roller equipment is rising, particularly among those who experience issues with full range of motion. These rollers can be used during warm-up or cool-down periods, to work on areas of the body that are trigger points, or muscles that need focused attention or deep tissue work.

## WEIGHT TRAINING

Strength training, also known as "weightlifting" or "bodybuilding," is another somewhat timeless fitness trend that has never fallen out of favor. Strength training involves lifting weights, either free weights or through the use of weight-lifting machines, in a manner that targets specific muscles or groups of muscles. In strength training, various weights are lifted in repetitions known as sets, with periods of rest between sets. Strength training can be performed at a gym or at home, using traditional weights and/or weightlifting machines.

Bodyweight training, also known as "calisthenics," is a minimalist form of exercise that requires no special equipment. Bodyweight training uses a person's own body mass as resistance, for example, exercises such as push-ups, sit-ups, and jumping jacks. This type of exercise was once the most popular form of physical training in the U.S. Although it never completely fell out of favor, bodyweight training has at various times been eclipsed by newer activities and workouts based around gym equipment. Bodyweight training is experiencing a resurgence in popularity among those looking for a "back to basics" approach to fitness.

## PERSONAL TRAINERS, FITNESS COACHES, AND WELLNESS

Personal training continues to be a popular trend in fitness. Modern fitness enthusiasts are demanding fitness training services provided by educated, certified, experienced fitness professionals. Consumers of personal training services have become more aware of the benefits of working with a certified trainer, and many consumers look for trainers that have certain credentials or qualifications. Group personal training has gained popularity among those looking for a more cost-effective way to access the services of a personal trainer. In group personal training, a small group of people share the cost of personal training sessions. Under this arrangement, the personal trainer divides her or his time in the training session among all the group members. Online fitness training is another option that is growing in popularity among those who wish to access the services of a personal trainer at a time or place that is most convenient for them.

Wellness coaching is a form of personal fitness training that uses a more integrative approach to behavior modification. Wellness coaching often focuses on disease prevention, rehabilitation, and health maintenance. Sessions can occur in person, by phone or video, or other format, including individual one-on-one sessions or group meetings.

## Latest Trends in Fitness and Exercise

Wellness tourism is a relatively new trend among fitness enthusiasts. The term "wellness" encompasses the total state of a person's health, including physical, mental, and social aspects, with particular focus on proactive measures that promote, maintain, and improve one's overall healthiness. Wellness tourism, also known as "fitness tourism," is any form of recreational travel that supports the goals of total personal wellness. Wellness tourism focuses on disease prevention and enhancement of healthy lifestyles through visits to spas, hot springs, and other therapeutic retreat centers.

## CONTINUING TRENDS

Programs that combine exercise and weight loss continue to be popular choices for many fitness enthusiasts. These programs combine physical fitness coaching with nutrition and dietary instruction to promote a more rounded approach to health and well-being.

Circuit training is another form of workout that has remained popular among fitness enthusiasts. Circuit training involves a selection of exercises that are done in sequence, normally to promote strength and endurance. One circuit is the completion of all the exercises in the program. Circuit training can include virtually any form of exercise, such as weightlifting, aerobics, and so on.

Yoga remains one of the most popular and enduring fitness trends in recent years. Sometimes practiced for stress reduction and relaxation, yoga can also be a form of exercise centered on stretching the body and assuming specific poses for specific amounts of time.

### References

1. Brown, Jill S. "Top Fitness Trends for 2016: Does Your Favorite Make the List?" Huffington Post, November 23, 2015.
2. Roberts. Amy. "Forecast: The Top 10 Fitness Trends in 2016," *Men's Fitness*, 2016.
3. Thompson, Walter R. "Worldwide Survey of Fitness Trends for 2016: 10th Anniversary Edition," ACSM's *Health and Fitness Journal*, November/December 2015.

# Part 4 | **Physical Limitations: Impact and Coping**

# Chapter 34 | Impact of Disability on Family and Caregivers

## MY FAMILY MEMBER HAS AN ILLNESS OR DISABILITY

If you have a family member with an illness or disability, you may face some stressful times or have extra responsibilities. But, as you probably know, some great things can come from it too!

### My Parent, Guardian, or Grandparent Has an Illness or Disability

If your parent, guardian, or grandparent has a disability or illness, your life may be a little different from your friends' lives. You may have to do more chores, cook dinner, or help your parent, guardian, or grandparent eat or get dressed.

Having a parent, guardian, or grandparent with an illness or disability can be tough. For example, your parent, guardian, or grandparent may not be able to come to your sports games. But, they will probably want to hear how the game went as soon as you get home. And you most likely feel more at ease with different types of people because you are used to seeing differences at home. The lessons you learn will be with you for life and will help you to be a better person.

### My Sister or Brother Has an Illness or Disability

If you have a sibling with an illness or disability, you may feel:

- Guilty because you do not have the same struggle

This chapter contains text excerpted from the following sources: Text under the heading "My Family Member Has an Illness or Disability" is excerpted from "My Family Member Has an Illness or Disability," girlshealth.gov, Office on Women's Health (OWH), October 31, 2013. Reviewed November 2019; Text under the heading "Family Caregiver Guide to Assistive Technologies and Home Modifications" is excerpted from "Accelerating Adoption of Assistive Technology to Reduce Physical Strain among Family Caregivers of the Chronically Disabled Elderly Living at Home. Appendix B. Family Caregiver Guide to Assistive Technologies and Home Modifications," Office of the Assistant Secretary for Planning and Evaluation (ASPE), January 12, 2012. Reviewed November 2019; Text under the heading "How to Treat People with Illnesses and Disabilities" is excerpted from "How to Treat People with Illnesses and Disabilities," girlshealth.gov, Office on Women's Health (OWH), October 31, 2013. Reviewed November 2019.

- Lonely because you think no one gets what you are going through or because you feel that you do not get to spend much time with your parents or guardians
- Jealous of all the attention your sister or brother gets

You may also feel:

- Proud of your sister or brother
- Glad that you have the chance to be helpful to someone who needs it
- Having such different emotions all at the same time might seem strange. But, all these feelings are normal

## FAMILY CAREGIVER GUIDE TO ASSISTIVE TECHNOLOGIES AND HOME MODIFICATIONS

Caregivers give much-needed support for older adults with disabilities or illness living at home. But, often caregiving can be a physical strain. When you take care of yourself, you can better help your family member or friend. Many assistive technologies (AT) and home modifications (HM) may help make life easier for you and protect your safety and the safety of your family member.

### Example AT/HM Needed by Family Caregivers and Older Adults

- Bathing/toileting aids: grab bars, raised toilet seats, shower benches
- AT/HM for mobility: wheelchairs, walkers, canes, ramps, stairlifts
- Transfer aids: lifting devices, hoists
- Electronic systems for health record tracking, care coordination, emergency response, monitoring
- Devices for dressing, food preparation (shoe horns, jar openers)
- Hearing and vision aids
- Medical supplies (incontinence supplies)
- AT for cognitive impairments (activities, games, devices for memory and communication)
- Medication management aids (automated dispensers, pillboxes)
- Home repairs-repairing handrails, floors for safety
- Home renovations: downstairs bedroom, downstairs bathroom, ramp
- No-cost home mods (removing clutter or home hazards)
- Vehicle mods/accessible car

## HOW TO TREAT PEOPLE WITH ILLNESSES AND DISABILITIES

Treat a friend with a disability or illness just like you would any other friend. Your friend may want to talk about their condition; then again, your friend may not. You can let them know you care by telling them you will listen any time they feel like talking. If you are meeting someone new, you may need to figure out how to act. You can ask the person if she wants any help and talk about the usual things you talk about with anyone new.

## How to Treat Someone with a Health Issue

- Before you give help, ask if the person needs it. The person may want to do things for herself/himself.
- It is okay to ask friends or classmates about their illnesses or disabilities. But, do not be offended if your friend does not want to talk about it.
- Do not be afraid to ask questions if you are not sure how to act.
- Invite friends or classmates with illnesses or disabilities to sleepovers and birthday parties, and to hang out. Think about ways to make sure they can be included in the things you do.
- Ask your parents not to park in places reserved for people with disabilities.
- When you go to restaurants and shopping malls, check to see if a friend with an illness or disability could be there with you. If not, you can be a good friend by asking the manager to put in ramps, get raised numbers for the elevators, or have Braille menus printed.
- Kids with illnesses or disabilities can have it tough sometimes. Be friendly and welcoming to them. And if you see them being bullied, get help.

## How to Handle Specific Disabilities

- Remember that just because people use wheelchairs, it does not mean they are sick. Many people who use wheelchairs are otherwise healthy and strong.
- When you are talking with a friend in a wheelchair, try to come down to her or his level—kneel down or pull up a chair.
- Do not lean on a wheelchair or touch it without asking. Do not push it without asking either.
- It is okay to use words such as "see," "hear," "walk," and "run" when you are talking with friends who have disabilities.
- It is okay to ask people who have speech problems to repeat what they said if you did not understand the first time. You can also try repeating what you think they said and they can reply "yes" or "no."
- If you are talking with someone who has a speech problem, try to ask questions that require only short answers or a nod of the head.
- If an interpreter is helping you speak to a person with hearing disability, talk to the person with hearing disability, not the interpreter.
- If a hearing person with a disability is going to be reading your lips, they need to see your face. Make sure you have their attention before

you start talking. Keep your hands away from your face and avoid chewing gum. Use short, simple sentences. You might try writing instead if that is easier.

- Do not speak loudly when talking to people with visual disabilities. They hear as well as you do.
- If you need to guide a person with a visual disability, give the person your arm instead of grabbing on to them.
- When you are talking with a person with a visual disability, tell her/him when you are leaving or she/he would not know.
- Do not pet or play with service dogs without first asking the owner if it is okay.
- Remember that just because a person has a learning disability, it does not mean they are stupid. They could be really bright and just may learn differently from you.
- When you are talking with someone with limited intellectual abilities, be patient. Give that person time to process what you have said and respond. You might keep your sentences short and simple. If you are in a public area with many distractions, consider moving to a quiet or private location.
- If an adult has an intellectual disability, still treat them as an adult.

# Chapter 35 | Change in Family Relationships after a Disability

## WHAT DO YOU NEED TO KNOW?

The changes in your loved one will affect the entire family. Tasks they once did may no longer be possible. You and other family members may be faced with responsibilities. These could include housework, yard work or managing money.

Some family members may not be able or willing to help. This is often difficult to accept. Some people have a harder time than others dealing with illness. Some may be overwhelmed with taking on tasks. Try to forgive those who cannot help. With time, they may come around. Seek help from other family members and friends. Talk to your healthcare team about other resources in your area.

## WHAT IS YOUR LOVED ONE'S ROLE IN THE FAMILY?

Your loved one may be different physically, mentally and emotionally. A lot may have changed. What has not changed is that your loved one is still part of the family. Even if your loved one cannot fulfill past roles, she or he can still contribute.

- Find roles and things that your loved one can do—This will boost confidence.
- Encourage your loved one to do as much as possible—Help when you need to. But, avoid being too protective.
- Be patient—The stroke can make it hard to do simple tasks.
- Help your loved one relearn skills in small steps—Start with easy tasks. Slowly, add skills.
- Have a daily routine—Allow short, frequent times in the day to practice skills.

This chapter includes text excerpted from "RESCUE Factsheet—Changes in Relationships," U.S. Department of Veterans Affairs (VA), January 5, 2011. Reviewed November 2019.

## WHAT IS THE EFFECT ON FAMILY RELATIONSHIPS?

The stress of caregiving can strain family relationships. Family members may need to sacrifice time and money to help with care. This can lead to feelings of anger and resentment. Arguments over care and money can cause misunderstandings and hurt feelings.

## HELPFUL TIPS TO IMPROVE FAMILY RELATIONSHIPS

- **Hold family meetings**—Come together to discuss concerns. Be open and honest about your feelings. Allow others to do the same.
- **Show appreciation**—Caregiving can be a thankless job at times. Be sure to tell each other thank you. Everyone deserves to feel appreciated.
- **Work together**—Include family members in decision making. They will be more likely to want to be involved in care.

## WHAT IS THE EFFECT ON RELATIONSHIPS WITH FRIENDS?

Recovery is a long and often slow process. After the crisis stage is over, people return to their own lives. Friends may not call or come by as often. Some may assume that you do not need to be bothered. Others may be afraid of how to interact with the stroke survivor.

Caregiving can be a lonely job. It is hard for anyone who is not going through it to understand. Friends may want to help but may not know-how. Reach out to your friends. Tell your friends specific ways they can help. If your friends shy away, find others who can support you. Start by finding a support group for caregivers in your area.

# Chapter 36 | Impact of Disability on Society

More than 20 million of the 69.6 million families in the United States include at least one family member who has a disability. Specific psychological, social, political, and economic factors impact these individuals with a disability, their families, and their communities, and increase the likelihood of impoverishment, social exclusion, and limited accessibility.

When someone has a functional disability, social participation is possible only when the environment is supportive. If there is a lack of environmental support, then the distance between what the environment offers and what this person needs in order to participate fully creates obstacles that prevents full participation.

## FAMILY

Families that live with and care for a person with a disability are impacted in both positive and negative ways. Disability sometimes creates stronger bonds between family members, but can also strain relationships between spouses and other parent-child relationships. Families often face a lifetime of added expenses associated with the disorder too, as well as caregiver fatigue.

## RISK OF POVERTY

A study conducted by the London School of Commerce confirmed that presence of a disability increases the risk of impoverishment. The risk of individuals with a disability and their family members slipping into poverty is twice that of a individuals without a disability or household. Lack of paid employment is the primary cause of this risk. And, while the Americans with Disability Act (ADA) prohibits discrimination against people with disabilities, a disproportionate number of people with a disability nevertheless struggle to find meaningful employment.

## SOCIAL EXCLUSION

Communication differences, social norms, and individual comfort levels can contribute to an environment in which a person with a disability faces social exclusion and shunning.

In ancient cultures, a person with a disability was often shunned, left in the forest, or sent to a mental institution. Many villagers believed that people with a disability were possessed by evil spirits or that the disability was punishment for their parents' sins.

The Rehabilitation Act of 1973 enshrined into law the civil rights of disabled Americans, yet many people with a disability still face significant restrictions and discrimination in their day-to-day lives.

Factors that impact how people view disabilities include:

- **Ableism:** A form of discrimination that favors able-bodied people over people with a disability
- **Attitudes:** A form of discrimination in which a person's biases negatively color their reactions to and acceptance of people with a disability
- **Stereotypes:** A fixed or oversimplified bias about people with a disability that results in a generalized negative view about all people with a disability
- **Stigma:** A social marker, attitude, and/or belief that sets individuals with a disability apart from others and encourages prejudice, discrimination, and shunning

## ATTITUDES AND AWARENESS

Disability is a legal classification applied to disorders that is employed to justify and allocate specific services, resources, and advocacy efforts. This classification system, however, sometimes leads others to assume that all people with the same disability share the exact same abilities, experiences, and characteristics.

## CHALLENGING ATTITUDES

There are many ways to shift individual and public biases toward people with disabilities. Practicing the following strategies requires little effort but makes a big difference in the lives of people with a disability:

- Treat each individual with equal respect. A disability does not define a person's character and each of us is worthy of the same respect.
- Educate people who share negative and offensive views about people with a disability.
- Interact with people with a disability. Ask them about their disability. Most of people with a disability will not mind sharing this information with you.

### Impact of Disability on Society

- Increase your knowledge about disabilities and the struggles that people with disabilities face. This will help you to better understand the obstacles, challenges, and hassles faced in the day-to-day life of people with a disability.

The best way to spread awareness and educate a large number of people is through participating in advocacy activities and efforts to raise awareness.

## References


1. "Impairment, Disability, or Handicap?" World Health Organization (WHO), March 12, 2014.
2. Josephine, Alexa. "Social Impacts of Disability," The Classroom, December 19, 2003.

# Chapter 37 | Health Promotion in People with Disability

The Centers for Disease Control and Prevention's (CDC) Disability and Health Branch currently provides funds to two National Centers on Disability under the cooperative agreement CDC-RFA-DD16-1602, entitled National Centers on Health Promotion for People with Disabilities. This is a 5-year project, from April 1, 2016, to March 31, 2021. The purpose of this cooperative agreement is to fund and support national organizations that work with people with mobility limitations and/or intellectual disabilities and have national reach through a network of 15 or more state/local programs, chapters and/or affiliates across the United States. The National Centers on Disability develop, implement, evaluate, and report on activities aimed at reducing health differences between people with and without disabilities, and improving the health of people with mobility limitations and/or intellectual disabilities across their lifespans.

## NATIONAL CENTER ON HEALTH, PHYSICAL ACTIVITY, AND DISABILITY

The National Center on Health, Physical Activity and Disability (NCHPAD) primarily focus on improving the health, wellness, and quality of life of people with disabilities. NCHPAD supports local, state and national organizations in adopting guidelines, recommendations and adaptations that promote the inclusion of children and adults with mobility limitations in public health practices. Specifically, NCHPAD's goal is to develop the infrastructure to support the accessibility and inclusion of people with disabilities in existing and future public health promotion programs geared toward improving their physical activity, nutrition, and healthy weight management.

This chapter includes text excerpted from "National Centers on Health Promotion for People with Disabilities," Centers for Disease Control and Prevention (CDC), October 28, 2019.

### Key Activities:

The Centers for Disease Control and Prevention and NCHPAD will work together to:

- Identify models, programs, practices, and policies that have been shown to work, and adapt them for children and adults with mobility limitations
- Develop customized training materials to teach partners about the tools and resources that accommodate people with different types of mobility limitations
- Help local providers implement adaptations to their existing programs, practices, strategies, and services
- Expand and publicize the best practices related to inclusive physical activity, nutrition, and obesity prevention strategies in community settings

## SPECIAL OLYMPICS

Special Olympics provides year-round sports training and athletic competition in a variety of Olympic type sports for children and adults with intellectual disabilities. Special Olympics provides athletes with continuing opportunities to develop physical fitness, demonstrate courage, experience joy, and participate in a sharing of gifts, skills, and friendships with their peers, families, and the broader community. CDC's Disability and Health Branch has funded the Special Olympics Healthy Athletes® (since 2002) and Healthy Communities (starting in 2012) programs to provide Special Olympics athletes with increased access to free health screenings, education, and referrals for follow-up healthcare, as well as year-round health promotion and disease prevention programs.

### Key Activities:

The Centers for Disease Control and Prevention and Special Olympics work together to:

- Train healthcare professionals to conduct and support Healthy Athletes® screening events throughout the United States, which provide free health screenings, education, and referrals for Special Olympics athletes who need follow-up healthcare
- Increase the availability of data during and after screening events to enhance the capacity to evaluate effectiveness; this can be achieved by improving data collection through the use of digital health technology
- Provide disability awareness training to healthcare professionals, community wellness partners, schools, and other collaborators who have limited or no experience working with people with intellectual disabilities

# Chapter 38 | Use of Yoga, Meditation, and Chiropractic for Physical Limitations

Yoga is an ancient spiritual practice that emerged in India from six philosophical schools of thought, or Shastras. The traditional purpose of yoga has been the attainment of self-knowledge by transcendence of the ego, characterized by inward transformation. Research confirms that yoga can offer people who are disabled overall health benefits and help to prevent disease when it is practiced alongside other regular medical treatments and therapies. Yoga should also be practiced in combination with a healthy diet and exercise.

Yoga is practiced as a spiritual discipline in Hinduism, Buddhism, and Jainism, each of which focus on self-enlightenment, or self-actualization, as the ultimate goal in life. There are many different styles of yoga—Anusara, Ashtanga, Bikram, Hatha, Iyengar, Jivamukti, Kripalu, Kundalini, Sivananda, and Vinyasa; however, Hatha yoga is one of the most popular forms practiced in the West.

## HATHA YOGA

Hatha yoga is known as a "discipline of force." The style is primarily known for its therapeutic value of bringing healing to the mind and the body. The practice emphasizes mastery over the body by achieving a spiritual state in which the mind is withdrawn from external factors. Hatha yoga helps practitioners develop strength, flexibility, relaxation, and mental concentration.

Hatha yoga involves postures and asanas that stem from ancient beliefs. The asanas are ideal for meditation and help the body rise above bodily consciousness. It is important to maintain a straight spine while practicing postures and asanas, as this allows the energy to flow freely upward and a state of immobility causes one to become aware of the inner energies of the body.

## HEALTH BENEFITS OF YOGA

Research has confirmed the benefits of yoga for people with a disability, including the following:

- Yoga is considered safe for people with high blood pressure, heart disease, and body aches and pains—including lower back pain.
- Yoga significantly decreases the secretion of cortisol—the hormone responsible for stress—and improves overall mental health.
- Research has shown that, among those practicing yoga, feelings of anxiety have been drastically reduced.
- Yoga improves heart health by lowering cholesterol levels. When complemented by changes in diet and lifestyle, yoga can also lower blood pressure and reduce the risk of heart disease.
- Findings also show that yoga can reduce chronic inflammation.
- Yoga helps to improve the quality of sleep, reduces pain and fatigue, and enhances your spiritual well-being.
- Studies have shown that yoga improves the physical function of people affected by arthritis and joint-related pain.
- Yoga improves flexibility and balance and, when incorporated with breathing exercises, improves lung function.
- There is increasing evidence that yoga can help to relieve migraines when the vagus nerve is stimulated.
- Some studies have shown that yoga can be an effective method for practicing mindfulness and helping to control one's eating habits.
- Yoga increases strength in the upper body, builds endurance, and helps in weight loss.

## YOGA INSTRUCTION FOR CHILDREN WITH DISABILITIES

Yoga is also proven to be therapeutic for children with disabilities, especially those with Down syndrome, cerebral palsy, autism, attention deficiency disorder (ADD), attention deficit hyperactivity disorder (ADHD), and learning difficulties.

### References

1. "13 Benefits of Yoga That Are Supported by Science," Healthline Media, n.d.
2. "Teaching Yoga to Children with Special Needs," Yoga U, n.d.
3. "Hatha Yoga," Ananda Sangha Worldwide, n.d.
4. "Yoga for Children and Young People's Mental Health and Well-Being: Research Review and Reflections on the Mental Health Potentials of Yoga," National Center for Biotechnology Information (NCBI), April 2, 2014.

5. "The Origin of Yoga in Daily Life," Yoga in Daily Life, n.d.
6. "Yoga—A Guide," Focus on Disability, n.d.
7. Pizer, Ann. "Most Popular Types of Yoga Explained," Verywell, May 25, 2018.

# Part 5 | Populations with Distinctive Physical Rehabilitation Concerns

# Chapter 39 | How to Exercise with Limited Mobility

Everybody, including people with disabilities, needs physical activity for good health. However, nearly half of adults with disabilities who are able to be physically active do not get any aerobic physical activity.

Physical activity plays an important role in maintaining health, well-being, and quality of life (QOL). According to the 2008 Physical Activity Guidelines for Americans (PAG), physical activity can help control weight, improve mental health, and lower the risk for early death, heart disease, type 2 diabetes, and some cancers. For people with disabilities, it can help improve the ability to do activities of daily living and be self-sufficient.

In the United States, about one in five people have a disability. A disability is any condition of the body or mind that makes it more difficult for the person with the condition to do certain activities and interact with the world around them. Disability does not equal poor health, and most adults with disabilities are able to participate in regular physical activity and avoid being inactive. However, nearly half of all adults with disabilities do not get any aerobic physical activity. Aerobic physical activity is when the body's large muscles move in a rhythmic manner for a sustained period of time, thus improving heart and lung fitness. Examples of aerobic activities that might be available to adults with disabilities include walking, water aerobics, swimming, hand-crank bicycling, and various wheelchair athletics.

## HEALTHCARE PROVIDERS PLAY A ROLE

Healthcare providers are in a key position to influence physical activity participation among their adult patients with disabilities. First, adults with disabilities are more likely than those without disabilities to visit a healthcare provider on a regular basis. In addition, they are more likely to be physically active if their provider recommends it.

This chapter includes text excerpted from "Physical Activity Is for Everybody," Centers for Disease Control and Prevention (CDC), October 18, 2017.

Here are some easy steps healthcare providers can follow to encourage people with disabilities to be physically active:

## Remember That Physical Activity Guidelines Are for Everybody

- Doctors and other health professionals should recommend physical activity, based on the 2008 Physical Activity Guidelines, to their patients with disabilities. Adults of all sizes and abilities can benefit from being physically active, including those with disabilities.
- Adults should get at least 2-½ hours of aerobic physical activity each week at a moderate-intensity level.
- When adults with disabilities are not able to meet the above guidelines, they should engage in regular physical activity according to their abilities and should avoid being inactive.

## Ask about Physical Activity

Doctors will ask the following questions regarding physical activity participation by their patients with disabilities:

- How much physical activity are you currently doing each week?
    - How often?
    - How long?
    - At what intensity level?
- What types of physical activity do you enjoy, now or in the past?
- How can you add more physical activity to your life?

## Discuss Barriers to Physical Activity

Adults with disabilities face barriers to getting aerobic physical activity. Discuss the following barriers with your patients with disabilities to help them find ways to be more active:

- Knowing about and getting to programs, places, and spaces where they can be physically active;
- Having social support for physical activity (such as, setting up a buddy system, making contracts with others to complete specified levels of physical activity, or setting up walking groups or other groups to provide friendship and support);
- Having limited information about accessible facilities and programs; and
- Finding fitness and health professionals who can provide physical activity options that match their specific abilities.

## Recommend Physical Activity Options

- Engage in the amount and types of physical activity that are right for them;

## How to Exercise with Limited Mobility

- Find opportunities to increase regular physical activity in ways that meet their needs and abilities;
- Start slowly, based on their abilities and fitness level (for example, be active for at least 10 minutes at a time, and slowly increase activity over several weeks, if necessary);
- Include aerobic physical activities that make them breathe harder and their heart beat faster for important health benefits, such as reducing the risk of heart disease, stroke, diabetes, and some cancers;
- Know that most aerobic physical activities may need to be modified, adapted, or may need additional assistance or equipment; and
- Avoid being physically inactive. Some physical activity is better than none.

# Chapter 40 | Early Intervention among Children

## WHAT IS EARLY INTERVENTION?

- Early intervention is the term used to describe the services and supports that are available to babies and young children with developmental delays and disabilities and their families.
- Early intervention may include speech therapy, physical therapy, and other types of services based on the needs of the child and family.
- Early intervention can have a significant impact on a child's ability to learn skills and overcome challenges and can increase success in school and life.
- Early intervention programs are available in every state and territory. These publicly funded programs provide services for free or at a reduced cost for any child who is eligible.

## HOW DO I FIND OUT IF MY CHILD IS ELIGIBLE FOR SERVICES?

Eligibility for early intervention services is based on an evaluation of your child's skills and abilities.

If you, your child's doctor, or other care provider is concerned about your child's development, ask to be connected with your state or territory's early intervention program to find out if your child can get services to help. If your doctor is not able to connect you, you can reach out to yourself. A doctor's referral is not necessary.

This chapter contains text excerpted from the following sources: Text beginning with the heading "What Is Early Intervention?" is excerpted from "What Is Early Intervention?" Centers for Disease Control and Prevention (CDC), February 8, 2019; Text beginning with the heading "Talk to Your Child's Doctor" is excerpted from "Concerned about Your Child's Development?" Centers for Disease Control and Prevention (CDC), February 8, 2019.

- If your child is under age 3: Call your state or territory's early intervention program and say: "I have concerns about my child's development and I would like to have my child evaluated to find out if she/he is eligible for early intervention services."
- Children 3 years old or older: If your child is age 3 or older, call any local public elementary school (even if your child does not go to school there) and say: "I have concerns about my child's development and I would like to have my child evaluated through the school system for preschool special education services." If the person who answers is unfamiliar with preschool special education, ask to speak with the school or district's special education director.

## TALK TO YOUR CHILD'S DOCTOR

As a parent, you know your child best. If your child is not meeting the milestones for her or his age, or if you think there could be a problem with the way your child plays, learns, speaks, acts, and moves; talk to your child's doctor and share your concerns. Do not wait. Acting early can make a real difference!

## ASK FOR A REFERRAL

If you or the doctor think there might be a delay, ask the doctor for a referral to a specialist who can do a more in-depth evaluation of your child.

Doctors your child might be referred to include:

- **Developmental pediatricians.** These doctors have special training in child development and children with special needs.
- **Child neurologists.** These doctors work on the brain, spine, and nerves
- **Child psychologists or psychiatrists.** These doctors know about the human mind.

# Chapter 41 | **Physical Activity during Pregnancy**

Physical activity during pregnancy benefits a woman's overall health. Moderate-intensity physical activity by healthy women during pregnancy increases or maintains cardiorespiratory fitness, reduces the risk of excessive weight gain and gestational diabetes, and reduces symptoms of postpartum depression. Reduced risk of excessive weight gain during pregnancy can also reduce the risk of excessive postpartum weight retention, future obesity, and an infant born with high birth weight. Strong scientific evidence shows that the risks of moderate-intensity activity done by healthy women during pregnancy are very low, and do not increase risk of low birth weight, preterm delivery, or early pregnancy loss. Some evidence suggests that physical activity may reduce the risk of pregnancy complications, such as preeclampsia, reduce the length of labor and postpartum recovery, and reduce the risk of having a cesarean section.

During a normal postpartum period, regular physical activity continues to benefit a woman's overall health. Studies show that moderate-intensity physical activity during the period following the birth of a child increases a woman's cardiorespiratory fitness and improves her mood. Such activity does not appear to have adverse effects on breast milk volume, breast milk composition, or infant growth.

Physical activity also helps women achieve and maintain a healthy weight during the postpartum period and, when combined with caloric restriction, helps promote weight loss.

This chapter contains text excerpted from the following sources: Text in this chapter begins with excerpts from "Physical Activity Guidelines for Americans—2nd Edition," Office of Disease Prevention and Health Promotion (ODPHP), U.S. Department of Health and Human Services (HHS), December 15, 2015. Reviewed November 2019; Text beginning with the heading "Keeping Fit during Pregnancy" is excerpted from "Staying Healthy and Safe," Office on Women's Health (OWH), U.S. Department of Health and Human Services (HHS), March 14, 2019; Text beginning with the heading "Follow These Tips When You Do Muscle Strengthening Activities" is excerpted from "Stay Active during Pregnancy: Quick Tips," Office of Disease Prevention and Health Promotion (ODPHP), U.S. Department of Health and Human Services (HHS), June 24, 2019.

## KEY GUIDELINES FOR WOMEN DURING PREGNANCY AND THE POSTPARTUM PERIOD

- Women should do at least 150 minutes (2 hours and 30 minutes) of moderate-intensity aerobic activity a week during pregnancy and the postpartum period. Preferably, aerobic activity should be spread throughout the week.
- Women who habitually engaged in vigorous-intensity aerobic activity or who were physically active before pregnancy can continue these activities during pregnancy and the postpartum period.
- Women who are pregnant should be under the care of a healthcare provider who can monitor the progress of the pregnancy. Women who are pregnant can consult their healthcare provider about whether or how to adjust their physical activity during pregnancy and after the baby is born.

Women who are pregnant should be under the care of a healthcare provider with whom they can discuss whether or how to adjust their physical activity during pregnancy and after the baby is born. Unless a woman has medical reasons to avoid physical activity during pregnancy or the postpartum period, she can begin or continue light intensity to moderate-intensity aerobic and muscle-strengthening physical activity. When beginning physical activity during pregnancy, women should increase the amount of physical activity gradually over time. Women who habitually did vigorous-intensity activity or a lot of aerobic or muscle-strengthening physical activity before pregnancy can continue to be physically active during pregnancy and after giving birth. They generally do not need to drastically reduce their activity levels, provided that they remain healthy and discuss with their healthcare provider whether and how to adjust activity levels during this time.

During pregnancy, perceived exertion is often a better indicator of intensity than heart rate or estimated absolute energy requirements of specific activities. On a rating of perceived exertion scale of 0 to 10, where 0 is sitting and 10 is the greatest effort possible, moderate-intensity activity would be an effort of 5 to 6. Another way to gauge moderate intensity is with a talk test, where carrying on a conversation (but not singing) is still possible. Women should avoid doing exercises that involve lying on their back after the first trimester of pregnancy because this position can restrict blood flow to the uterus and fetus. They should also avoid participating in contact or collision sports and activities with high risk of falling or abdominal trauma, such as soccer, basketball, horseback riding, or downhill skiing.

## KEEPING FIT DURING PREGNANCY

Fitness goes hand in hand with eating right to maintain your physical health and well-being during pregnancy. Pregnant or not, physical fitness helps keep the heart, bones, and mind healthy. Healthy pregnant women should get at least 2 hours and 30 minutes of moderate-intensity aerobic activity a week. It is best to spread your workouts throughout the week. If you regularly engage in a vigorous-intensity aerobic activity or high amounts of activity, you can keep up your activity level as long as your health does not change and you talk to your doctor about your activity level throughout your pregnancy.

### Special Benefits of Physical Activity during Pregnancy

- Exercise can ease and prevent aches and pains of pregnancy including constipation, varicose veins, backaches, and exhaustion.
- Active women seem to be better prepared for labor and delivery and recover more quickly.
- Exercise may lower the risk of preeclampsia and gestational diabetes during pregnancy.
- Fit women have an easier time getting back to a healthy weight after delivery.
- Regular exercise may improve sleep during pregnancy.
- Staying active can protect your emotional health. Pregnant women who exercise seem to have better self-esteem and a lower risk of depression and anxiety.
- Results from a large study suggest that women who are physically active during pregnancy may lower their chances of preterm delivery.

## GETTING STARTED

For most healthy moms to be who do not have any pregnancy-related problems, exercise is a safe and valuable habit. Even so, talk to your doctor or midwife before exercising during pregnancy. She or he will be able to suggest a fitness plan that is safe for you. Getting a doctor's advice before starting a fitness routine is important for both inactive women and women who exercised before pregnancy.

If you have one of these conditions, your doctor will advise you not to exercise:

- Risk factors for preterm labor
- Vaginal bleeding
- Premature rupture of membranes (when your water breaks early, before labor)

## BEST ACTIVITY FOR PREGNANT WOMEN

Low impact activities at a moderate level of effort are comfortable and enjoyable for many pregnant women. Walking, swimming, dancing, cycling, and low impact aerobics are some examples. These sports also are easy to take up, even if you are new to physical fitness.

Some higher intensity sports are safe for some pregnant women who were already doing them before becoming pregnant. If you jog, play racquet sports, or lift weights, you may continue with your doctor's okay.

Keep these points in mind when choosing a fitness plan:

- Avoid activities in which you can get hit in the abdomen such as kickboxing, soccer, basketball, or ice hockey.
- Steer clear of activities in which you can fall such as horseback riding, downhill skiing, and gymnastics.
- Do not scuba dive during pregnancy. Scuba diving can create gas bubbles in your baby's blood that can cause many health problems.

## TIPS TO BE SAFE AND HEALTHY PHYSICAL ACTIVITY

Follow these tips for safe and healthy fitness:

- When you exercise, start slowly, progress gradually, and cool down slowly.
- You should be able to talk while exercising. If not, you may be overdoing it.
- Take frequent breaks.
- Do not exercise on your back after the first trimester. This can put too much pressure on an important vein and limit blood flow to the baby.
- Avoid jerky, bouncing, and high impact movements. Connective tissues stretch much more easily during pregnancy. So these types of movements put you at risk of joint injury.
- Be careful not to lose your balance. As your baby grows, your center of gravity shifts making you more prone to falls. For this reason, activities such as jogging, using a bicycle, or playing racquet sports might be riskier as you near the third trimester.
- Do not exercise at high altitudes (more than 6,000 feet). It can prevent your baby from getting enough oxygen.
- Make sure you drink lots of fluids before, during, and after exercising.
- Do not workout in extreme heat or humidity.
- If you feel uncomfortable, short of breath, or tired, take a break and take it easier when you exercise again.

Stop exercising and call your doctor as soon as possible if you have any of the following:

- Dizziness
- Headache
- Chest pain
- Calf pain or swelling
- Abdominal pain

- Blurred vision
- Fluid leaking from the vagina
- Vaginal bleeding
- Less fetal movement
- Contractions

## WORK OUT YOUR PELVIC FLOOR (KEGEL EXERCISES)

Your pelvic floor muscles support the rectum, vagina, and urethra in the pelvis. Toning these muscles with Kegel exercises will help you push during delivery and recover from birth. It also will help control bladder leakage and lower your chance of getting hemorrhoids.

Pelvic muscles are the same ones used to stop the flow of urine. Still, it can be hard to find the right muscles to squeeze. You can be sure you are exercising the right muscles if when you squeeze them you stop urinating. Or you can put a finger into the vagina and squeeze. If you feel pressure around the finger, you have found the pelvic floor muscles. Try not to tighten your stomach, legs, or other muscles.

Kegel exercises:

1. Tighten the pelvic floor muscles for a count of three, then relax for a count of three.
2. Repeat 10 to 15 times, 3 times a day.
3. Start Kegel exercises lying down. This is the easiest position. When your muscles get stronger, you can do Kegel exercises sitting or standing as you like.

## FOLLOW THESE TIPS WHEN YOU DO MUSCLE STRENGTHENING ACTIVITIES

- Do not strain to lift heavy weights. Instead, do more repetitions (lifts) with lighter weights. You can also use water bottles or cans of food as weights.
- Make sure you are not holding your breath. Breathe out as you lift the weight, and breathe in as you lower it.

## AVOID HIGH-RISK ACTIVITIES

- Avoid doing any activities while lying on your back after the first trimester (12 weeks).
- Stay away from activities that increase your risk of falling, such as downhill skiing or horseback riding.
- Avoid playing sports where you could get hit in the stomach, such as basketball or soccer.
- Do not scuba dive while you are pregnant.

# Chapter 42 | The Importance of Sports for People with a Disability

Recruitment is one of the biggest challenges regarding physical activity programs for people with disabilities. With the help of a fitness coordinator and student disability services, a variety of adaptive programs—chair aerobics, yoga, aquatics, archery, rock climbing, skiing, and an introduction to wheelchair basketball were developed at the Kent State University (KSU). Hardly any of the students voluntarily signed up for any of the programs, and the rest had to be encouraged. Some students were simply not interested in these types of activities, but others, just had a lack of knowledge—not knowing these programs existed, and not knowing that they could participate in sports and exercise activities even if they do have a physical disability. Also, sports and exercise are generally introduced early to children. But, due to the competitive nature of sports, children with disabilities often did not get to reap the benefits of physical activity at all or were exposed to them much later in their lives.

Temple University in Philadelphia has one of the most creative programming ideas. It is called the "workout buddy program," and is one of the many available from their adaptive recreation department. The goal of the workout buddy program is to provide an opportunity for students with disabilities to experience various sports and exercise activities. Students with disabilities who want to participate are partnered up with a fellow student or volunteer, and they participate together in whatever activity they choose— tandem walking/jogging, hand-cycling, aquatics, weight training, cardiovascular conditioning, etc.

This chapter contains text excerpted from the following sources: Text in this chapter begins with excerpts from "Encouraging Individuals with Disabilities to Participate in Physical Activity," Office of Disease Prevention and Health Promotion (ODPHP), U.S. Department of Health and Human Services (HHS), August 31, 2011. Reviewed November 2019; Text beginning with the heading "Physical Activity Comes in Many Forms" is excerpted from "Sports and Recreation," girlshealth.gov, Office on Women's Health (OWH), December 26, 2014. Reviewed November 2019.

Since many individuals with disabilities are not aware of adaptive sports/recreation programs, there needs to be introductory programs that expose young individuals with disabilities to various physical activities. They also need to learn about how exercise and sports can benefit them physically and emotionally, and understand that participating in physical activity improves their health and well-being. Universities and colleges in particular should be providing such programs for their students since the setting is ideal for fostering new experiences and self-growth.

## PHYSICAL ACTIVITY COMES IN MANY FORMS

Types of exercise include:

- Swimming laps
- Taking a walk
- Playing wheelchair basketball
- Walking up the stairs

## IMPORTANT PHYSICAL ACTIVITY TIPS

Before you start any physical activity program, talk to your doctor to make sure that it is okay. Your doctor will help you be active in the safest way possible.

Make sure you stop being physically active or playing a sport if you feel pain, feel sick, feel dizzy, or are short of breath.

Make sure to drink plenty of water before, during, and after you are physically active.

## HOW TO FIND ACTIVITIES AND SPORTS

Your community probably has many places where you can take part in activities you love and even try new ones. To start, call your city's recreation department, your own school, health clubs, the local girls scout council, and nearby colleges. They might have pools, sports teams, exercise rooms, and more. You can also call the local Chamber of Commerce to find out where else you can find programs in your area.

Another place to try calling is your nearby Center for Independent Living (CIL). CILs are agencies staffed mainly by people with disabilities. They know all about resources in your community for people with disabilities.

## QUESTIONS TO ASK ABOUT FITNESS OR EXERCISE PROGRAMS

- Where are you located?
- What sports teams, games, programs, or exercise equipment do you offer?
- How much does it cost?
- How can I apply for financial help if I need it?
- What are the times and dates of your programs?

- How do you register?
- Are your facilities and programs accessible to people with disabilities?
- Do you have any adaptive equipment or tools that people with disabilities can use?
- Do you have anyone on the staff who can help people with disabilities use your facilities? (These people are sometimes called "inclusion aides.")
- Do you have any programs that are just for people with disabilities?
- Can teenagers use the facility?

## TIPS FOR PLAYING SPORTS DIFFERENTLY TO MEET YOUR NEEDS

- **Soccer**: Walk instead of running if you need to, or hold the ball in your lap if you use a wheelchair.
- **Volleyball**: Use a larger ball that is softer or brightly colored, or allow the ball to bounce on the ground before hitting it.
- **Bowling**: Use two hands instead of one, or use a ramp.
- **Tennis**: Use a racquet with a large head, or do not use a net.

For many sports, you could try using an inclusion aide. An inclusion aide is a person who helps people with disabilities participate in sports and other activities. For example, if you are interested in horseback riding but have an illness or disability that makes this hard for you to do alone, an inclusion aide would assist you.

# Chapter 43 | Early Mobilization and Rehabilitation in Critically Ill Patients

## THE IMPORTANCE OF EARLY MOBILITY IN THE INTENSIVE CARE UNIT

A high proportion of survivors of critical illness suffer from significant physical, cognitive, and psychological disabilities. Profound neuromuscular weakness secondary to critical illness, prolonged bed rest, and immobility leads to impaired physical function. Physical impairment affects approximately 50 percent of the intensive care unit (ICU) patients, with at least half of discharged patients unable to return to premorbid levels of activity. Cognitive impairment, including impaired executive function, memory, language, and attention, is widespread; almost 80 percent of ICU survivors suffer from cognitive impairment early after discharge, with deficits often lasting from months to years. The prevalence of psychiatric morbidity, including clinically significant depression, anxiety, and posttraumatic stress disorder, remains high among ICU survivors. Evidence suggests that mobilization mitigates the physical, cognitive, and psychological complications of critical illness. Mobilization has also been linked to decreased time on the ventilator, decreased hospital length of stay and improved functional outcomes. The mobilization of ICU patients is safe and feasible. However, ICU patients are typically perceived as being too sick to tolerate activity. As a result, they have limited exposure to physical rehabilitation. In addition to this culture

This chapter contains text excerpted from the following sources: Text under the heading "The Importance of Early Mobility in the Intensive Care Unit" is excerpted from "Early Mobility Guide for Reducing Ventilator-Associated Events in Mechanically Ventilated Patients," Agency for Healthcare Research and Quality (AHRQ), U.S. Department of Health and Human Services (HHS), January 2017; Text under the heading "Key Interventions of Early Mobility" is excerpted from "Introduction and Evidence for Early Mobility: A Protocol to Get Patients Out of Bed Faster: Facilitator Guide," Agency for Healthcare Research and Quality (AHRQ), U.S. Department of Health and Human Services (HHS), February 2017.

of immobility, variability in research and published protocols make translating evidence into practice challenging. The implementation of an early mobilization program requires a multidisciplinary approach, including collaboration between nurses, rehabilitation therapists, respiratory therapists, physicians, and administrators. This chapter integrates available resources to help you educate and engage all stakeholders, proposes protocols to standardize the screening and mobilization of your patients, and provide tools to collect data and evaluate your progress.

## KEY INTERVENTIONS OF EARLY MOBILITY

These are the five key daily early mobility interventions that can be used to improve the mobilization of your mechanically ventilated patients. These interventions begin with using a multidisciplinary and coordinated approach that includes the joint participation of nurses, doctors, physical, occupational, and respiratory therapists, and technicians and administrators to create what the Society of Critical Care Medicine calls, "a culture of mobility." This approach also works to achieve consistent mobility for all of your patients.

The second intervention is interrupting daily sedation and minimizing sedative use. Heavily sedated patients are not able to safely participate in a mobility program, and so targeting light sedation and interrupting sedation daily enable them to remain alert and cooperative.

Using structured assessments of sedation and delirium through validated scales might more effectively target light sedation levels for your patient and mitigate and treat delirium. By doing this, patients can be effectively and reliably mobilized.

The fourth intervention is to screen every day for the highest level of mobility your patients achieve. Implementing a standard algorithm to screen patients can help determine which patients may safely participate in a mobilization program.

And then the final intervention: employing a nurse-driven protocol to achieve the highest level of mobility. As we know, traditionally nurses mobilize patients once they have recovered from their acute illness. However, shifting the focus of nurse-driven mobilization to the phase of acute illness when they are very sick and integrating a systematic protocol into routine nursing care can promote recovery.

# Chapter 44 | Physical Therapy for Healthy Aging

Regular physical activity is essential for healthy aging. Adults aged 65 years and older gain substantial health benefits from regular physical activity, and these benefits continue to occur throughout their lives. Promoting physical activity for older adults is especially important because this population is the least physically active of any age group.

Older adults are a varied group. Most, but not all, have one or more chronic conditions, and these conditions vary in type and severity. All have experienced a loss of physical fitness with age, some more than others. This diversity means that some older adults can run several miles, while others struggle to walk several blocks.

## KEY GUIDELINES FOR OLDER ADULTS

The following guidelines are the same for adults and older adults:

- All older adults should avoid inactivity. Some physical activity is better than none, and older adults who participate in any amount of physical activity gain some health benefits.
- For substantial health benefits, older adults should do at least 150 minutes (2 hours and 30 minutes) a week of moderate-intensity, or 75 minutes (1 hour and 15 minutes) a week of vigorous-intensity aerobic physical activity, or an equivalent combination of moderate and vigorous-intensity aerobic activity. Aerobic activity should be performed in episodes of at least 10 minutes, and preferably, it should be spread throughout the week.
- For additional and more extensive health benefits, older adults should increase their aerobic physical activity to 300 minutes (5 hours) a week of moderate-intensity, or 150 minutes a week of vigorous-intensity aerobic physical activity, or an equivalent combination of moderate

This chapter includes text excerpted from "Active Older Adults," Office of Disease Prevention and Health Promotion (ODPHP), U.S. Department of Health and Human Services (HHS), October 7, 2008. Reviewed November 2019.

and vigorous-intensity activity. Additional health benefits are gained by engaging in physical activity beyond this amount.
- Older adults should also do muscle-strengthening activities that are moderate or high intensity and involve all major muscle groups on 2 or more days a week, as these activities provide additional health benefits.

The following Guidelines are just for older adults:
- When older adults cannot do 150 minutes of moderate-intensity aerobic activity a week because of chronic conditions, they should be as physically active as their abilities and conditions allow.
- Older adults should do exercises that maintain or improve balance if they are at risk of falling.
- Older adults should determine their level of effort for physical activity relative to their level of fitness.
- Older adults with chronic conditions should understand whether and how their conditions affect their ability to do regular physical activity safely.

## HOW MUCH TOTAL ACTIVITY A WEEK?

Older adults should aim to do at least 150 minutes (2 hours and 30 minutes) of moderate-intensity physical activity a week, or an equivalent amount (75 minutes or 1 hour and 15 minutes) of vigorous-intensity activity. Older adults can also do an equivalent amount of activity by combining moderate and vigorous-intensity activity. As is true for younger people, greater amounts of physical activity provide additional and more extensive health benefits to people aged 65 years and older.

No matter what its purpose—walking the dog, taking a dance or exercise class, or bicycling to the store—aerobic activity of all types counts toward the Guidelines.

## MUSCLE-STRENGTHENING ACTIVITIES

At least two days a week, older adults should do muscle-strengthening activities that involve all the major muscle groups. These are the muscles of the legs, hips, chest, back, abdomen, shoulders, and arms.

Muscle-strengthening activities make muscles do more work than they are accustomed to during activities of daily life. Examples of muscle-strengthening activities include lifting weights, working with resistance bands, doing calisthenics using body weight for resistance (such as push-ups, pull-ups, and sit-ups), climbing stairs, carrying heavy loads, and heavy gardening.

Muscle-strengthening activities count if they involve a moderate to a high level of intensity, or effort, and work the major muscle groups of the body.

Whatever the reason for doing it, any muscle-strengthening activity counts toward meeting the guidelines. For example, muscle-strengthening activity done as part of a therapy or rehabilitation program can count. No specific amount of time is recommended for muscle strengthening, but muscle-strengthening exercises should be performed to the point at which it would be difficult to do another repetition without help. When resistance training is used to enhance muscle strength, one set of 8 to 12 repetitions of each exercise is effective, although 2 or 3 sets may be more effective. The development of muscle strength and endurance is progressive over time. This means that gradual increases in the amount of weight or the days per week of exercise will result in stronger muscles.

## BALANCE ACTIVITIES FOR OLDER ADULTS AT RISK OF FALLS

Older adults are at increased risk of falls if they have had falls in the recent past or have trouble walking. In older adults at increased risk of falls, strong evidence shows that regular physical activity is safe and reduces the risk of falls. Reduction in falls is seen for participants in programs that include balance and moderate-intensity muscle-strengthening activities for 90 minutes (1 hour and 30 minutes) a week plus moderate-intensity walking for about 1 hour a week.

Preferably, older adults at risk of falls should do balance training 3 or more days a week and do standardized exercises from a program demonstrated to reduce falls. Examples of these exercises include backward walking, sideways walking, heel walking, toe walking, and standing from a sitting position. The exercises can increase in difficulty by progressing from holding onto stable support (like furniture) while doing the exercises to doing them without support. It is not known whether different combinations of type, amount, or frequency of activity can reduce falls to a greater degree. Tai chi exercises also may help prevent falls.

## INACTIVE OLDER ADULTS

Older adults should increase their amount of physical activity gradually. It can take months for those with a low level of fitness to gradually meet their activity goals. To reduce injury risk, inactive or insufficiently active adults should avoid vigorous aerobic activity at first. Rather, they should gradually increase the number of days a week and duration of moderate-intensity aerobic activity. Adults with a very low level of fitness can start out with episodes of activity less than 10 minutes and slowly increase the minutes of light-intensity aerobic activity, such as light-intensity walking.

Older adults who are inactive or who do not yet meet the Guidelines should aim for at least 150 minutes a week of relatively moderate-intensity physical activity. Getting at least 30 minutes of relatively moderate-intensity physical activity on 5 or more days each week is a reasonable way to meet these Guidelines. Doing muscle-strengthening activity on 2 or 3 nonconsecutive days each week is also an acceptable and appropriate goal for many older adults.

## ACTIVE OLDER ADULTS

Older adults who are already active and meet the Guidelines can gain additional and more extensive health benefits by moving beyond the 150 minutes a week minimum to 300 or more minutes a week of relatively moderate-intensity aerobic activity. Muscle-strengthening activities should also be done at least 2 days a week.

# Part 6 | **Rehabilitation for Major Diseases or Conditions**

# Chapter 45 | Cancer

## ONCOLOGY PROGRAM

The oncology program is designed to address the rehabilitation needs of cancer patients. Approximately 50 percent of the referrals to physical therapy are from the National Cancer Institute (NCI). Physicians and therapists treat patients involved in Phase 1 research studies, where scientists are determining the safety of medications to Phase 4 research studies, where safety and efficacy of chemotherapeutic agents are established. Services are provided to reduce the impairments of cancer, improve patient function and minimize disability. These services improve quality of life (QOL) as they relate to rehabilitation medicine and physical therapy.

## IS PHYSICAL ACTIVITY BENEFICIAL FOR CANCER SURVIVORS?

Research indicates that physical activity may have beneficial effects on several aspects of cancer survivorship specifically, weight gain, quality of life, cancer recurrence or progression, and prognosis (likelihood of survival). Most of the evidence for the potential benefits of physical activity in cancer survivors comes from people diagnosed with breast, prostate, or colorectal cancer.

### Weight Gain

Both reduced physical activity and the side effects of cancer treatment can contribute to weight gain after a cancer diagnosis. In a cohort study (a type of epidemiologic study), weight gain after breast cancer diagnosis was linked to worse survival. In a 2012 meta-analysis of randomized controlled clinical trials examining physical activity in cancer survivors, physical activity was found to reduce both body mass index and body weight.

This chapter contains text excerpted from the following sources: Text under the heading "Oncology Program" is excerpted from "Physical Therapy—Clinical Services," Clinical Center (CC), National Institutes of Health (NIH), August 7, 2019; Text beginning with the heading "Is Physical Activity Beneficial for Cancer Survivors?" is excerpted from "Physical Activity and Cancer," National Cancer Institute (NCI), January 27, 2017; Text beginning with the heading "What Is Palliative Care?" is excerpted from "Palliative Care in Cancer," National Cancer Institute (NCI), October 20, 2017; Text under the heading "Exercise Rehabilitation in Patients with Cancer" is excerpted from "Exercise Rehabilitation in Patients with Cancer," U.S. Department of Health and Human Services (HHS), March 6, 2012.

## Quality of Life

A 2012 Cochrane Collaboration systematic review of controlled clinical trials of exercise interventions in cancer survivors indicated that physical activity may have beneficial effects on overall health-related QOL and on specific QOL issues, including body image/self-esteem, emotional well-being, sexuality, sleep disturbance, social functioning, anxiety, fatigue, and pain. In a 2012 meta-analysis of randomized controlled trials examining physical activity in cancer survivors, physical activity was found to reduce fatigue and depression and to improve physical functioning, social functioning, and mental health.

## Recurrence, Progression, and Survival

Being physically active after a cancer diagnosis is linked to better cancer-specific outcomes for several cancer types.

### Breast Cancer

Consistent evidence from epidemiologic studies link physical activity after diagnosis with better breast cancer outcomes. For example, a large cohort study found that women who exercised moderately (the equivalent of walking 3 to 5 hours per week at an average pace) after a breast cancer diagnosis had approximately 40 to 50 percent lower risk of breast cancer recurrence, death from breast cancer, and death from any cause compared with more sedentary women. The potential physical activity benefit with regard to death from breast cancer was most apparent in women with hormone receptor-positive tumors.

Another prospective cohort study found that women who had breast cancer and who engaged in recreational physical activity roughly equivalent to walking at an average pace of 2 to 2.9 mph for 1 hour per week had a 35 to 49 percent lower risk of death from breast cancer compared with women who engaged in less physical activity.

### Colorectal Cancer

Evidence from multiple epidemiologic studies suggests that physical activity after a colorectal cancer diagnosis is associated with reduced risks of dying from colorectal cancer. In a large prospective cohort of patients with colorectal cancer, those who engaged in leisure-time physical activity had a 31 percent lower risk of death than those who did not, independent of their leisure-time physical activity before diagnosis.

### Prostate Cancer

Limited evidence from a few epidemiologic studies have suggested a possible link between physical activity and better outcomes among men diagnosed with prostate cancer. In onstudy, men with nonmetastatic prostate cancer who engaged in vigorous activity for at least 3 hours per week had a 61 percent lower risk of death from prostate cancer compared with men who engaged in vigorous activity for less than 1 hour per week. Another study of men with localized prostate cancer found that higher levels of physical activity were associated with reduced overall and prostate cancer-specific mortality.

Findings from epidemiologic studies cannot completely exclude reverse causation as a possible explanation of the link between physical activity and better cancer outcomes. That is, people who feel good are more likely to exercise and be physically active than people who do not feel good.

## WHAT IS KNOWN ABOUT THE RELATIONSHIP BETWEEN PHYSICAL ACTIVITY AND CANCER RISK?

There is substantial evidence that higher levels of physical activity are linked to lower risks of several cancers.

### Colon Cancer

Colon cancer is one of the most extensively studied cancers in relation to physical activity. A 2009 meta-analysis of 52 epidemiologic studies that examined the association between physical activity and colon cancer risk found that the most physically active individuals had a 24 percent lower risk of colon cancer than those who were the least physically active. A pooled analysis of data on leisure-time physical activity (activities done at an individual's discretion generally to improve or maintain fitness or health) from 12 prospective U.S. and European cohort studies reported a risk reduction of 16 percent when comparing individuals who were most active to those where least active. Incidence of both distal colon and proximal colon cancers is lower in people who are more physically active than in those who are less physically active. Physical activity is also associated with a decreased risk of colon adenomas (polyps), a type of colon polyp that may develop into colon cancer. However, it is less clear whether physical activity is associated with lower risks that polyps that have been removed will come back.

### Breast Cancer

Many studies show that physically active women have a lower risk of breast cancer than inactive women; in a 2013 meta-analysis of 31 prospective studies, the average breast cancer risk reduction associated with physical activity was 12 percent. Physical activity has been associated with a reduced risk of breast cancer in both premenopausal and postmenopausal women; however, the evidence for an association is stronger for postmenopausal breast cancer. Women who increase their physical activity after menopause may also have a lower risk of breast cancer than women who do not.

### Endometrial Cancer

Many studies have examined the relationship between physical activity and the risk of endometrial cancer (cancer of the lining of the uterus). In a meta-analysis of 33 studies, the average endometrial cancer risk reduction associated with high versus low physical activity was 20 percent. There is some evidence that the association between physical activity and endometrial cancer risk may reflect the effect of physical activity on obesity, a known risk factor for endometrial cancer.

For a number of other cancers, there is more limited evidence of a relationship with physical activity. In a study of over 1 million individuals, leisure-time physical activity was linked to reduced risks of esophageal adenocarcinoma, liver cancer, gastric cardia cancer (a type of stomach cancer), kidney cancer, myeloid leukemia, myeloma, and cancers of the head and neck, rectum, and bladder. These results are generally corroborated by large cohort studies or meta-analyses.

Nearly all of the evidence linking physical activity to cancer risk comes from observational studies, in which individuals report on their physical activity and are followed for years for diagnoses of cancer. Data from observational studies can give researchers clues about the relationship between physical activity and cancer risk, but such studies cannot definitively establish that being physically inactive causes cancer (or that being physically active protects against cancer). That is because people who are not physically active may differ from active people in ways other than their level of physical activity. These other differences, rather than the differences in physical activity, could explain their different cancer risk. For example, if someone does not feel well, they may not exercise much, and sometimes people do not feel well because they have undiagnosed cancer.

## HOW MIGHT PHYSICAL ACTIVITY BE LINKED TO REDUCED RISKS OF CANCER?

Exercise has a number of biological effects on the body, some of which have been proposed to explain associations with specific cancers, including:

- Lowering the levels of hormones, such as insulin and estrogen, and of certain growth factors that have been associated with cancer development and progression
- Helping to prevent obesity and decreasing the harmful effects of obesity, particularly the development of insulin resistance (failure of the body's cells to respond to insulin)
- Reducing inflammation
- Improving immune system function
- Altering the metabolism of bile acids, resulting in decreased exposure of the gastrointestinal (GI) tract to these suspected carcinogens
- Reducing the amount of time it takes for food to travel through the digestive system, which decreases GI tract exposure to possible carcinogens.

## WHAT IS PALLIATIVE CARE?

Palliative care is care given to improve the quality of life of patients who have a serious or life-threatening disease, such as cancer. Palliative care is an approach to care that addresses the person as a whole, not just their disease. The goal is to prevent or treat, as early as possible, the symptoms and side effects of the disease and its treatment, in addition to any related psychological, social, and spiritual problems. Palliative care is also called "comfort care," supportive care, and symptom management. Patients may receive palliative care in the hospital, an outpatient clinic, a long-term care facility, or at home under the direction of a physician.

## WHO GIVES PALLIATIVE CARE?

Palliative care is usually provided by palliative care specialists, healthcare practitioners who have received special training and/or certification in palliative care. They provide holistic care to the patient and family or caregiver focusing on the physical, emotional, social, and spiritual issues cancer patients may face during the cancer experience.

Often, palliative care specialists work as part of a multidisciplinary team that may include doctors, nurses, registered dieticians, pharmacists, chaplains, psychologists, and social workers. The palliative care team works in conjunction with your oncology care team to manage your care and maintain the best possible quality of life for you.

Palliative care specialists also provide caregiver support, facilitate communication among members of the healthcare team, and help with discussions focusing on goals of care for the patient.

## WHAT ISSUES ARE ADDRESSED IN PALLIATIVE CARE?

The physical and emotional effects of cancer and its treatment may be very different from person to person. Palliative care can address a broad range of issues, integrating an individual's specific needs into care. A palliative care specialist will take the following issues into account for each patient:

- **Physical.** Common physical symptoms include pain, fatigue, loss of appetite, nausea, vomiting, shortness of breath, and insomnia.
- **Emotional and coping.** Palliative care specialists can provide resources to help patients and families deal with the emotions that come with a cancer diagnosis and cancer treatment. Depression, anxiety, and fear are only a few of the concerns that can be addressed through palliative care.
- **Spiritual.** With a cancer diagnosis, patients and families often look more deeply for meaning in their lives. Some find the disease brings them closer to their faith or spiritual beliefs, whereas others struggle to

understand why cancer happened to them. An expert in palliative care can help people explore their beliefs and values so that they can find a sense of peace or reach a point of acceptance that is appropriate for their situation.

- **Caregiver needs.** Family members are an important part of cancer care. Like the patient, they have changing needs. It is common for family members to become overwhelmed by the extra responsibilities placed upon them. Many find it hard to care for a sick relative while trying to handle other obligations, such as work, household duties, and caring for other family members. Uncertainty about how to help their loved one with medical situations, inadequate social support, and emotions such as worry and fear can also add to caregiver stress.
- **These challenges can compromise caregivers' own health.** Palliative care specialists can help families and friends cope and give them the support they need.
- **Practical needs.** Palliative care specialists can also assist with financial and legal worries, insurance questions, and employment concerns. Discussing the goals of care is also an important component of palliative care. This includes talking about advance directives and facilitating communication among family members, caregivers, and members of the oncology care team.

## WHEN IS PALLIATIVE CARE USED IN CANCER CARE?

Palliative care may be provided at any point along the cancer care continuum, from diagnosis to the end of life. When a person receives palliative care, she or he may continue to receive cancer treatment.

## EXERCISE REHABILITATION IN PATIENTS WITH CANCER

Emerging evidence indicates that patients with cancer have considerable impairments in cardiorespiratory fitness, which is likely to be a result of the direct toxic effects of anticancer therapy as well as the indirect consequences secondary to therapy (for example, deconditioning). This reduced cardiorespiratory fitness is associated with heightened symptoms, functional dependence, and possibly with an increased risk of cardiovascular morbidity and mortality. Current understanding of the complex interaction between the effects of the tumor and cancer-associated therapies on the organ components that govern cardiorespiratory fitness, and the effects of exercise training on these parameters is limited; further research will be critical for further progress of exercise-based rehabilitation in the oncology setting. The efficacy and adaptations to exercise training to prevent and/or mitigate dysfunction in conjunction with exercise prescription considerations for clinical use are also discussed.

## Cancer

Structured exercise training is established as the cornerstone of primary and secondary disease prevention in multiple clinical settings. In stark contrast, the role of exercise following a diagnosis of cancer has, until recently, received comparably less attention. The precise reasons for this are unknown but likely stem from the prevailing dogma that a cancer diagnosis is associated with poor prognosis, immune deficiency, and other severe debilitating side effects that preclude participation in, and benefit from, exercise training. Modern cancer management typically involves aggressive and prolonged combination locoregional and/or systemic therapy that causes a plethora of acute and long-term toxic effects leading to considerable functional morbidity and an increased risk of mortality from noncancer-related causes. Exercise training is a pleiotropic therapeutic strategy with the capacity to act across multiple organ systems to facilitate attenuation and/or prevention of cancer therapy-associated morbidity as well as improve clinical outcomes in patients with cancer. The purpose of this article is to review the current evidence regarding the level, mechanisms, and clinical importance of diminished cardiorespiratory fitness in patients with cancer.

# Chapter 46 | Depression Associated with Injury

It is common for patients to suffer from depression in the aftermath of an injury that involves a lengthy recovery time. The symptoms of depression usually present in the patient either immediately or within the first year following an injury.

Evidence shows that people who have a well-balanced life and are surrounded by friends and family are less likely to succumb to postinjury depression than people who have less support. Patients who suffer from mild anxiety and mood swings are also more prone to depression following an injury. A patient's psychological well-being is not always considered as part of a treatment plan for a physical injury, yet psychological care is vital to a person who has suffered a life-threatening injury and psychological well-being impacts a patient's ability to recover.

## EFFECTS OF DEPRESSION

The more a person's identity is based on their physical form or ability, the higher their chances of suffering from acute postinjury depression. Physical injuries can affect a person's day-to-day life by constraining their physical functionality.

This in turn affects a person's mental well-being and can lead to depression. The injury may also trigger certain other mental-health issues, such as addiction, changes in sleep patterns, loss of appetite, a lack of motivation, and anxiety and panic attacks. Depression also is more likely to affect women, due to hormones and other biological factors. Athletes are also more likely to suffer a decrease in self-esteem and self-worth following a physical injury. In rare cases, postinjury depression can even be fatal and lead to suicide.

## SYMPTOMS OF POSTINJURY DEPRESSION

The major characteristics of postinjury depression are persistent feelings of sadness and general discontent. If left untreated, postinjury depression can result in a range of behavioral changes and physical symptoms including:

- Chronic anxiety

- Loss of concentration
- Decline in self-esteem
- Reduced sexual interest
- Isolation
- Feelings of despair and loneliness
- Harmful coping strategies
- Increasing fatigue
- Insomnia or hypersomnia (difficulty falling/staying asleep or excessive sleeping)
- Suicidal thoughts
- Significant weight loss

## OVERCOMING DEPRESSION

With appropriate psychological care, a person can recover from mental stress in the aftermath of an injury and before it turns into long-term depression. Since depression is often accompanied by psychological myopia, which focuses a patient's thinking on negative thoughts, one path to healing involves shifting the focus to pleasant memories instead of dwelling on painful recollections of the injury. Concentrating on the future and directing one's thoughts toward getting better also has a positive effect on people dealing with postinjury depression.

## ACCEPTANCE

Acceptance and commitment therapy (ACT) has proven to enhance psychological coping during sports-injury rehabilitation. It is crucial to understand that healing takes time and that it is acceptable to rest while your body recuperates. Engaging yourself in tasks that you are capable of doing will help you make use of your time, establish routines, and help you feel productive.

## MEDITATION AND MINDFULNESS

It is vital to calm and relax yourself when dealing with postinjury depression. Meditation helps reduce mental stress and can be vital in helping to optimize your body's healing process. You can also cope with depression by being mindful and self-aware of your present situation. This may involve writing down your feelings or starting a journal. You also can occupy yourself with a good book to keep your mind focused.

## SUPPORT

Activities that were easily performed when one was healthy can become difficult to perform in the aftermath of a physical injury that compromises one's normal functional capability. If you require help, either emotional or physical, do not hesitate to ask for it. Try to be as socially active as possible and engage in activities that make you feel connected socially.

## PROFESSIONAL HELP

It is important to seek professional help if your depression spirals out of control or lasts for more than six weeks. Studies show that psychological interventions by trained mental-health professionals are known to improve self-esteem and stabilize moods, which in turn can help you heal physically within a shorter period of time.

## TREATMENT OPTIONS

Various forms of treatment options are available for treating postinjury depression, including:

- **Psychotherapy.** Psychotherapy involves changing your thinking patterns and learning the coping and stress-reduction skills that are needed to help you overcome your depression. Cognitive behavioral therapy (CBT) is a form of psychotherapy that deals specifically with modifying dysfunctional behaviors, emotions, and thoughts. CBT focuses on the attitudes and beliefs of the patient and helps in the development of personal coping strategies. Using CBT alongside interpersonal psychotherapy provides optimal results.
- **Medications.** Antidepressants and other suitable drugs are designed to help restore emotional balance and relieve feelings of anxiety and restlessness. Your doctor may prescribe one or more of these drugs to alleviate the symptoms of depression. Drugs alone cannot be used as a permanent cure for depression, however. Instead, they must be used in addition to therapies such as CBT. Your medication also must be monitored by a doctor. Significant improvement may be observed anywhere from three to six months after starting such therapy.
- **Peer support.** Participating in a support group can provide you with beneficial emotional support. Support groups can be found either in your local area or on online forums. Social contact is of immense importance for the maintenance of good health. It improves your general outlook and enhances your ability to cope with depression.

Depression associated with injuries can be diagnosed and treated. Collaborative interventions, when administered at the appropriate time, maximize functional outcomes in affected people and enable them to return to their preinjury level of functioning as early as possible.

### References

1. Muska, Scott. "What a Physical Injury Taught Me about My Mental Health," NBC News Digital, October 23, 2017.
2. "Injury and Depression—How Connected Is the Body and Mind?" Harley Therapy Blog, November 30, 2017.

3. "How to Battle Depression during Injury," Lotsa Helping Hands, April 11, 2015.
4. "How to Overcome Depression after a Sports Injury," U.S. News, July 21, 2014.
5. Richmond, Therese S. "The Effect of Post-Injury Depression on Return to Pre-Injury Function: A Prospective Cohort Study," March 2, 2009.
6. "12 Ways to Deal with Injury Depression," Tina Muir, April 17, 2017.
7. Smith, Kathleen. "Chronic Pain and Depression," Psycom.net, September 19, 2019.
8. Ellis, Rachel Reiff. "Post-Trauma Treatment: Healing More than the Body," WebMD, November 29, 2018.

# Chapter 47 | Obesity and Disability

## ABOUT OVERWEIGHT AND OBESITY

Overweight and obesity are both labels for ranges of weight that are greater than what is generally considered healthy for a given height. The terms also identify ranges of weight that have been shown to increase the likelihood of certain diseases and other health problems. Behavior, environment, and genetic factors can affect whether a person is overweight or obese.

### Adults

For adults, overweight and obesity ranges are determined by using weight and height to calculate a number called the "body mass index" (BMI). BMI is used because, for most people, it correlates with their amount of body fat.

- An adult who has a BMI between 25 and 29.9 is considered overweight.
- An adult who has a BMI of 30 or higher is considered obese.

### Children

Among children of the same age and sex, overweight is defined on the Centers for Disease Control and Prevention (CDC) growth charts as a BMI at or above the 85th percentile and lower than the 95th percentile. Obesity is defined as having a BMI at or above the 95th percentile.

## THE OBESITY EPIDEMIC

Obesity affects different people in different ways and may increase the risk for other health conditions among people with and without disabilities.

### People with Disabilities

- Children and adults with mobility limitations and intellectual or learning disabilities are at greatest risk for obesity.

This chapter includes text excerpted from "Disability and Obesity," Centers for Disease Control and Prevention (CDC), September 6, 2019.

- 20 percent of children 10 through 17 years of age who have special healthcare needs are obese compared with 15 percent of children of the same ages without special healthcare needs.
- Annual healthcare costs of obesity that are related to disability are estimated at approximately $44 billion.

### In the United States

- More than one-third of adults—more than 72 million people—are obese.
- Obesity rates are significantly higher among some racial and ethnic groups. Non-Hispanic Blacks or African Americans have a 51 percent higher obesity prevalence and Hispanics have a 21 percent higher obesity prevalence than Non-Hispanic Whites.
- A CDC Vital Signs report, titled "State-Specific Obesity Prevalence among Adults United States, 2009," points out that people who are obese incurred $1,429 per person extra in medical costs compared to people of normal weight.
- Annual healthcare costs of obesity for all adults in the United States were estimated to be as high as $147 billion dollars for 2008.

## CHALLENGES FACING PEOPLE WITH DISABILITIES

People with disabilities can find it more difficult to eat healthy, control their weight, and be physically active. This might be due to:

- A lack of healthy food choices
- Difficulty with chewing or swallowing food, or its taste or texture
- Medications that can contribute to weight gain, weight loss, and changes in appetite
- Physical limitations can reduce a person's ability to exercise
- Pain
- A lack of energy
- A lack of accessible environments (for example, sidewalks, parks, and exercise equipment) that can enable exercise
- A lack of resources (for example, money, transportation, and social support from family, friends, neighbors, and community members)

### What Can Be Done?

Obesity is a complex problem that requires a strong call for action, at many levels, for both adults as well as children. More efforts are needed, and federal initiatives are helping to change our communities into places that strongly support healthy eating and active living.

### Obesity and Disability

All people can:

- Eat more fruits and vegetables and fewer foods high in fat and sugar.
- Drink more water instead of sugary drinks.
- Watch less television.
- Support breastfeeding.
- Promote policies and programs at school, at work, and in the community that make the healthy choice the easy choice.
- Be more physically active.

## HEALTH CONSEQUENCES OF OVERWEIGHT AND OBESITY

Overweight and obesity increases the risk of a number of other conditions, including:

- Coronary heart disease (CHD)
- Type 2 diabetes
- Cancers (endometrial, breast, and colon)
- High blood pressure
- Lipid disorders (for example, high total cholesterol or high levels of triglycerides)
- Stroke
- Liver and gallbladder disease
- Sleep apnea and respiratory problems
- Osteoarthritis (OA) (a degeneration of cartilage and its underlying bone within a joint)
- Gynecological problems (abnormal periods, infertility)

# Chapter 48 | Vestibular and Balance Disorders

## WHAT IS A BALANCE DISORDER?

A balance disorder is a condition that makes you feel unsteady or dizzy. If you are standing, sitting, or lying down, you might feel as if you are moving, spinning, or floating. If you are walking, you might suddenly feel as if you are tipping over.

Everyone has a dizzy spell now and then, but the term "dizziness" can mean different things to different people. For one person, dizziness might mean a fleeting feeling of faintness, while for another it could be an intense sensation of spinning (vertigo) that lasts a long time.

About 15 percent of American adults (33 million) had a balance or dizziness problem in 2008. Balance disorders can be caused by certain health conditions, medications, or a problem in the inner ear or the brain. A balance disorder can profoundly affect daily activities and cause psychological and emotional hardship.

## WHAT ARE THE SYMPTOMS OF A BALANCE DISORDER?

If you have a balance disorder, your symptoms might include:

- Dizziness or vertigo (a spinning sensation)
- Falling or feeling as if you are going to fall
- Staggering when you try to walk
- Lightheadedness, faintness, or a floating sensation
- Blurred vision
- Confusion or disorientation

This chapter contains text excerpted from the following sources: Text beginning with the heading "What Is a Balance Disorder?" is excerpted from "Balance Disorders," National Institute on Deafness and Other Communication Disorders (NIDCD), March 6, 2018; Text under the heading "Science Capsule: Balance or Vestibular Disorders in Adults" is excerpted from "Science Capsule: Balance or Vestibular Disorders in Adults," National Institute on Deafness and Other Communication Disorders (NIDCD), January 27, 2017.

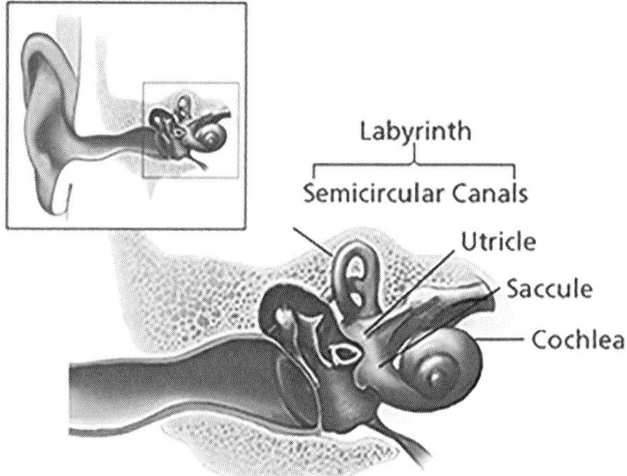


**Figure 48.1.** Structures of the Balance System inside the Inner Ear

## WHAT CAUSES BALANCE DISORDERS

Causes of balance problems include medications, ear infection, a head injury, or anything else that affects the inner ear or brain. Low blood pressure can lead to dizziness when you stand up too quickly. Problems that affect the skeletal or visual systems, such as arthritis or eye muscle imbalance, can also cause balance disorders. Your risk of having balance problems increases as you get older.

Unfortunately, many balance disorders start suddenly and with no obvious cause.

## WHAT ARE SOME TYPES OF BALANCE DISORDERS?

There are more than a dozen different balance disorders. Some of the most common are:

- **Benign paroxysmal positional vertigo (BPPV) or positional vertigo**: A brief, intense episode of vertigo triggered by a specific change in the position of the head. You might feel as if you are spinning when you bend down to look under something, tilt your head to look up or over your shoulder, or roll over in bed. BPPV occurs when loose otoconia tumble into one of the semicircular canals and affect how the cupula works. This keeps the cupula from flexing properly, sending incorrect information about your head's position to your brain, and causing vertigo. BPPV can result from a head injury, or can develop just from getting older.
- **Labyrinthitis**: An infection or inflammation of the inner ear that causes dizziness and loss of balance. It is often associated with an upper respiratory infection, such as the flu.

- **Ménière disease**: Episodes of vertigo, hearing loss, tinnitus (a ringing or buzzing in the ear), and a feeling of fullness in the ear. It may be associated with a change in fluid volume within parts of the labyrinth, but the cause or causes are still unknown.
- **Vestibular neuronitis**: An inflammation of the vestibular nerve that can be caused by a virus, and primarily causes vertigo.
- **Perilymph fistula**: A leakage of inner ear fluid into the middle ear. It causes unsteadiness that usually increases with activity, along with dizziness and nausea. Perilymph fistula can occur after a head injury, dramatic changes in air pressure (such as when scuba diving), physical exertion, ear surgery, or chronic ear infections. Some people are born with perilymph fistula.
- **Mal de Debarquement syndrome (MdDS)**: A feeling of continuously rocking, swaying, or bobbing, typically after an ocean cruise or other sea travel, or even after prolonged running on a treadmill. Usually, the symptoms go away within a few hours or days after you reach land or stop using the treadmill. Severe cases, however, can last months or even years, and the cause remains unknown.

## HOW ARE BALANCE DISORDERS DIAGNOSED?

Diagnosis of a balance disorder is difficult. To find out if you have a balance problem, your primary doctor may suggest that you see an otolaryngologist and an audiologist. An otolaryngologist is a physician and surgeon who specializes in diseases and disorders of the ear, nose, neck, and throat. An audiologist is a clinician who specializes in the function of the hearing and vestibular systems.

You may be asked to participate in a hearing examination, blood tests, a video nystagmogram (a test that measures eye movements and the muscles that control them), or imaging studies of your head and brain. Another possible test is called "posturography." For this test, you stand on a special movable platform in front of a patterned screen.

Posturography measures how well you can maintain steady balance during different platform conditions, such as standing on an unfixed, movable surface. Other tests, such as rotational chair testing, brisk head-shaking testing, or even tests that measure eye or neck muscle responses to brief clicks of sound, may also be performed. The vestibular system is complex, so multiple tests may be needed to best evaluate the cause of your balance problem.

## HOW ARE BALANCE DISORDERS TREATED?

The first thing an otolaryngologist will do if you have a balance problem is determine if another health condition or a medication is to blame. If so, your doctor will treat the condition, suggest a different medication, or refer you to a specialist if the condition is outside her or his expertise.

If you have BPPV, your otolaryngologist or audiologist might perform a series of simple movements, such as the Epley maneuver, to help dislodge the otoconia from the semicircular canal. In many cases, one session works; other people need the procedure several times to relieve their dizziness.

If you are diagnosed with Ménière disease, your otolaryngologist may recommend that you make some changes to your diet and, if you are a smoker, that you stop smoking. Antivertigo or antinausea medications may relieve your symptoms, but they can also make you drowsy. Other medications, such as gentamicin (an antibiotic) or corticosteroids may be used. Although gentamicin may reduce dizziness better than corticosteroids, it occasionally causes permanent hearing loss. In some severe cases of Ménière disease, surgery on the vestibular organs may be needed.

Some people with a balance disorder may not be able to fully relieve their dizziness and will need to find ways to cope with it. A vestibular rehabilitation therapist can help you develop an individualized treatment plan.

Talk to your doctor about whether it is safe to drive, and about ways to lower your risk of falling and getting hurt during daily activities, such as when you walk up or downstairs, use the bathroom or exercise. To reduce your risk of injury from dizziness, avoid walking in the dark. Wear low-heeled shoes or walking shoes outdoors. If necessary, use a cane or walker and modify conditions at your home and workplace, such as adding handrails.

## WHEN SHOULD I SEEK HELP IF I THINK I HAVE A BALANCE DISORDER?

To help you decide whether to seek medical help for dizziness or balance problems, ask yourself the following questions. If you answer "yes" to any of these questions, talk to your doctor:

- Do I feel unsteady?
- Do I feel as if the room is spinning around me, even for a very brief time?
- Do I feel as if I am moving when I know I am sitting or standing still?
- Do I lose my balance and fall?
- Do I feel as if I am falling?
- Do I feel lightheaded or as if I might faint?
- Do I have blurred vision?
- Do I ever feel disoriented—losing my sense of time or location?

## SCIENCE CAPSULE: BALANCE OR VESTIBULAR DISORDERS IN ADULTS

Balance disorders are associated, as mentioned, with falling, which is the leading cause of injury deaths among older adults. One in three Americans aged 65 and older falls each year, and falls can result in severe trauma and even loss of life. Each year, more than 4 million older U.S. adults go to emergency departments for fall-related injuries at a cost of $4 billion. The National Institute on Deafness and Other Communication Disorders (NIDCD) supports a longitudinal study that measures vestibular function in older adults. The NIDCD is also sponsoring the AVERT (Acute video-oculography for Vertigo in Emergency Rooms for rapid Triage) clinical trial to help diagnose vertigo, dizziness, and other balance problems. The team of researchers is using a diagnostic medical device (video-oculography, or VOG) in the triage of patients who go to an emergency room with complaints of vertigo and/or dizziness. The device measures abnormal eye movements to differentiate benign causes of the dizziness or imbalance from dangerous causes (like stroke). This study offers the potential for improving standard of care in the diagnosis and treatment of patients with vertigo or dizziness, leading to better outcomes at lower cost.

# Part 7 | **Disability Inclusion and Support Services**

# Chapter 49 | **Disability Inclusion**

### Chapter Contents

## Section 49.1 | What Is Disability Inclusion?

This section includes text excerpted from "Disability Inclusion," Centers for Disease Control and Prevention (CDC), September 4, 2019.

Including people with disabilities in everyday activities and encouraging them to have roles similar to their peers who do not have a disability is disability inclusion. This involves more than simply encouraging people; it requires making sure that adequate policies and practices are in effect in a community or organization.

Inclusion should lead to increased participation in socially expected life roles and activities—such as being a student, worker, friend, community member, patient, spouse, partner, or parent.

Socially expected activities may also include engaging in social activities, using public resources such as transportation and libraries, moving about within communities, receiving adequate healthcare, having relationships, and enjoying other day-to-day activities.

### DISABILITY INCLUSION AND THE HEALTH OF PEOPLE WITH DISABILITIES

Disability inclusion allows for people with disabilities to take advantage of the benefits of the same health promotion and prevention activities experienced by people who do not have a disability. Examples of these activities include:

- Education and counselling programs that promote physical activity, improve nutrition or reduce the use of tobacco, alcohol or drugs, and
- Blood pressure and cholesterol assessment during annual health exams, and screening for illnesses such as cancer, diabetes, and heart disease

Including people with disabilities in these activities begins with identifying and eliminating barriers to their participation.

### WHY IS THIS IMPORTANT?

Disability affects approximate 61 million, or nearly 1 in 4 (26%) people in the United States living in communities. Disability affects more than one billion people worldwide.

According to the United Nations Convention on the Rights of Persons with Disabilities, people "with disabilities include those who have long-term physical, mental, intellectual or sensory [such as hearing or vision] impairments which in interaction with various barriers may hinder their full and effective participation in society on an equal basis with others."

People with disabilities experience significant disadvantages when it comes to health, such as:

- Adults with disabilities are three times more likely to have heart disease, stroke, diabetes, or cancer than adults without disabilities.
- Adults with disabilities are more likely than adults without disabilities to be current smokers.
- Women with disabilities are less likely than women without disabilities to have received a breast cancer x-ray test (mammogram) during the past two years.

Although disability is associated with health conditions (such as arthritis, mental, or emotional conditions) or events (such as injuries), the functioning, health, independence, and engagement in society of people with disabilities can vary depending on several factors:

- Severity of the underlying impairment
- Social, political, and cultural influences and expectations
- Aspects of natural and built surroundings
- Availability of assistive technology and devices
- Family and community support and engagement

Disability inclusion means understanding the relationship between the way people function and how they participate in society and making sure everybody has the same opportunities to participate in every aspect of life to the best of their abilities and desires.

## Section 49.2 | **Disability Barriers to Inclusion**

This section includes text excerpted from "Common Barriers to Participation Experienced by People with Disabilities," Centers for Disease Control and Prevention (CDC), September 4, 2019.

Nearly everyone faces hardships and difficulties at one time or another. But, for people with disabilities, barriers can be more frequent and have greater impact. The World Health Organization (WHO) describes barriers as being more than just physical obstacles. Here is the WHO definition of barriers:

> Factors in a person's environment that, through their absence or presence, limit functioning and create disability. These include aspects such as:
>
> - A physical environment that is not accessible
> - Lack of relevant assistive technology (assistive, adaptive, and rehabilitative devices)
> - Negative attitudes of people towards disability

- Services, systems, and policies that are either nonexistent or that hinder the involvement of all people with a health condition in all areas of life

Often there are multiple barriers that can make it extremely difficult or even impossible for people with disabilities to function. Here are the seven most common barriers. Often, more than one barrier occurs at a time.

- Attitudinal
- Communication
- Physical
- Policy
- Programmatic
- Social
- Transportation

## ATTITUDINAL BARRIERS

Attitudinal barriers are the most basic and contribute to other barriers. For example, some people may not be aware that difficulties in getting to or into a place can limit a person with a disability from participating in everyday life and common daily activities. Examples of attitudinal barriers include:

- **Stereotyping**: People sometimes stereotype those with disabilities, assuming their quality of life (QOL) is poor or that they are unhealthy because of their impairments.
- **Stigma, prejudice, and discrimination**: Within society, these attitudes may come from people's ideas related to disability—People may see disability as a personal tragedy, as something that needs to be cured or prevented, as a punishment for wrongdoing, or as an indication of the lack of ability to behave as expected in society.

Society's understanding of disability is improving as we recognize "disability" as what occurs when a person's functional needs are not addressed in her or his physical and social environment. By not considering disability a personal deficit or shortcoming, and instead of thinking of it as a social responsibility in which all people can be supported to live independent and full lives, it becomes easier to recognize and address challenges that all people–including those with disabilities–experience.

## COMMUNICATION BARRIERS

Communication barriers are experienced by people who have disabilities that affect hearing, speaking, reading, writing, and or understanding, and who use different ways to communicate than people who do not have these disabilities. Examples of communication barriers include:

- Written health promotion messages with barriers that prevent people with vision impairments from receiving the message. These include:
  - Use of small print or no large-print versions of material, and
  - No Braille or versions for people who use screen readers.
- Auditory health messages may be inaccessible to people with hearing impairments, including—
  - Videos that do not include captioning, and
  - Oral communications without accompanying manual interpretation (such as American Sign Language).
- The use of technical language, long sentences, and words with many syllables may be significant barriers to understanding for people with cognitive impairments.

## PHYSICAL BARRIERS

Physical barriers are structural obstacles in natural or manufactured environments that prevent or block mobility (moving around in the environment) or access. Examples of physical barriers include:

- Steps and curbs that block a person with mobility impairment from entering a building or using a sidewalk
- Mammography equipment that requires a woman with mobility impairment to stand and
- Absence of a weight scale that accommodates wheelchairs or others who have difficulty stepping up

## POLICY BARRIERS

Policy barriers are frequently related to a lack of awareness or enforcement of existing laws and regulations that require programs and activities be accessible to people with disabilities. Examples of policy barriers include:

- Denying qualified individuals with disabilities the opportunity to participate in or benefit from federally funded programs, services, or other benefits
- Denying individuals with disabilities access to programs, services, benefits, or opportunities to participate as a result of physical barriers, and
- Denying reasonable accommodations to qualified individuals with disabilities, so they can perform the essential functions of the job for which they have applied or have been hired to perform

## PROGRAMMATIC BARRIERS

Programmatic barriers limit the effective delivery of a public-health or healthcare program for people with different types of impairments. Examples of programmatic barriers include:

- Inconvenient scheduling
- Lack of accessible equipment (such as mammography screening equipment)
- Insufficient time set aside for medical examination and procedures
- Little or no communication with patients or participants and
- Provider's attitudes, knowledge, and understanding of people with disabilities

## SOCIAL BARRIERS

Social barriers are related to the conditions in which people are born, grow, live, learn, work and age or social determinants of health that can contribute to decreased functioning among people with disabilities. Here are examples of social barriers:

- People with disabilities are far less likely to be employed. In 2017, 35.5 percent of people with disabilities, ages 18 to 64 years, were employed, while 76.5 percent of people without disabilities were employed, about double that of people with disabilities.
- Adults age 18 years and older with disabilities are less likely to have completed high school compared to their peers without disabilities (22.3% compared to 10.1%).
- People with disabilities are more likely to have income of less than $15,000 compared to people without disabilities (22.3% compare to 7.3%).
- Children with disabilities are almost four times more likely to experience violence than children without disabilities.

## TRANSPORTATION BARRIERS

Transportation barriers are due to a lack of adequate transportation that interferes with a person's ability to be independent and to function in society. Examples of transportation barriers include:

- Lack of access to accessible or convenient transportation for people who are not able to drive because of vision or cognitive impairments, and
- Public transportation may be unavailable or at inconvenient distances or locations

## Section 49.3 | **Disability and Health Inclusion Strategies**

This section includes text excerpted from "Disability and Health Inclusion Strategies," Centers for Disease Control and Prevention (CDC), September 4, 2019.

Inclusion of people with disabilities into everyday activities involves practices and policies designed to identify and remove barriers such as physical, communication, and attitudinal, that hamper individuals' ability to have full participation in society, the same as people without disabilities. Inclusion involves:

- Getting fair treatment from others (nondiscrimination)
- Making products, communications, and the physical environment more usable by as many people as possible (universal design)
- Modifying items, procedures, or systems to enable a person with a disability to use them to the maximum extent possible (reasonable accommodations) and
- Eliminating the belief that people with disabilities are unhealthy or less capable of doing things (stigma, stereotypes)

Disability inclusion involves input from people with disabilities, generally through disability-focused and independent living organizations, in a program or structural design, implementation, monitoring, and evaluation.

### NATIONAL POLICY AND LEGISLATION

Three federal laws protect the rights of people with disabilities and ensure their inclusion in many aspects of society:

- Section 504 of the Rehabilitation Act of 1973
- The Americans with Disabilities Act (ADA) of 1990, which was followed by the ADA Amendments Act of 2008 in an attempt to restore the original intent of the legislation
- The Patient Protection and Affordable Care Act in 2010

#### Section 504 of the Rehabilitation Act

Section 504 of the Rehabilitation Act of 1973 is a federal law that protects individuals from discrimination based on disability. The nondiscrimination requirements of the law apply to employers and organizations that receive financial assistance from federal departments or agencies. Section 504 forbids organizations and employers from denying individuals with disabilities an equal opportunity to receive program benefits and services. It defines the rights of individuals with disabilities to participate in, and have access to, program benefits and services.

## Americans with Disabilities Act

The Americans with Disabilities Act (ADA) of 1990, as amended, protects the civil rights of people with disabilities, and has helped remove or reduce many barriers for people with disabilities. The legislation required the elimination of discrimination against people with disabilities. The ADA has expanded opportunities for people with disabilities by reducing barriers, changing perceptions, and increasing participation in community life.

ADA guarantees equal opportunity for individuals with disabilities in several areas:

- Employment
- Public accommodations such as restaurants, hotels, theaters, doctors' offices, pharmacies, retail stores, museums, libraries, parks, private schools, and day care centers
- Transportation
- State and local government services
- Telecommunications such as telephones, televisions, and computers

## People with Disabilities and the Patient Protection and Affordable Care Act

On March 23, 2010, President Obama signed into law the Patient Protection and Affordable Care Act, commonly referred to as ACA.

For people with disabilities, the ACA:

- Provides more healthcare choices and enhanced protection for Americans with disabilities
- Provides new healthcare options for long-term support and services
- Improves the Medicaid home- and community-based services option
- Provides access to high-quality and affordable healthcare for many people with disabilities
- Mandates accessible preventive screening equipment
- Designates disability status as a demographic category and mandates data collection to assess health disparities

## UNIVERSAL DESIGN

The intent of universal design is to simplify life for everyone by making products, communications, and the physical environment more usable by as many people as possible at little or no extra cost. Universal design benefits people of all ages and abilities. The Center for Universal Design at North Carolina State University has developed seven principles for universal design:

- **Equitable use.** The design is useful and marketable to people with diverse abilities.

For example:

- Power doors with sensors at entrances that are convenient for all users

- **Flexibility in use.** The design accommodates a wide range of individual preferences and abilities.

  For example:

  - An automated teller machine (ATM) that has enhancements in the way it looks, feels, or sounds so that people with vision or hearing impairments can use it
  - A tapered card opening for ease in inserting or removing a bank card, and
  - A palm rest to aid those with arm mobility or strength limitations

- **Simple and intuitive use.** Use of the design is easy to understand, regardless of the user's experience, knowledge, language skills, or current concentration level.

  For example:

  - Including an instruction manual with clear drawings and no text

- **Perceptible information.** The design communicates necessary information effectively to the user, regardless of the current light, visual, or sound conditions or the person's abilities to read, see, or hear.

  For example:

  - Alarm systems that can be both seen and heard
  - Routinely making captioning available in all television or video presentations

- **Tolerance for error.** The design minimizes hazards and the harmful consequences of accidental or unintended actions.

  For example:

  - Ground-fault interrupter (GFI) electrical outlet that reduces the risk of shock in bathrooms and kitchens

- **Low physical effort.** The design can be used efficiently and comfortably with minimum fatigue.

  For example:

  - Easy-to-use handles that make opening doors easier for people of all ages and abilities

- **Size and space for approach and use.** Appropriate size and space is provided for approach, reach, manipulation, and use regardless of person's body size, posture, or mobility.

  For example:

  - Counters and service windows low enough for everyone to reach, including people who use wheelchairs

- Curb cuts or sidewalk ramps, essential for people in wheelchairs, but are used by all people, and also convenient for people pushing baby strollers

## ACCESSIBILITY

Accessibility is when the needs of people with disabilities are specifically considered, and products, services, and facilities are built or modified so that they can be used by people of all abilities. Here are a few examples of accessibility:

- Parking spaces are close to entrances
- Floor spaces and hallways are free of equipment and other barriers
- Staff and healthcare professionals can use sign language or have access to someone who can use sign language

## REASONABLE ACCOMMODATIONS

Accommodations are alterations that have been made to items, procedures, or systems that enable a person with a disability to use them to the maximum extent possible. An accommodation can also be a modification to an existing environment or process to increase the participation by an individual with an impairment or activity limitation. Braille, large print, or audiobooks are examples of accommodations for people who are blind or who have visual limitations otherwise. For people with a communication disability or who have difficulty hearing, accommodations may take the form of having an American Sign Language interpreter available during meetings or presentations or exchanging written messages. Communication accommodations do not have to be elaborated, but they must be able to convey information effectively.

# Section 49.4 | **Disability Inclusion in Programs and Activities**

This section includes text excerpted from "Including People with Disabilities in Public Health Programs and Activities," Centers for Disease Control and Prevention (CDC), September 4, 2019.

The Centers for Disease Control and Prevention (CDC) operates on the principle that people with disabilities are best served by public health when they are included in all public health programs and activities such as:

- Education and counseling programs that promote physical activity, improve nutrition or reduce the use of tobacco, alcohol or drugs

- Blood pressure and cholesterol assessment during annual health exams, and screening for illnesses such as cancer, diabetes, and heart disease

People with disabilities need public-health programs and healthcare services for the same reasons anyone does—to be healthy, active, and engaged as part of the community.

The CDC's approach is to:

- Work across public-health systems to encourage including accessibility features for all people with disabilities
- Focus on specific functional populations (for example, those with vision or hearing loss, or mobility limitation) as a whole, with accommodations as necessary
- Develop and implement public-health programs for people with specific conditions

A public-health strategy is to use prevention efforts to help make the broadest health impact possible on the health of populations, in this case, people with disabilities. Public health is directed at improving the health of communities or populations, and is distinguishable from clinical health, which is directed at the health of the individual.

## DISABILITY AND HEALTH PROGRAMS

The CDC supports state-based disability and health programs dedicated to improve the health of people with disabilities, which broadens expertise and information-sharing among states. Nineteen of these state-based programs promote equity in health, prevent chronic disease (such as diabetes, asthma, and high blood pressure), and increase the quality of life (QOL) for people with disabilities. Each program customizes its activities to meet its state's needs.

These state programs represent a network of standardized programs committed to helping people with disabilities benefit from public-health services to the greatest extent possible. The states serve as communities of practice and play a much-needed role in identifying effective practices, policies, and services for people with disabilities.

State-based disability and health programs also inform policy and practice. Such programs ensure that individuals with disabilities are included in disease prevention and health promotion activities within the state.

The purpose of the National Centers on Disability is to improve the quality of life of individuals living with disabilities by providing health information, education, and consultation to healthcare professionals, people with disabilities, caregivers, media, researchers, policymakers, and the public.

## Disability Inclusion

The National Centers on Disability accomplish these goals by implementing the following activities:

- Serve as a resource for increasing knowledge and changing attitudes and practices as it relates to people with disabilities
- Educate policymakers about differences in health among people with disabilities
- Build collaborations with consumers, local health organizations, the CDC, and other relevant partners
- Share information about programs, methods, materials, and lessons learned
- Measure and document the National Centers on Disability's impact using common methods of evaluation and reporting activities, such as the population reached by activities, and outcomes/impact indicators, and
- Identify the health needs of people with disabilities

# Chapter 50 | Rehabilitative and Assistive Technology

**Chapter Contents**

## Section 50.1 | **Assistive Technology: An Overview**

This section contains text excerpted from the following sources: Text in this section begins with excerpts from "Rehabilitative and Assistive Technology," *Eunice Kennedy Shriver* National Institute of Child Health and Human Development (NICHD), October 24, 2018; Text under the heading "Assistive Technology Program" is excerpted from "Assistive Technology," Administration for Community Living (ACL), September 4, 2019.

Rehabilitative and assistive technology refers to tools, equipment, or products that can help people with disabilities successfully complete activities at school, home, work, and in the community. Disabilities are disorders, diseases, health conditions, or injuries that affect a person's physical, intellectual, or mental well-being and functioning. Rehabilitative and assistive technologies can help people with disabilities function more easily in their everyday lives and can also make it easier for a caregiver to care for a person with disabilities. The term "rehabilitative technology" refers to aids that help people recover their functioning after injury or illness. "Assistive technologies" may be as simple as a magnifying glass to improve vision or as complex as a digital communication system.

Some of these technologies are made possible through rehabilitative engineering research, which applies engineering and scientific principles to study how people with disabilities function in society. It includes studying barriers and designing solutions so that people with disabilities can interact successfully in their environments.

The *Eunice Kennedy Shriver* National Institute of Child Health and Human Development (NICHD) houses the National Center for Medical Rehabilitation Research (NCMRR), which is charged with advancing scientific knowledge on disabilities and rehabilitation, while also providing vital support and focus for the field of medical rehabilitation to help ensure the health, independence, productivity, and quality of life of all people. Through the NCMRR, NICHD supports the development and testing of rehabilitative and assistive technologies, with a focus on physical rehabilitation.

### ASSISTIVE TECHNOLOGY PROGRAM

The Office of Interagency Innovation within Administration for Community Living (ACL)'s Center for Innovation and Partnership oversees the state grant for the Assistive Technology Program and the Assistive Technology National Activities funded under the Assistive Technology Act (AT Act of 2004).

- The state grant for Assistive Technology (AT) Program supports state efforts to improve the provision of assistive technology to individuals with disabilities of all ages through comprehensive, statewide programs that are consumer-responsive. The state grant for Assistive Technology Program makes assistive technology devices and services more available and accessible to individuals with disabilities and their families. The program provides one grant to each state, the District of Columbia, Puerto Rico, and the outlying areas (American Samoa, the Commonwealth of the Northern Mariana Islands, Guam, and the U.S. Virgin Islands). The state grant for Assistive Technology Program is a formula grant program; there are no grant competitions. The amount of each state's annual award is based largely on state population.

- General contact information for state Assistive Technology Programs can be found in the State Assistive Technology Program Directory on the AT3 Center website (www.at3center.net/stateprogram). Specific program contact information, including Lead Agency and Implementing Entity, for the State Grant for AT programs is contained in the state plan.
- The Assistive Technology National Activities Program provides information and technical assistance through grants, contracts, or cooperative agreements, on a competitive basis, to individuals, service providers, states, protection and advocacy entities, and others to support and improve the implementation of the AT Act of 2004. Grants awarded under this program are competitive and open to public or private entities, including for-profit organizations and institutions of higher education with relevant expertise

In Financial Year (FY) 2005, Congress amended the AT Act to eliminate the separate Alternative Financing Program authorization and instead authorized a AT state grant program that is inclusive of financing activities, including alternative financing loan programs. Each state grant for Assistive Technology Program includes financing activities. In FY 2015, FY 2016, FY 2017, FY 2018, and FY 2019 Congress appropriated funding separate and apart from the Assistive Technology Act for the purposes of making alternative financing program grants.

## Section 50.2 | Types of Assistive Devices and Rehabilitative Technologies

This section contains text excerpted from the following sources: Text under the heading "Assistive Devices" is excerpted from "What Are Some Types of Assistive Devices and How Are They Used?" *Eunice Kennedy Shriver* National Institute of Child Health and Human Development (NICHD), October 24, 2018; Text under the heading "Rehabilitative Technologies" is excerpted from "What Are Some Types of Rehabilitative Technologies?" *Eunice Kennedy Shriver* National Institute of Child Health and Human Development (NICHD), October 24, 2018.

### ASSISTIVE DEVICES

- Mobility aids, such as wheelchairs, scooters, walkers, canes, crutches, prosthetic devices, and orthotic devices
- Hearing aids to help people hear or hear more clearly
- Cognitive aids, including computer or electrical assistive devices, to help people with memory, attention, or other challenges in their thinking skills
- Computer software and hardware, such as voice recognition programs, screen readers, and screen enlargement applications, to help people with mobility and sensory impairments use computers and mobile devices
- Tools such as automatic page-turners, book holders, and adapted pencil grips to help learners with disabilities participate in educational activities
- Closed captioning to allow people with hearing problems to watch movies, television programs, and other digital media
- Physical modifications in the built environment, including ramps, grab bars, and wider doorways to enable access to buildings, businesses, and workplaces
- Lightweight, high-performance mobility devices that enable persons with disabilities to play sports and be physically active
- Adaptive switches and utensils to allow those with limited motor skills to eat, play games, and accomplish other activities
- Devices and features of devices to help perform tasks such as cooking, dressing, and grooming; specialized handles and grips, devices that extend reach, and lights on telephones and doorbells are a few examples

### REHABILITATIVE TECHNOLOGIES

- **Robotics**. Specialized robots help people regain and improve function in arms or legs after a stroke.
- **Virtual reality**. People who are recovering from an injury can retrain themselves to perform motions within a virtual environment.

- **Musculoskeletal modeling and simulations**. These computer simulations of the human body can pinpoint underlying mechanical problems in a person with a movement-related disability. This technique can help improve assistive aids or physical therapies.
- **Transcranial magnetic stimulation (TMS)**. TMS sends magnetic impulses through the skull to stimulate the brain. This system can help people who have had a stroke recover movement and brain function.
- **Transcranial direct current stimulation (tDCS)**. In tDCS, a mild electrical current travels through the skull and stimulates the brain. This can help recover movement in patients recovering from a stroke or other conditions.
- **Motion analysis**. Motion analysis captures a video of human motion with specialized computer software that analyzes the motion in detail. The technique gives healthcare providers a detailed picture of a person's specific movement challenges to guide proper therapy.

## Section 50.3 | Augmentative Communication Devices

This section includes text excerpted from "Assistive Devices for People with Hearing, Voice, Speech, or Language Disorders," National Institute on Deafness and Other Communication Disorders (NIDCD), March 6, 2017.

The simplest Augmentative and Alternative Communication (AAC) device is a picture board or touch screen that uses pictures or symbols of typical items and activities that make up a person's daily life. For example, a person might touch the image of a glass to ask for a drink. Many picture boards can be customized and expanded based on a person's age, education, occupation, and interests.

Keyboards, touch screens, and sometimes a person's limited speech may be used to communicate desired words. Some devices employ a text display. The display panel typically faces outward so that two people can exchange information while facing each other. Spelling and word prediction software can make it faster and easier to enter information.

Speech-generating devices go one step further by translating words or pictures into speech. Some models allow users to choose from several different voices, such as male or female, child or adult, and even some regional accents. Some devices employ a vocabulary of prerecorded words while others have an unlimited vocabulary, synthesizing speech as words are typed in. Software programs that convert personal computers into speaking devices are also available.

### AUGMENTATIVE AND ALTERNATIVE COMMUNICATION DEVICES FOR TELEPHONE

For many years, people with hearing loss have used text telephone or telecommunications devices, called "TTY" or "TDD machines," to communicate by phone. This same technology also benefits people with speech difficulties. A TTY machine consists of a typewriter keyboard that displays typed conversations onto a readout panel or printed on paper. Callers will either type messages to each other over the system or, if a call recipient does not have a TTY machine, use the national toll-free telecommunications relay service at 711 to communicate. Through the relay service, a communications assistant serves as a bridge between two callers, reading typed messages aloud to the person with hearing while transcribing what is spoken into type for the person with hearing loss.

With electronic communication devices, however, TTY machines have almost become a thing of the past. People can place phone calls through the telecommunications relay service using almost any device with a keypad, including a laptop, personal digital assistant, and a cell phone. Text messaging has also become a popular method of communication, skipping the relay service altogether.

Another system uses voice recognition software and an extensive library of video clips depicting American Sign Language (ASL) to translate a signer's words into text or computer-generated speech in real-time. It is also able to translate spoken words back into sign language or text.

Finally, for people with mild to moderate hearing loss, captioned telephones allow you to carry on a spoken conversation, while providing a transcript of the other person's words on a readout panel or computer screen as a backup.

## Section 50.4 | Home Modifications—Personal Emergency Response Systems

This section includes text excerpted from "Personal Emergency Response Systems: Health Information for Older People," Federal Trade Commission (FTC), October 15, 2008. Reviewed November 2019.

Personal emergency response systems (PERS), also known as "medical emergency response systems," let you call for help in an emergency by pushing a button. A PERS has three components: a small radio transmitter, a console connected to your telephone, and an emergency response center that monitors calls.

Transmitters are light-weight, battery-powered devices. You can wear one around your neck, on a wrist band, on a belt, or in your pocket. When you need help, you press the transmitter's help button, which sends a signal to the console. The console automatically dials one or more emergency telephone numbers.

Most PERS are programmed to telephone an emergency response center. The center will try to find out the nature of your emergency. They also may review your medical history and check who should be notified.

You can purchase, rent, or lease a PERS. Keep in mind that Medicare, Medicaid, and most insurance companies typically do not pay for the equipment, and the few that pay require a doctor's recommendation. Some hospitals and social service agencies may subsidize the device for low-income users. If you buy a PERS, expect to pay an installation fee and a monthly monitoring charge. Rentals are available through national manufacturers, local distributors, hospitals, and social service agencies, and fees often include the monitoring service. Read the contract carefully before you sign, and make a note of extra charges, such as cancellation fees.

Your local Area Agency on Aging may be able to tell you what systems are available in your area. See if friends, neighbors, or relatives have recommendations. When you have a list of agencies you are considering, check with your local consumer protection agency, state Attorney General, and Better Business Bureau to see if any complaints have been filed against them. Questions you can ask a PERS company include:

- Is the monitoring center open 24/7? What kind of training does staff receive?
- What is the average response time, and who gets alerted?
- Will I be able to use the same system with other response centers if I move? What if I move to another city or state?
- What is your repair policy? What happens if I need a replacement?
- What are the initial costs? What costs are ongoing? What kind of services and features will I get?

## Section 50.5 | **Power-Driven Mobility Devices**

This section includes text excerpted from "Wheelchairs, Mobility Aids, and Other Power-Driven Mobility Devices," ADA.gov, U.S. Department of Justice (DOJ), January 31, 2014. Reviewed November 2019.

People with mobility, circulatory, respiratory, or neurological disabilities use many kinds of devices for mobility. Some use walkers, canes, crutches, or braces. Some use manual or power wheelchairs or electric scooters. In addition, advances in technology have given rise to new devices, such as Segways®, that some people with disabilities use as mobility devices, including many veterans injured while serving in the military. And more advanced devices will inevitably be invented, providing more mobility options for people with disabilities.

## WHEELCHAIRS

Most people are familiar with the manual and power wheelchairs and electric scooters used by people with mobility disabilities. The term "wheelchair" is defined in the new rules as "a manually-operated or power-driven device designed primarily for use by an individual with a mobility disability for the main purpose of indoor or of both indoor and outdoor locomotion."

## OTHER POWER-DRIVEN MOBILITY DEVICES

In recent years, some people with mobility disabilities have begun using less traditional mobility devices such as golf cars or Segways®. These devices are called "other power-driven mobility device" (OPDMD) in the rule. OPDMD is defined in the new rules as "any mobility device powered by batteries, fuel, or other engines that is used by individuals with mobility disabilities for the purpose of locomotion, including golf cars, electronic personal assistance mobility devices such as the Segway® personal transporter (PT), or any mobility device designed to operate in areas without defined pedestrian routes, but that is not a wheelchair. When an OPDMD is being used by a person with a mobility disability, different rules apply under the Americans with Disabilities Act (ADA) than when it is being used by a person without a disability

## CHOICE OF DEVICE

People with disabilities have the right to choose whatever mobility device best suits their needs. For example, someone may choose to use a manual wheelchair rather than a power wheelchair because it enables her to maintain her upper body strength. Similarly, someone who is able to stand may choose to use a Segway® rather than a manual wheelchair because of the health benefits gained by standing. A facility may be required to allow a type of device that is generally prohibited when being used by someone without a disability when it is being used by a person who needs it because of a mobility disability. For example, if golf cars are generally prohibited in a park, the park may be required to allow a golf car when it is being used because of a person's mobility disability, unless there is a legitimate safety reason that it cannot be accommodated.

## REQUIREMENTS REGARDING MOBILITY DEVICES AND AIDS

Under the new rules, covered entities must allow people with disabilities who use wheelchairs (including manual wheelchairs, power wheelchairs, and electric scooters) and manually-powered mobility aids such as walkers, crutches, canes, braces, and other similar devices into all areas of a facility where members of the public are allowed to go.

In addition, covered entities must allow people with disabilities who use any OPDMD to enter the premises unless a particular type of device cannot be accommodated because of legitimate safety requirements. Such safety requirements must be based on actual risks, not on speculation or stereotypes about a particular type of device or how it might be operated by people with disabilities using them.

- For some facilities—such as a hospital, a shopping mall, a large home improvement store with wide aisles, a public park, or an outdoor amusement park—covered entities will likely determine that certain classes of OPDMDs being used by people with disabilities can be accommodated. These entities must allow people with disabilities using these types of OPDMDs into all areas where members of the public are allowed to go.
- In some cases, even in facilities such as those described above, an OPDMD can be accommodated in some areas of a facility, but not in others because of legitimate safety concerns. For example, a cruise ship may decide that people with disabilities using Segways® can generally be accommodated, except in constricted areas, such as passageways to cabins that are very narrow and have low ceilings.
- For other facilities—such as a small convenience store, or a small town manager's office—covered entities may determine that certain classes of OPDMDs cannot be accommodated. In that case, they are still required to serve a person with a disability using one of these devices in an alternate manner if possible, such as providing curbside service or meeting the person at an alternate location.

## Section 50.6 | **Research Plan on Rehabilitation**

This section includes text excerpted from "Research Plan on Rehabilitation," *Eunice Kennedy Shriver* National Institute of Child Health and Human Development (NICHD), 2016. Reviewed November 2019.

About 53 to 57 million Americans—about 1 in 5, or 22.2 percent of adults—have a disability of some kind. About 33 million Americans have a disability that makes it difficult for them to carry out daily activities, ranging from attending school or work to daily physical care. Approximately 2.2 million people in the United States depend on a wheelchair for day-to-day tasks and mobility; additionally, 6.5 million people use a cane, a walker, or crutches. Cognitive disability is frequently cited as a disability, with 15.2 million Americans estimated to have difficulty with mental or emotional functioning (6%). Disabilities associated with sensory abilities are widespread. About 36 million American adults (17%) report having some degree of hearing loss; nearly one-half of adults ages 75 years and older have hearing loss. About 3.6 million Americans have a visual impairment, and more than 1 million of them are legally blind. Nearly 7.5 million people in the United States have trouble using their voices, and between 6 million and 8 million people in the United States have some form of language impairment.

When setting national health priorities as part of the Healthy People 2020 initiative, the U.S. Department of Health and Human Services (HHS) documented that individuals with disabilities are more likely to experience health disparities. They are more likely to experience delays or difficulties in accessing healthcare, have fewer preventive tests or procedures (e.g., Pap tests or mammograms), spend less time on fitness activities, and have higher rates of tobacco use and obesity than the general population. Although the Agency for Healthcare Research and Quality (AHRQ) found a high rate of improvement in quality indicators for healthcare in those without disability over a 10-year period, only 20 to 35 percent of these quality indicators improved for individuals with activity limitations.

Disability affects not only those who experience these challenges firsthand but also those who support or care for people with disabilities. Based on a 2015 study, the American Association of Retired Persons (AARP) estimates that the United States is home to approximately 43.5 million caregivers. Most caregivers are adults age 50 and older. People who provide care can experience emotional stress, poor health, decreased opportunity to work, financial strain, and decreased ability to participate in social or community roles.

The extent of disability in the United States and its widespread public health impact on those with disabilities and their families and communities requires a response aimed at improving function, activity, and participation for these people with disabilities. The primary aims of rehabilitation research at the National Institutes of Health (NIH) are to improve rehabilitation and habilitation approaches for individuals with disabilities and to gain knowledge about the underlying diseases that cause disability. For the purpose of this plan, rehabilitation research includes the study of mechanisms, interventions, and methods that improve, restore, or replace lost, underdeveloped, or deteriorating function for people with disabilities in the context of their environment. The function includes a person's use of body systems, the ability to complete activities and participate in society, and satisfaction with their quality of life.

Rehabilitation research faces a number of challenges that have parallels in other areas of medicine. Those who could benefit from the research have limitations in transportation, mobility, finances, and access to information that can interfere with their participation in studies. These factors place significant limitations on researchers' ability to conduct appropriately powered studies. Outcome metrics rely on more subjective self-report and individual clinician measurements that can vary over time. Although evidence-based therapy is urgently needed, conducting a tightly controlled study can be difficult. Finding a well-matched comparison group for the treatment group poses significant challenges. Masking the treatment and control conditions, which is useful to ensure an impartial analysis of the results, can be problematic. Despite incredible progress over the past 20 years, new directions and challenges are apparent and underlie the need for new priorities to drive rehabilitation science.

# Chapter 51 | Benefits for Children with Disabilities

## SUPPLEMENTAL SECURITY INCOME PAYMENTS FOR CHILDREN WITH DISABILITIES

Supplemental Security Income (SSI) is a monthly payment to people with low income and limited resources who are 65 or older, or blind, or disabled. Your child, if younger than age 18, can qualify if they have a medical condition or combination of conditions that meets the U.S. Social Security Administration (SSA)'s definition of disability for children, and if her or his income and resources fall within the eligibility limits. The amount of the SSI payment is different from state to state because some states add to the SSI payment. Your local Social Security office can tell you more about your state's total SSI payment.

## SUPPLEMENTAL SECURITY INCOME RULES ABOUT INCOME AND RESOURCES

The SSA considers your child's income and resources when deciding if your child is eligible for SSI. They also consider the income and resources of family members living in the child's household. These rules apply if your child lives at home. They also apply if your child is away at school but returns home from time to time and is subject to your control. If your child's income and resources, or the income and resources of family members living in the child's household, are more than the amount allowed, the SSA will deny the child's application for SSI payments. The SSA limits the monthly SSI payment to $30 when a child is in a medical facility, and health insurance pays for her or his care.

## SUPPLEMENTAL SECURITY INCOME RULES ABOUT DISABILITY

Your child must meet all of the following requirements to be considered disabled and, therefore, medically eligible for SSI:

- The child, who is not blind, must not be working or earning more than $1,220 a month in 2019. A child who is blind must not be working

This chapter includes text excerpted from "Benefits for Children with Disabilities," U.S. Social Security Administration (SSA), January 2019.

or earning more than $2,040. (This earnings amount usually changes every year.)

- The child must have a medical condition, or a combination of conditions, that result in "marked and severe functional limitations." This means that the condition(s) must very seriously limit the child's activities.
- The child's condition(s) must have been disabling, or be expected to be disabling, for at least 12 months; or the condition(s) must be expected to result in death.

## PROVIDING INFORMATION ABOUT YOUR CHILD'S CONDITION

When you apply for SSI payments for your child based on a disability, the SSA will ask you for detailed information about the child's medical condition and about how it affects the child's ability to perform daily activities. They also will ask you to give permission to the doctors, teachers, therapists, and other professionals who have information about your child's condition to send the information to the SSA. If you have any of your child's medical or school records, please bring them with you. This will help speed up the decision-making process.

## WHAT HAPPENS NEXT

The SSA Supplemental Security Income program sends all of the SSI information you provide to the Disability Determination Services office in your state. Doctors and other trained staff in that state agency will review the information and will request your child's medical and school records, and any other information needed to decide if your child meets SSI criteria for disability. If the state agency cannot make a disability determination using only the medical information, school records, and other facts they have, they may ask you to take your child for a medical examination or test. They will pay for the exam or test.

## STATE AGENCY MAY MAKE IMMEDIATE SUPPLEMENTAL SECURITY INCOME PAYMENTS TO YOUR CHILD

The state agency may take three to five months to decide if your child meets SSI criteria for disability. For some medical conditions, however, they make SSI payments right away, and for up to six months, while the state agency decides if your child has a qualifying disability. Following are some of the conditions that may qualify:

- Total blindness
- Total deafness
- Cerebral palsy
- Down syndrome
- Muscular dystrophy
- Severe intellectual disability (child age 4 or older)

- Symptomatic human immunodeficiency virus (HIV) infection
- Birth weight below 2 pounds, 10 ounces—SSI experts evaluate low birth weight in infants from birth to attainment of age 1 and failure to thrive in infants and toddlers from birth to attainment of age 3. SSI experts use the infant's birth weight as documented by an original or certified copy of the infant's birth certificate or by a medical record signed by a physician.

If your child has one of the qualifying conditions, they will get SSI payments right away. If the state agency ultimately decides that your child's disability is not severe enough for SSI, you would not have to pay back the SSI payments that your child got.

## WHAT HAPPENS WHEN YOUR CHILD TURNS AGE 18

In the SSI program, a child becomes an adult at age 18, and the SSI program uses different medical and nonmedical rules when deciding if an adult can get SSI disability payments. For example, the SSA does not count the income and resources of family members, except for a spouse, when deciding whether an adult meets the financial limits for SSI. The SSA counts only the adult's and spouse's income and resources. The SSA also uses the disability rules for adults when deciding whether an adult is disabled.

If your child is already receiving SSI payments, the SSA must review the child's medical condition when they turn age 18. The SSA usually does this review during the one-year period that begins on your child's 18th birthday. The SSA will use the adult disability rules to decide whether your 18-year-old is eligible for SSI.

Even if your child was not eligible for SSI before her or his 18th birthday because you and your spouse had too much income or too many resources, they may become eligible for SSI at age 18.

# Chapter 52 | **Community Support for Parents with Disabilities**

**Chapter Contents**

## Section 52.1 | **Personal Assistance Services**

**This section includes text excerpted from "Chapter 13: Supporting Parents with Disabilities and Their Families in the Community," National Council on Disability (NCD), September 27, 2012. Reviewed November 2019.**

An African proverb, "It takes a village to raise a child," recognizes the reality that parents, whether or not they have a disability, cannot and should not parent alone. Indeed, parents without disabilities rely on a variety of formal and informal supports to help them with their child-rearing responsibilities. Elizabeth Lightfoot, PhD (Associate Professor and Director of the Doctoral Program, School of Social Work, University of Minnesota) and Traci LaLiberte, PhD (Executive Director, Center for Advanced Studies in Child Welfare, School of Social Work, University of Minnesota) say, "Formal supports that are typically used among North American parents include paid day care, housecleaning, paid tutoring, or even takeout restaurants. Typical informal supports include grandparents providing a night out for parents (respite care), neighbors shoveling snow off the driveway of a new parent (chore services), or parents joining together for carpooling to soccer practice (transportation services)." Parents with disabilities must have similar supports available to them and their families.

### PERSONAL ASSISTANCE SERVICES

Personal assistance services (PAS) are a crucial support for more than 13.2 million people with disabilities. PAS help people with activities of daily living (ADLs), such as eating, bathing, dressing, and toileting, as well as with instrumental activities of daily living (IADLs), such as grocery shopping, cooking, and cleaning. PAS typically fall into two categories: informal (unpaid) services provided by family members, friends, or neighbors; and formal services that are typically paid by public funding, private insurance, or out of pocket.

Personal assistance services have the potential to be of great help to parents with disabilities and their families. In a national survey of 1,200 parents with disabilities conducted for Through the Looking Glass (TLG) by Linda Barker and Vida Maralami, nearly four-fifths (79%) reported a need for some type of personal assistance, and more than half (57%) reported needing help with parenting tasks. This survey revealed that parents with various disabilities would benefit from PAS: Approximately 60 percent of parents with psychiatric or physical disabilities reported that they would benefit from assistance with parenting activities, and approximately 50 percent of those with sensory or developmental disabilities said they would benefit.

According to this survey, parents with disabilities need assistance with a variety of parenting tasks. They need the most help enjoying recreational activities with their children (43%). 40 percent reported needing assistance with "chasing and retrieving their children" and 40 percent reported needing assistance with traveling outside their home. Other areas in which parents reported needing assistance were lifting/carrying children, organizing supplies/clothing, disciplining children, playing with children, bathing children, childproofing the home, and advocating for children.

Cost is the most significant barrier for parents with disabilities who need PAS to help them with parenting activities. Pursuant to the Social Security Act, states may elect, as an optional benefit, to provide personal care services. According to the Centers for Medicare & Medicaid Services (CMS) State Medicaid Manual:

> Personal care services (also known in States by other names such as personal attendant services, personal assistance services, or attendant care services, etc.) covered under a state's program may include a range of human assistance provided to persons with disabilities and chronic conditions of all ages which enable them to accomplish tasks that they would normally do for themselves if they did not have a disability. Assistance may be in the form of hands-on assistance (actually performing a personal care task for a person) or cuing so that the person performs the task by herself/him. Such assistance most often relates to performance of ADLs and IADLs. ADLs include eating, bathing, dressing, toileting, transferring, and maintaining continence. IADLs capture more complex life activities and include personal hygiene, light housework, laundry, meal preparation, transportation, grocery shopping, using the telephone, medication management, and money management. Personal care services can be provided on a continuing basis or on episodic occasions.

Government-funded PAS does not allow attendants who are assisting parents with disabilities to also care for their children without a disability, which creates a significant challenge for these parents. According to the survey, only 10 percent of respondents who needed parenting help used government-funded PAS for parenting tasks. The rest of the respondents reported finding other ways to address this need. The most common solution, reported by 68 percent of parents, was to get unpaid help from family or friends, although 43 percent reported paying for extra assistance out of pocket. Equally troublesome—and a clear sign of their devotion to their children—35 percent of parents reported going without some personal care or household help they needed for themselves. Finally, 19 percent of the parents reported that they felt unable to provide their children with all the care they needed.

Personal assistance services have the potential to greatly assist parents with their disabilities and their families, and the benefits of PAS go beyond improving quality of life (QOL)—they have been found to be cost-effective, too. Several states have conducted small pilot projects in which foster care money is put toward well-coordinated aid to parents in crisis—because of substance abuse, disabilities, or other challenges—in hopes of keeping their children out of the foster care system. Santa Clara, one of the first California counties to try the new approach, calculated that for every dollar it spent on the intensive program, it saved $1.72 in federal, state, and county funds earmarked for foster care, not counting court costs involved in arranging foster care. Adaptive parenting equipment and home modification can also prove cost-effective by reducing the need for PAS hours.

The importance of PAS for parenting was emphasized by several of the parents who spoke to the National Council on Disability (NCD). Rachel, a widowed mother and wheelchair user with a physical disability, often uses PAS to assist her in parenting. Although she acknowledges that she is not supposed to, she has her attendant help with parenting activities such as meal preparation, transporting her daughter, recreation activities, and being available if her daughter has a behavioral incident. Rachel, who is on a limited income, pays her attendant extra for this assistance and wishes Medicaid allowed PAS hours to be used for parenting. Some parents with disabilities expressed the need for PAS to assist them with parenting on an intermittent basis—something like respite care.

## Section 52.2 | **Peer Supports**

This section includes text excerpted from "Supporting Parents with Disabilities and Their Families in the Community," National Council on Disability (NCD), September 27, 2012. Reviewed November 2019.

Most parents and prospective parents rely heavily on their peer-support network. Peer support provides the opportunity to exchange ideas and experiences with others who are facing similar situations. Peer-support networks also provide parenting role models.

The importance of peer supports for parents and prospective parents with disabilities may be even greater because of the limited information available on parenting with a disability. As one expectant mother with a disability said, "Perhaps what I have found the most helpful during my pregnancy has been the advice and input from other women with disabilities who have 'been there, done that.' I am fortunate to call many women with disabilities my colleagues and friends, and pregnancy has been a special time for me to reach out to those who are also mothers. Speaking with mothers with disabilities has helped me gain perspective on the experience of pregnancy. Even though physically our experiences are different, other women with disabilities have faced the same societal and attitudinal barriers that I am currently dealing with." Nearly all the parents who spoke with National Council on Disability (NCD) mentioned the importance of peer supports, often noting that peers were more supportive than their families of their quest to become parents.

Most parents, and people who are considering becoming parents, do not have to look far to find positive role models. However, parents and potential parents with disabilities do not have the same opportunities. Researchers have found that parents who are blind or have low vision often try to parent according to "sighted ways of functioning" when they do not have role models with similar disabilities. According to one mother, "The kind of support one can get from other mothers with visual impairments is not available in the sighted community." Research has found that parents with intellectual disabilities tend to be isolated and to have limited social networks.

Some disability organizations have begun to create networks for parents with disabilities. For example, parents who are deaf are included in forums and presentations on families at national and worldwide organizations for people who are deaf or hard of hearing, including the World Federation of the Deaf (WFD), the National Association of the Deaf (NAD), Deaf Seniors of America, and Deaf Way. Similarly, in 2000, the Committee on Parental Concerns and the National Federation of the Blind (NFB) announced dual sponsorship of a mailing list for parents with a visual impairment. This mailing list creates a forum for parents with a visually impairment to share their experiences and offer peer-based support and information. The National Multiple Sclerosis Society provides parenting information for its consumers. Through the Looking Glass (TLG) has developed a national parent-to-parent network as part of its national centers for parents with disabilities. The organization has also facilitated peer-support groups for parents with diverse disabilities for 30 years. Although some communities have found it difficult to establish groups for parents with intellectual disabilities, a particularly successful group established 11 years ago has led to the design of a training module—designing support groups for parents with intellectual disabilities—to support replication elsewhere.

Peer professional staffing in programs that serve parents with disabilities—such as the programs at TLG—is an important vehicle for conveying the wisdom of peers and providing role models. Publications by parents with disabilities, including publications by parents who compile input from other parents, are another such vehicle.

Throughout the world, families headed by parents with intellectual disabilities tend to be less affluent and more isolated. As a result, the community connections and discretionary income necessary to create memory-making family trips, outings, and recreation are often limited or nonexistent. This situation has an effect on the quality of family life. Hanna Björg Sigurjónsdóttir of the University of Iceland designed and recently concluded a three-year project that funded the creation of family peer groups facilitated by professionals in the community. Sigurjónsdóttir summarized the project as follows: "The groups engaged in family days and weekends, the aim of which was for parents and children to get to know each other across families and for family members within each family to enjoy each other's company, have fun together, and build up collective memories. The project is responsive to the families' needs and makes it possible to focus on issues that they are dealing with currently in their lives as parents. The year culminated with a community family snow trip that provided a chance for activities, celebration, and fun. The parents and children were also able to invite members of their extended families or close family friends, to provide them with an opportunity to give something back to those who often provided their social support system." American sensibility tends to view such a program as a privilege, but other nations approach the idea of community integration and family support with creativity and an eye for quality of life that is completely absent from our own approach.

The Internet, especially social networking sites such as Facebook, has greatly assisted parents with disabilities who want to connect with their peers. Many of the parents who spoke with NCD use the Internet to connect with other parents with disabilities. But, although the Internet provides wonderful opportunities to connect with other parents with disabilities, its usefulness has limits. For instance, a 2010 survey conducted by the Kessler Foundation and the National Organization on Disability (NOD) found that 85 percent of adults without disabilities access the Internet compared with only 54 percent of adults with disabilities—a gap of 31 percent. For some parents with intellectual and other cognitive disabilities that affect reading ability, the Internet remains largely inaccessible.

Despite increasing opportunities for peer support, many of the parents who spoke with NCD desire a more formal and organized network. For instance, Ken, a father with HIV infection, hemophilia, and hepatitis C, told NCD that while Facebook has helped him connect, he wishes there were a more established group, similar to the national organization parents, families and friends of lesbians and gays (commonly referred to as "PFLAG"). Ken also expressed an interest in having a conference for parents with disabilities and their families. He said that he and his wife, a wheelchair user, are always looking for "concrete examples of how it is been done." Kathryn, a mother who is a little person and a wheelchair user, wishes more peer supports and social gatherings were available for parents with disabilities and their families. Kathryn also believes that the lack of role models is a significant barrier for parents with disabilities. Lindsay, a mother with physical disabilities and an acquired brain injury, has found very few role models for parents with acquired brain injuries.

Raising children can be very stressful. For parents with disabilities, limited peer supports often leaves them discouraged and lacking necessary information. Peer-support networks can be easily developed or expanded at a minimal cost and would be supportive for many parents. NCD recommends broader dissemination of national networks and listservs, blogs, and so on. A primary national network should include peer staffing, provide peer-to-peer links, gather information, and provide links to other networking efforts, including those in state websites. This network should also maintain an accessible website and "warm line" (during business hours) with cross-disability, legal, and crisis-intervention expertise. State sites should include peer staffing and peer-to-peer networking and should link to the national network. State sites could also maintain accessible websites and warm lines with cross-disability and crisis-intervention expertise, and links to resources in their regions. Peer-support groups could be located in independent living centers and programs that specialize in parents with disabilities or deafness. These local parent support groups could provide ongoing peer connections that are important for the alleviation of isolation in communities. Collaboration among national, state, and local services should be a priority, including training and dissemination of information.

# Chapter 53 | **Housing Support for People with Disabilities**

## HOUSING RESOURCES FOR PEOPLE WITH DISABILITIES

A variety of federal, state, and local housing programs can help you find and afford a place to live, modify an existing home for disabilities, or help you develop skills to live independently.

Each program has its own eligibility rules and application process.

### Rental Housing

- People with disabilities are eligible for all public housing programs, rental assistance or subsidized housing, and Housing Choice voucher programs.
- You may also be eligible for a Non-Elderly Disabled (NED) Voucher, which helps people who are not seniors and have a disability get housing in a development traditionally set aside for seniors.
- Your state and your local city or county governments can explain any housing aid and programs for people with disabilities in your area.
- Certain Developments Vouchers can help nonelderly families that include a person with a disability find affordable rentals in housing developments limited to elderly residents.

### Homeownership

- If you are buying a home, Homeownership Vouchers can help pay mortgage and homeownership expenses.
- The U.S. Department of Agriculture (USDA) Rural Development program offers loans and grants for homeowners in rural areas

This chapter includes text excerpted from "Housing Help," USA.gov, April 10, 2019.

for removing health hazards and making home modifications to accommodate a household member with a physical disability.
- If you are a veteran with a service-connected or age-related disability, you may be eligible for a housing grant to build or modify a home for your needs.

### Independent Living Skills

- State and local independent living centers can help you develop skills to live on your own with a disability.
- Contact your state to find out how its department of human services or disability office may be able to assist with modifications, housing counseling, locating rental housing, and independent living skills.

### How Do I Complain?

You may require things like ramps, grab bars, or service animals. It is illegal for housing providers to deny someone housing because of a disability or refuse to make reasonable accommodations for a tenant with a disability.

## U.S. DEPARTMENT OF VETERANS AFFAIRS LOANS TO BUY, REFINANCE, OR IMPROVE A HOME

The U.S. Department of Veterans Affairs (VA) offers home loans and grants. These programs help service members, veterans, and surviving spouses buy, refinance, or modify their home. The VA guarantees part of the loan, meaning they will cover a portion of the loan if you default. This allows lenders, such as banks and mortgage companies, to offer you more favorable terms.

### How to Apply for a U.S. Department of Veterans Affairs Loan

- Find out if you qualify for a VA home loan you must meet the credit and income requirements and get a Certificate of Eligibility (COE).
- Apply for a VA home loan or housing-related assistance—You can apply online, through your lender, or by mail.

### U.S. Department of Veterans Affairs Loans for Homebuying and Refinancing

- If you are planning to buy a home, check into the variety of home loans offered by the VA. The most common are VA purchase loans. This type requires no down payment and no private mortgage insurance.
- If you have an existing VA home loan, you can apply for an Interest Rate Reduction Refinance Loan (IRRRL) to save money with a better interest rate.

## U.S. Department of Veterans Affairs Loans and Grants for Home Improvements

- You can get a VA cash-out to refinance loan to get money from your home's equity. This can help you pay for home improvements, college costs, and more.

If you have a service-connected or age-related disability, you may be eligible for a veteran housing grant. These grants help you modify your home for disabilities related to military service or aging.

# Chapter 54 | Financial Support for People with Disabilities

## HELP WITH MEDICAL BILLS

### Medicaid and Medicaid and the Children's Health Insurance Program (Healthcare for Children)

Medicaid and the Children's Health Insurance Program (CHIP) provides help with paying medical costs for children of families who cannot afford health insurance or do not get it through their work.

### Social Security and Medicare

Local Social Security Administration (SSA) offices help those on Social Security and Medicare find help. People over 65, people with disabilities under 65, and people with end-stage kidney disease are eligible for Medicare.

### Medicaid for Adults

#### What Help Is Available?

You may qualify for Medicaid, a joint federal and state program that helps with medical costs for some people with limited income from the Centers for Medicare & Medicaid Services (CMS).

#### Am I Eligible?

Each state has different rules about eligibility and applying for Medicaid for adults.

This chapter includes text excerpted from "Financial Assistance and Support Services for People with Disabilities," USA.gov, October 29, 2019.

#### How Do I Apply?

Each state has different application requirements for Medicaid for adults. Call your state Medicaid program to see if you qualify and to learn how to apply.

### Health Insurance through the Health Insurance Marketplace

#### What Help Is Available?

HealthCare.gov helps you find insurance options, compare care, learn about preventive services, and more. If your employer does not offer insurance, you are self-employed, or you prefer to purchase your own insurance, you and your family can get health, dental, and vision insurance through the Health Insurance Marketplace.

#### Am I Eligible?

Everyone is eligible for health insurance through the Marketplace. You may also qualify for subsidies to help pay your premiums. If you have experienced certain life changes, like loss of a job or childbirth, you may be eligible to make changes to your health insurance in a Special Enrollment Period.

#### How Do I Apply?

How you apply for a plan in the Health Insurance Marketplace depends on what plan you choose.

#### How Do I Complain or Where Do I Call for Extra Help?

Visit the Health Insurance Marketplace's top questions section for additional help with finding or applying for healthcare. To file a complaint, call 800-318-2596 (Toll-free TTY: 855-889-4325).

### Is There Anything Else I Need to Know?

If you need more help getting or paying for medical care, try these resources:

- Contact your state or local social services agencies to find out if you qualify for any healthcare programs in your area.
- Community clinics offer free or low-cost medical services including prenatal care.
- Research institutes including the National Cancer Institute (NCI) and the National Institutes of Health (NIH) often list clinical trials and studies that are seeking participants for research on medications and certain medical conditions.
- Find out how you may be able to lower the cost of your prescription drugs and medical devices.
- Charity care programs help uninsured patients who cannot afford to pay their medical bills and do not qualify for government aid. The patient services department of your local hospital can help you find out

if you are eligible. Reach out to the hospital before your medical service and explain your situation. If you do not qualify, the hospital may offer you a payment plan.

- Learn about your dental coverage options from local and state health programs, government insurance plans, dental schools, and dental clinical trials for people with limited incomes.
- You may qualify for financial assistance programs to help with eye exams, surgery, prescriptions, or glasses.

If you are uninsured or underinsured and must seek emergency medical treatment:

Under the Emergency Medical Treatment and Labor Act (EMTALA), you are guaranteed access to an emergency medical evaluation, even if you cannot pay. The act requires hospitals that receive Medicare funding and that provide emergency services to evaluate anyone who comes to their emergency room and requests treatment. If the evaluation confirms that you have an emergency medical condition, including active labor, they are then required to provide stabilizing treatment for you regardless of your ability to pay.

## GET HELP MODIFYING YOUR VEHICLE FOR DISABILITIES

If you are thinking of adapting your vehicle for your disability, these tips on modifying or buying a vehicle can help.

### Get Financial Help Buying a Vehicle or Modifying It for Disabilities

Start by contacting your state vocational rehabilitation agency. The agency can point you to state grant and loan programs that may help cover costs. You can also look into other ways to pay. Depending on your situation and where you live, these can include:

- Local nonprofit organizations
- Your car insurance
- Workers' compensation
- Vehicle manufacturers
- Tax assistance

If you are a service member or veteran with a disability, you may qualify for help from the U.S. Department of Veterans Affairs (VA) to help pay for vehicle modifications.

### Find and Get Help Paying for a Driver Rehabilitation Specialist

A driver rehabilitation specialist (DRS) will identify the best vehicle modifications for you. They will give you advice on buying an adapted vehicle. To find a qualified DRS in your area, check with your local rehabilitation center.

#### Get Help Paying for an Evaluation

You may be able to find sources to cover part or the entire cost of your DRS evaluation.

Check with your:

- State vocational rehabilitation agency
- State workers' compensation official
- Health insurance company

### Find a Qualified Mobility Dealer

Your DRS or rehabilitation agency can help you locate a qualified mobility equipment dealer to:

- Make sure you buy a vehicle that can be modified to meet your needs
- Modify your vehicle

### Get Training for Your Vehicle's New Disability Equipment

Your DRS can provide hands-on training in using your new equipment, which may be complex. Your vocational rehabilitation agency or workers' compensation may pay for the training.

# Chapter 55 | Insurance Benefits for People with Disabilities

## SHORT- AND LONG-TERM DISABILITY INSURANCE

If you cannot work because you get sick or injured, disability insurance will pay part of your income. You may be able to get insurance through your employer. You can also buy your own policy.

There are two types of disability policies:

- Short-term policies may pay for up to two years. Most last for a few months to a year
- Long-term policies may pay benefits for a few years or until the disability ends

Employers who offer coverage may provide short-term coverage, long-term coverage, or both.

If you plan to buy your own policy, shop around and ask:

- How is disability defined?
- When do benefits begin?
- How long do benefits last?
- How much money will the policy pay?

### Federal Disability Programs

Two U.S. Social Security Administration (SSA) programs pay benefits to people with disabilities which is Social Security Disability Insurance (SSDI) and Supplemental Security Insurance (SSI).

This chapter includes text excerpted from "Benefits and Insurance for People with Disabilities," USA.gov, September 12, 2019.

## SOCIAL SECURITY BENEFITS FOR PEOPLE WITH DISABILITIES

If you have a disability, two programs from the SSA may be able to help.

### Social Security Disability Insurance and Supplemental Security Insurance Programs for People with Disabilities

- SSDI is for people who have become disabled after earning enough Social Security work credits within a certain time.
- SSI is for people with disabilities or who are 65 or older with little to no income and resources. SSI is not Social Security. Although the names sound similar and the Social Security Administration runs the program, it does not fund SSI.

#### Definition of Disability

To qualify for either program, you must meet the SSA's definition of disability:

- You cannot work.
- Your disability is expected to last for at least one year or result in death.
- Your impairment is on the SSA's list of disabling medical conditions.

The SSA uses a step-by-step process to decide if you have a disability. Partial and short-term disabilities do not meet the SSA's standard. They are not eligible for benefits.

### Applying for Social Security Disability Insurance

#### Work Requirements

When you work and pay Social Security taxes, you earn Social Security "work credits." You earn up to four times a year depending on your income. To be eligible for SSDI, you must have earned a certain number of work credits, some of them recently. The number of work credits you need depends on your age when you stopped working due to your disability.

#### Benefits for Family Members

Your spouse or former spouse and your children may be eligible for benefits when you start getting SSDI.

You can apply for benefits online, by phone, or in person.

- If your application is denied, you can appeal the decision.
- If it is approved, you will have a five-month waiting period for benefits to start. You will receive benefits for the sixth full month after the date SSA finds your disability began.
- You will be enrolled in Medicare two years after you begin receiving SSDI payments.

#### Returning to Work

You can usually return to work without losing your SSDI if you earn less than a "substantial" amount. In 2019, the SSA considered average earnings of $1,220 or more per month "substantial."

You can try out your ability to return to work for at least nine months. You would not lose your SSDI benefits or Medicare coverage.

### Applying for Supplemental Security Income

Supplemental Security Income (SSI) benefits are for adults and children with a disability and little income or resources. Seniors 65 and older without a disability may be eligible if they meet the income limits. People who are eligible to receive SSDI may be eligible for SSI too.

In most states, people who receive SSI also receive Medicaid coverage. Many states also provide supplemental payments to certain SSI recipients.

Adults can apply for SSI by phone, in person at a local Social Security office, or in some cases online. To apply for SSI for a child, you can start the process online but will need to complete it either in person or by phone. You can appeal if your claim is denied.

SSI work incentives help you go to work by reducing your risk of losing your SSI or Medicaid coverage. You can earn $65 a month without it affecting your cash benefit. Beyond that, your SSI payment will go down $1 for every $2 you earn.

When your earnings plus any other income exceed your state's SSI income limits, you would not receive SSI. Your payments will start again for any month your income drops to less than the SSI limits.

#### Defining Disability for Supplemental Security Income

Adults under 65 must meet SSA's definition of disability. For a child, disability means:

- Having a physical or mental impairment that causes marked and severe functional limitations
- The disability is expected to last for at least one year or result in death.

## HEALTH INSURANCE AND HEALTH RESOURCES FOR PEOPLE WITH DISABILITIES

### Health Coverage for People with Disabilities

If you have a disability, you have a number of options for health coverage through the government.

- Medicaid provides free or low-cost medical benefits to people with disabilities.
- Medicare provides medical health insurance to people under 65 with certain disabilities and any age with end-stage renal disease (permanent kidney failure requiring dialysis or a kidney transplant).

- The Affordable Care Act (ACA) Marketplace offers options to people who have a disability, do not qualify for disability benefits, and need health coverage.

### Health Resources for People with Disabilities

Federal, state, and local government agencies and programs can help with your health needs if you have a disability.

- Explore the Disability and Health section of Centers for Diseases Control and Prevention (CDC) website (cdc.gov) for articles, programs, tips for healthy living and more.
- Know about assistance and benefits for people with disabilities from the SSA.
- Contact your local city or county government to find out what medical and health services are available locally for people with disabilities.
- Your state social service agency can help you locate medical and health programs.

## U.S. DEPARTMENT OF VETERAN AFFAIRS DISABILITY COMPENSATION BENEFITS

Veterans who have a service-related injury or illness may be entitled to the U.S. Department of Veteran Affairs (VA) disability compensation. It is a tax-free monthly benefit.

Visit VA.gov to learn:

- Which conditions qualify you for benefits
- How the claims process works
- Where to file your claim
- How to appeal a decision you disagree with. The process changed in February 2019.

Survivors of veterans may receive compensation benefits in certain situations.

# Chapter 56 | Transport Facilities for People with Disabilities

**Chapter Contents**

## Section 56.1 | **Adapting Motor Vehicles for People with Disabilities**

This section includes text excerpted from "NHTSA Adapting Motor Vehicles for People with Disabilities," National Highway Traffic Safety Administration (NHTSA), September 29, 2007. Revised November 2019.

The introduction of technology continues to broaden opportunities for people with disabilities to drive vehicles with adaptive devices. Taking advantage of these opportunities, however, can be a time consuming and sometimes frustrating.

The information is based on the experience of driver rehabilitation specialists and other professionals who work with individuals who require adaptive devices for their motor vehicles. It is centered around a proven process—evaluating your needs, selecting the right vehicle, choosing a qualified dealer to modify your vehicle, being trained, maintaining your vehicle—that can help you avoid costly mistakes when purchasing and modifying a vehicle with adaptive equipment.

Also included is general information on cost savings, licensing requirements, and organizations to contact for help. Although it focuses on drivers of modified vehicles, it also contains important information for people who drive passengers with disabilities.

### INVESTIGATE COST SAVING OPPORTUNITIES AND LICENSING REQUIREMENTS

#### Cost Saving Opportunities

The costs associated with modifying a vehicle vary greatly. A vehicle modified with adaptive equipment can cost from $20,000 to $80,000. Therefore, whether you are modifying a vehicle you own or purchasing a vehicle with adaptive equipment, it pays to investigate public and private opportunities for financial assistance.

There are programs that help pay part or all of the cost of vehicle modification, depending on the cause and nature of the disability. For information, contact your state's Department of Vocational Rehabilitation or another agency that provides vocational services, and, if appropriate, the Department of Veterans Affairs (VA). You can find phone numbers for these state and federal agencies in a local phone book. Also, consider the following.

- Many nonprofit associations that advocate for individuals with disabilities have grant programs that help pay for adaptive devices
- If you have private health insurance or workers' compensation, you may be covered for adaptive devices and vehicle modification. Check with your insurance carrier.
- Many manufacturers have rebate or reimbursement plans for modified vehicles. When you are ready to make a purchase, find out if there is such a dealer in your area.

- Some states waive the sales tax for adaptive devices if you have a doctor's prescription for their use
- You may be eligible for savings when submitting your federal income tax return. Check with a qualified tax consultant to find out if the cost of your adaptive devices will help you qualify for a medical deduction.

### Licensing Requirements

All states require a valid learner's permit or driver's license to receive an on-the-road evaluation. You cannot be denied the opportunity to apply for a permit or license because you have a disability. However, you may receive a restricted license, based on your use of adaptive devices.

## EVALUATE YOUR NEEDS

Driver rehabilitation specialists perform comprehensive evaluations to identify the adaptive equipment most suited to your needs. A complete evaluation includes vision screening and, in general, assesses:

- Muscle strength, flexibility, and range of motion
- Coordination and reaction time
- Judgment and decision-making abilities
- Ability to drive with adaptive equipment

Upon completion of an evaluation, you should receive a report containing specific recommendations on driving requirements or restrictions, and a complete list of recommended vehicle modifications.

### Finding a Qualified Evaluator

To find a qualified evaluator in your area, contact a local rehabilitation center or call the Association for Driver Rehabilitation Specialists (ADRD). The phone number is in the resource section. The Association maintains a database of certified driver rehabilitation specialists throughout the country. Your insurance company may pay for the evaluation. Find out if you need a physician's prescription or other documentation to receive benefits.

### Being Prepared for an Evaluation

Consult with your physician to make sure you are physically and psychologically prepared to drive. Being evaluated too soon after an injury or other trauma may indicate the need for adaptive equipment you will not need in the future. When going for an evaluation, bring any equipment you normally use, e.g., a walker or neck brace. Tell the evaluator if you are planning to modify your wheelchair or obtain a new one.

### Evaluating Passengers with Disabilities

Evaluators also consult on compatibility and transportation safety issues for passengers with disabilities. They assess the type of seating needed and the person's ability to exit and enter the vehicle. They provide advice on the purchase of modified vehicles and recommend appropriate wheelchair lifts or other equipment for a vehicle you own. If you have a child who requires a special type of safety seat, evaluators make sure the seat fits your child properly. They also make sure you can properly install the seat in your vehicle.

## SELECT THE RIGHT VEHICLE

Selecting a vehicle for modification requires collaboration among you, your evaluator, and a qualified vehicle modification dealer. Although the purchase or lease of a vehicle is your responsibility, making sure the vehicle can be properly modified is the responsibility of the vehicle modification dealer. Therefore, take the time to consult with a qualified dealer and your evaluator before making your final purchase. It will save you time and money. Be aware that you will need insurance while your vehicle is being modified, even though it is off the road.

The following questions can help with vehicle selection. They can also help determine if you can modify a vehicle you own.

- Does the necessary adaptive equipment require a van, or will another passenger vehicle suffice?
- Can the vehicle accommodate the equipment that needs to be installed?
- Will there be enough space to accommodate your family or other passengers once the vehicle is modified?
- Is there adequate parking space at home and at work for the vehicle and for loading/unloading a wheelchair?
- Is there adequate parking space to maneuver if you use a walker?
- What additional options are necessary for the safe operation of the vehicle?

If a third party is paying for the vehicle, adaptive devices, or modification costs, find out if there are any limitations or restrictions on what is covered. Always get a written statement on what a funding agency will pay before making your purchase.

## CHOOSE A QUALIFIED DEALER TO MODIFY YOUR VEHICLE

Even a half-inch change in the lowering of a van floor can affect a driver's ability to use equipment or to have an unobstructed view of the road; so, take time to find a qualified dealer to modify your vehicle. Begin with a phone inquiry to find out about credentials, experience, and references. Ask questions about how they operate. Do they work with evaluators? Will they look at your vehicle before you purchase it? Do they require a prescription from a physician or other driver evaluation specialist? How long will it take before they can start work on your vehicle? Do they provide training on how to use the adaptive equipment?

If you are satisfied with the answers you receive, check references; then arrange to visit the dealer's facility. Additional information to consider is listed below.

- Are they members of the National Mobility Equipment Dealers Association (NMEDA) or another organization that has vehicle conversion standards?
- What type of training has the staff received?
- What type of warranty do they provide on their work?
- Do they provide ongoing service and maintenance?
- Do they stock replacement parts?

Once you are comfortable with the dealer's qualifications, you will want to ask specific questions, such as:

- How much will the modification cost?
- Will they accept third party payment?
- How long will it take to modify the vehicle?
- Can the equipment be transferred to a vehicle in the future?
- Will they need to modify existing safety features to install adaptive equipment?

While your vehicle is being modified, you will most likely need to be available for fittings. This avoids additional waiting time for adjustments once the equipment is fully installed. Without proper fittings, you may have challenges involving the safe operation of the vehicle and have to go back for adjustments.

Some state agencies specify the dealer you must use if you want reimbursement.

## OBTAIN TRAINING ON THE USE OF NEW EQUIPMENT

Both new and experienced drivers need training on how to safely use adaptive equipment. Your equipment dealer and evaluator should provide information and off-road instruction. You will also need to practice driving under the instruction of a qualified driving instructor until you both feel comfortable with your skills. Bring a family member or other significant person who drives to all your training sessions. It is important to have someone else who can drive your vehicle in case of an emergency.

Some state vocational rehabilitation departments pay for driver training under specified circumstances. At a minimum, their staff can help you locate a qualified instructor. If your evaluator does not provide on-the-road instructions, ask her or him for a recommendation. You can also inquire at your local motor vehicle administration office.

## MAINTAIN YOUR VEHICLE

Regular maintenance is important for keeping your vehicle and adaptive equipment safe and reliable. It may also be mandatory for compliance with the terms of your warranty. Some warranties specify a time period during which adaptive equipment must be inspected. These "check-ups" for equipment may differ from those for your vehicle. Make sure you or your modifier submits all warranty cards for all equipment to ensure coverage and so manufacturers can contact you in case of a recall.

# Section 56.2 | Passengers with Disabilities and the Air Carrier Access Act

This section contains text excerpted from the following sources: Text under the heading "About the Air Carrier Access Act" is excerpted from "Passengers with Disabilities," U.S. Department of Transportation (DOT), January 27, 2015. Reviewed November 2019; Text beginning with the heading "What Is an Assistive Device?" is excerpted from "Wheelchairs and Other Assistive Devices," U.S. Department of Transportation (DOT), November 15, 2017.

## ABOUT THE AIR CARRIER ACCESS ACT

The Air Carrier Access Act prohibits discrimination on the basis of disability in air travel. The U.S. Department of Transportation (DOT) has a rule defining the rights of passengers and the obligations of airlines under this law. This rule applies to all flights of U.S. airlines, and to flights to or from the United States by foreign airlines. The following are the main points of the DOT rule (Title 14 CFR Part 382).

### Prohibition of Discriminatory Practices

- Airlines may not refuse transportation to people on the basis of disability. Airlines may exclude anyone from a flight if carrying the person would be inimical to the safety of the flight. If a carrier excludes a person with a disability on safety grounds, the carrier must provide a written explanation of the decision.
- Airlines may not require advance notice that a person with a disability is traveling. Air carriers may require up to 48 hours' advance notice for certain accommodations that require preparation time (e.g., respirator hook-up, transportation of an electric wheelchair on an aircraft with less than 60 seats).
- Airlines may not limit the number of persons with disabilities on a flight

- Airlines may not require a person with a disability to travel with another person, except in certain limited circumstances where the rule permits the airline to require a safety assistant. If a passenger with a disability and the airline disagree about the need for a safety assistant, the airline can require the assistant, but cannot charge for the transportation of the assistant.
- Airlines may not keep anyone out of a specific seat on the basis of disability, or require anyone to sit in a particular seat on the basis of disability, except to comply with Federal Aviation Administration (FAA) or foreign-government safety requirements. FAA's rule on exit row seating says that airlines may place in exit rows only persons who can perform a series of functions necessary in an emergency evacuation.

## Accessibility of Facilities

- New aircraft with 30 or more seats must have movable aisle armrests on half the aisle seats in the aircraft
- New twin-aisle aircraft must have accessible lavatories
- New aircraft with 100 or more seats must have priority space for storing a passenger's folding wheelchair in the cabin
- Aircraft with more than 60 seats and an accessible lavatory must have an on-board wheelchair, regardless of when the aircraft was ordered or delivered. For flights on aircraft with more than 60 seats that do not have an accessible lavatory, airlines must place an on-board wheelchair on the flight if a passenger with a disability gives the airline 48 hours' notice that she or he can use an inaccessible lavatory, but needs an on-board wheelchair to reach the lavatory.
- Airlines must ensure that airport facilities and services that they own, lease or control are accessible in the manner prescribed in the rule

## Other Services and Accommodations

- Airlines are required to provide assistance with boarding, deplaning and making connections. Assistance within the cabin is also required, but not extensive personal services. Where level-entry boarding is not available, there must be ramps or mechanical lifts to service most aircraft with 19 or more seats at U.S. airports with over 10,000 annual enplanements.
- The items of passengers' with disabilities stored in the cabin must conform to FAA rules on the stowage of carry-on baggage. Assistive devices do not count against any limit on the number of pieces of carry-on baggage. Collapsible wheelchairs and other assistive devices

have priority for in-cabin storage space (including in closets) over other passengers' items brought on board at the same airport, if the passenger with a disability chooses to preboard.

- Wheelchairs and other assistive devices have priority over other items for storage in the baggage compartment
- Airlines must accept battery-powered wheelchairs, including the batteries, packaging the batteries in hazardous materials packages when necessary. The airline provides the packaging.
- Airlines must permit a passenger to use her/his portable oxygen concentrator during the flight if it is labeled as FAA-approved
- Airlines may not charge for providing accommodations required by the rule, such as hazardous materials packaging for batteries. However, they may charge for optional services such as providing oxygen.
- Other provisions concerning services and accommodations address treatment of mobility aids and assistive devices, passenger information, accommodations for persons with vision and hearing impairments, security screening, communicable diseases and medical certificates, and service animals.

### Administrative Provisions

- Training is required for airline and contractor personnel who deal with the traveling public
- Airlines must make available specially-trained "complaints resolution officials" to respond to complaints from passengers and must also respond to written complaints. A DOT enforcement mechanism is also available.
- Airlines must obtain an assurance of compliance from contractors who provide services to passengers

## WHAT IS AN ASSISTIVE DEVICE?

An assistive device is any piece of equipment that assists a passenger with a disability in coping with the effects of her or his disability. These devices are intended to assist passengers with a disability to hear, see, communicate, maneuver, or perform other functions of daily life. Assistive devices include (but are not limited to):

- Crutches, canes, and walkers
- Braces/prosthetics
- Wheelchairs
- Hearing aids
- Portable oxygen concentrators (POCs)
- Continuous positive airway pressure (CPAP) machines

- Prescription medications and any medical devices needed to administer those medications, such as syringes or auto-injectors

**Note:** If you are not sure if your device is an assistive device, contact your airline's disability or special assistance desk.

## THINGS TO KNOW

You may bring your assistive device with you on an airplane and stow it in the passenger compartment in the following locations:

- In an overhead compartment
- Under the seat in front of you
- In a designated stowage area if the device fits and is in accordance with FAA or foreign safety regulations

If the assistive device cannot be stowed in the passenger cabin as carry on baggage, the device can be stowed as cargo at no extra cost.

Airlines are required to transport only manual wheelchairs in the cabin of the aircraft. Most battery-powered wheelchairs are too large and too heavy to be safely stowed in the seating portion of the aircraft. Large and heavy powered wheelchairs are typically stowed in the cargo portion of the aircraft.

When your powered wheelchair is stowed in the cargo compartment, the airline must return your assistive device to you in a timely manner as close as possible to the door of the aircraft, unless you ask to pick it up in baggage claim.

Individuals with a collapsible or break-down wheelchair may stow their device in overhead compartments, under seats, or in the designated wheelchair stowage area if the device fits and is in accordance with the Federal Aviation Administration (FAA) safety regulations.

Airlines are required to accept for transport at least one manual wheelchair in aircraft with 100 or more seats.

If your wheelchair does not fit in the cabin of the aircraft, airline personnel are required to stow it in the cargo portion of the aircraft free of charge.

The airline must allow you to bring your portable oxygen concentrator (POC) on board the aircraft as long as it meets FAA requirements.

Airlines will require you to apply for special requirements to use of a POC onboard the airplane:

- Provide up to 48-hours advance notice that you will use your POC onboard
- Provide a medical certificate for the use of your POC onboard
- Bring a supply of fully charged batteries to power your device for no less than 150 percent of the duration of the flight
- Check-in one hour before the regular check-in time for the flight

Assistive devices do not count toward your baggage limit. However, if your bag also contains personal items, the airline can count your bag toward a baggage limit and it may be subject to a baggage fee.

## TIPS FOR TRAVELING WITH YOUR WHEELCHAIR AND OTHER ASSISTIVE DEVICES

### Before Your Trip

- Confirm with airliner that your wheelchair will fit in cargo hold if you are traveling on a small plane, such as a commuter aircraft or a regional jet
- Attach clear assembly and disassembly instructions to your wheelchair before you head to the airport. Having written instructions will assist airline personnel and contractors in case your wheelchair needs to be disassembled for transport.

### At the Airport

- If you travel with a battery-powered wheelchair, you must arrive at the airport 1 hour prior to the normal check-in time
- If your wheelchair or walker cannot be carried in the cabin, you can check it
- If you have a wheelchair or walker, you do not need to check them until you are at the gate
- You can request that your wheelchair or walker be returned to you on the jetway at your destination airport and not the baggage claim area. Airlines are required to return wheelchairs to users as closely as possible to the door of the aircraft if requested.
- Upon receiving your wheelchair, do a quick inspection before you use it. If there is any damage go immediately to the airline's customer service and file a claim.

### If Something Goes Wrong

- On domestic flights, U.S. carriers must fully compensate passengers for loss or damage to wheelchairs or other assistive devices, without regard to rules limiting liability for lost or damaged baggage
- On international flights, the Montreal convention provisions control payments for items including assistive devices
- If you believe your rights have been violated and the airline employee you find at first is unable to help you, ask to speak with a Complaints Resolution Official (CRO). A CRO is the airline's expert on disability accommodation issues. Airlines are required to make one available to you, at no cost, in person at the airport or by telephone during the times they are operating.

# Chapter 57 | Finding Meaningful Employment

**Chapter Contents**

## Section 57.1 | **Special Hiring Authorities and Programs**

This section includes text excerpted from "Careers at SSA: Individuals with Disabilities," U.S. Social Security Administration (SSA), October 27, 2016. Reviewed November 2019.

### SELECTIVE PLACEMENT PROGRAM/SCHEDULE A

Individuals with disabilities may apply through the competitive hiring process, or in some circumstances, under the noncompetitive hiring authority for individuals with disabilities (Schedule A).

For consideration under the noncompetitive hiring authority (Schedule A), send a resume, description of your career interests, your geographic preferences, and proof of disability to the Selective Placement Coordinator in your region

Veterans with a disability may also be considered under special hiring programs.

#### The ABCs of Schedule A for Applicants with Disabilities

In the noncompetitive hiring process, agencies may use a special authority to hire individuals with targeted disabilities without requiring them to compete for the job.

Individuals that may fall under this special hiring authority include individuals with intellectual disabilities, severe physical disabilities, or psychiatric disabilities.

### TICKET TO WORK PROGRAM

- The Ticket to Work program is voluntary. Through this program, individuals who receive Social Security disability benefits can increase self-sufficiency through a variety of support options.
- The Ticket to Work Program (choosework.ssa.gov) is a good fit for individuals who want to improve the earning potential and are committed to preparing for long-term success in the workplace
- The YourTicketToWork.SSA.gov website is for Employment Networks and State Vocational Rehabilitation agencies participating in the U.S. Social Security Administration (SSA)'s Ticket to Work and Self Sufficiency Program
- Visit the SSA's worksite (www.ssa.gov/work/home.html) for programmatic information about the Ticket to Work program
- Visit the SSA's worksite (choosework.ssa.gov/mycall) webpage for programmatic updates.

### VOCATIONAL REHABILITATION

The SSA supports the state vocational rehabilitation (VR) agencies in their efforts to help prepare people with disabilities for jobs and teach them job skills.

State VR agencies provide a range of services including:

- Vocational counseling and guidance
- Job placement assistance
- College/vocational training
- Supported employment services
- Skills training
- Job coaching/tutoring
- Transportation
- Interpreter services
- Services to transition-age youth
- Accommodations
- Assistive technology and rehabilitation technology services; referral services; support, advocacy, and follow-up services

## REASONABLE ACCOMMODATIONS

Reasonable accommodations are modifications or adjustments to a job or change in the work environment that enables a person with a disability to compete equally or perform the essential functions of the position.

Reasonable accommodation also includes adjustments to assure an individual with a disability has equal benefits and privileges of employment enjoyed by other similarly situated employees without disabilities.

The accommodation must be job-related e.g., hearing aids, prosthetic devices, wheelchairs, and transportation to work.

Accommodations also include:

- Assistive technology
- Readers and assistants
- Interpreter services
- Specialized training on the use of assistive devices
- Modified job duties and restructured worksites
- Provided accessible technology or other workplace adaptive equipment
- Reasonable accommodations can apply to the duties of the job and/or where or how job tasks are performed

## JOB SEARCH AND HIRING PROCESS

Know that the hiring officials are prohibited from asking questions about your disability unless the questions relate to your ability to perform the essential functions of the position and are consistent with the business needs of the position.

In addition to going to USAJOBS and researching jobs, an individual may also contact a Selective Placement Program Coordinator for employment help.

To review the Equal Employment Opportunity Commission's (EEOC) guidance about questions hiring officials can ask about an applicant's disability, please visit www.eeoc.gov/policy/docs/preemp.html for the "Enforcement Guidance: Preemployment Disability-Related Questions and Medical Examinations."

## Section 57.2 | **Ticket to Work**

This section contains text excerpted from the following sources: Text beginning with the heading "What Is the Ticket to Work Program?" is excerpted from "About Ticket to Work," U.S. Social Security Administration (SSA), August 5, 2017; Text under the heading "How It Works" is excerpted from "How It Works," U.S. Social Security Administration (SSA), September 19, 2014. Reviewed November 2019.

### WHAT IS THE TICKET TO WORK PROGRAM?

The U.S. Social Security Administration's (SSA) Ticket to Work program supports career development for social security disability beneficiaries age 18 through 64 who want to work. The Ticket program is free and voluntary. The Ticket program helps people with disabilities progress toward financial independence.

The Ticket program is a good fit for people who want to improve their earning potential and are committed to preparing for long-term success in the workforce. Ticket to Work offers beneficiaries with disabilities access to meaningful employment with the assistance of Ticket to Work employment service providers called "employment networks." If you are ready to go to work, there are people ready and waiting to help you!

The career development services and support you need are unique to you. The Ticket program can connect you with the right mix of free employment support services and approved service providers that will best fit your needs.

The Ticket program and Work Incentives allow you to keep your benefits while you explore employment, receive vocational rehabilitation services and gain work experience. Your cash benefits and Medicaid or Medicare often continue throughout your transition to work, and there are protections in place to help you return to benefits, if you find you are unable to continue working due to your disability.

### WHY TICKET TO WORK

If you receive Social Security disability benefits, then you know that getting those benefits took time, energy and patience. In determining your eligibility for disability benefits, the SSA found that you could not earn enough money to support yourself. With the right opportunities and supports, however, many people can earn a higher standard of living by going to work and leaving the benefit rolls.

Earning a living through employment is not something everyone can do, but it may be right for you. Many find that the rewards far outweigh the risks. Take the time to learn about the employment services and supports social security offers beneficiaries with disabilities through the Ticket to Work program . . . you may be surprised!

## HOW IT WORKS

Ticket to Work connects you with free employment services to help you decide if working is right for you, prepare for work, find a job or maintain success while you are working. If you choose to participate, you will receive services such as career counseling, vocational rehabilitation, and job placement and training from authorized Ticket to Work service providers, such as employment networks (EN) or your state vocational rehabilitation (VR) agency. The service provider you choose will serve as an important part of your "employment team" that will help you on your journey to financial independence.

### Who Qualifies

Everyone age 18 through 64 who receives Social Security Disability Insurance (SSDI) and/or supplemental security income (SSI) benefits because of her or his disability is eligible to participate in the Ticket to Work program. Participation in the Ticket to Work program is free and voluntary.

The SSA no longer sends paper Tickets in the mail, and you do not need a paper Ticket to participate. Your eligibility will be verified by the service provider with whom you choose to work. You can also find out about your eligibility status by calling the Ticket to Work helpline at 866-968-7842/866-833-2967 (Toll-free TTY).

### How to Get Started

If you decide to participate, getting started is easy! First, call the Ticket to Work helpline at 866-833-7842/866-833-2967 (Toll-free TTY) to verify your eligibility. The customer service representatives will explain to you how the program works and answer any questions or address any concerns you might have. They will also offer to mail you a list of service providers, or if you prefer, you can use the find help tool to get a customized list of providers that are available to help you.

The next step is deciding what service provider is right for you. You may work with either an employment network (EN) or your state vocational rehabilitation (VR) agency, depending on your needs. The "Finding an EN and Assigning Your Ticket Worksheet" can help you keep track of the ENs you are interested in and provides important questions for you to ask. You may also receive services from your VR agency and then receive ongoing services from an employment network.

Some ENs are also part of a state's public workforce system. These workforce ENs provide access to additional employment support services including training programs and special programs for youth in transition and veterans. A Ticket to Work participant who assigns their Ticket to a workforce EN will either work with a workforce EN directly or via other providers in the workforce system, including American job centers.

Once you and your service provider decide to work together, you will collaboratively develop a plan to help you reach your work goals. Your employment team will then help you make progress towards those goals and, eventually, a more financially independent future.

# Chapter 58 | **Speech-to-Speech Relay Service**

Speech-to-speech (STS) is one form of telecommunications relay service (TRS). TRS is a service that allows persons with hearing and speech disabilities to access the telephone system to place and receive telephone calls. STS enables persons with a speech disability to make telephone calls using their own voice (or an assistive voice device). Like all forms of TRS, STS uses Communications Assistants (CAs)—to relay the conversation back and forth between the person with the speech disability and the other party to the call. STS CAs are operators who are specifically trained in understanding a variety of speech disorders, which enables them to repeat what the caller says in a manner that makes the caller's words clear and understandable to the called party. The Commission's rules ensure that STS users have the same ease of reaching an STS CA as users of the other types of TRS.

## WHO USES SPEECH-TO-SPEECH

Often people with speech disabilities cannot communicate by telephone because the parties they are calling cannot understand their speech. People with cerebral palsy, multiple sclerosis, muscular dystrophy, Parkinson disease (PD) and those who are coping with limitations from a stroke or traumatic brain injury may have speech disabilities. People who stutter or have had a laryngectomy may also have difficulty being understood. In general, anyone with a speech disability or anyone who wishes to call someone with a speech disability can use STS.

## USING SPEECH-TO-SPEECH

A person can make an STS call from any telephone. You simply call the relay center by dialing 711, and indicate you wish to make an STS call. You are then connected to an STS CA who will repeat your spoken words, making the spoken words clear to the other party. Persons with speech disabilities may also receive

This chapter includes text excerpted from "Speech to Speech Relay Service," Federal Communications Commission (FCC), November 1, 2016. Reviewed November 2019.

STS calls. The calling party calls the relay center by dialing 711 and asks the CA to call the person with a speech disability. STS users have the option of muting their voices during an STS call (so that the party to whom they are speaking hears only the voice of the STS CA, and not the voice of the STS user). If you wish to use this option, please inform the STS CA to mute your voice for the other party to the call. If you choose this option, the STS CA will still be able to hear what you are saying, and will re-voice what you say to the other party.

# Part 8 | **Additional Help and Information**

# Chapter 59 | **Glossary of Terms Related to Physical Rehabilitation**

**activities of daily living (ADLs):** Basic personal activities which include bathing, eating, dressing, mobility, transferring from bed to chair, and using the toilet. ADLs are used to measure how dependent a person may be on requiring assistance in performing any or all of these activities.

**acute care:** Care that is generally provided for a short period of time to treat a certain illness or condition. This type of care can include short-term hospital stays, doctor's visits, surgery, and x-rays.

**addiction:** A chronic, relapsing disease characterized by compulsive drug seeking and use despite serious adverse consequences, and by long-lasting changes in the brain.

**Alzheimer disease (AD):** A progressive, irreversible disease characterized by degeneration of the brain cells and serve loss of memory, causing the individual to become dysfunctional and dependent upon others for basic living needs.

**anesthetic:** A drug that causes insensitivity to pain and is used for surgeries and other medical procedures.

**antibiotics:** Medicines that damage or kill bacteria and are used to treat some bacterial diseases.

**anxiety:** Feelings of fear, dread, and uneasiness that may occur as a reaction to stress. A person with anxiety may sweat, feel restless, and tense, and have a rapid heart beat.

**arthritis:** A disease that causes inflammation and pain in the joints.

**assessment:** The process of gathering evidence and documentation of a student's learning.

This glossary contains terms excerpted from documents produced by several sources deemed reliable.

**ataxia:** A condition in which the muscles fail to function in a coordinated manner.

**blood:** A tissue with red blood cells (RBCs), white blood cells (WBCs), platelets, and other substances suspended in fluid called "plasma." Blood takes oxygen and nutrients to the tissues, and carries away wastes.

**body mass index (BMI):** Body mass index is a measure of body weight relative to height. The BMI tool uses a formula that produces a score often used to determine if a person is underweight, at a normal weight, overweight, or obese.

**calcium:** A mineral that is an essential nutrient for bone health. It is also needed for the heart, muscles, and nerves to function properly and for blood to clot.

**cancer:** A term for diseases in which abnormal cells in the body divide without control. Cancer cells can invade nearby tissues and can spread to other parts of the body through the blood and lymphatic system, which is a network of tissues that clears infections and keeps body fluids in balance.

**cardiopulmonary resuscitation (CPR):** A group of treatments used when someone's heart and/or breathing stops. CPR is used in an attempt to restart the heart and breathing. It usually consists of mouth-to-mouth breathing and pressing on the chest to cause blood to circulate. Electric shock and drugs also are used to restart or control the rhythm of the heart.

**caregiver:** A caregiver is anyone who helps care for an elderly individual or person with a disability who lives at home. Caregivers usually provide assistance with activities of daily living and other essential activities like shopping, meal preparation, and housework.

**central nervous system (CNS):** The system consisting of the nerves in the brain and spinal cord.

**cerebellum:** A part of the brain that helps regulate posture, balance, and coordination. It is also involved in the processes of emotion, motivation, memory, and thought.

**cerebral cortex:** The gray matter that covers the surface of the cerebral hemispheres, whose functions include sensory processing and motor control along with language, reasoning, decision-making, and judgment.

**chest wall:** The system of structures outside the lungs that move as a part of breathing, including bones (the rib cage) and muscles (diaphragm and abdomen).

**cholesterol:** A waxy substance, produced naturally by the liver and also found in foods, that circulates in the blood and helps maintain tissues and cell membranes. Excess cholesterol in the body can contribute to atherosclerosis and high blood pressure.

**chronic illness:** Long-term or permanent illness (e.g., diabetes, arthritis) which often results in some type of disability and which may require a person to seek help with various activities.

**chronic pain:** Pain that can range from mild to severe, and persists or progresses over a long period of time.

**cognitive-behavioral therapy (CBT):** Cognitive-behavioral therapy helps people focus on how to solve their current problems. The therapist helps the patient learn how to identify distorted or unhelpful thinking patterns, recognize and change inaccurate beliefs, relate to others in more positive ways, and change behaviors accordingly.

**community-based services:** Services and service settings in the community, such as adult day services, home delivered meals, or transportation services. Often referred to as home- and community-based services, they are designed to help older people and people with disabilities stay in their homes as independently as possible.

**computed tomography (CT):** A procedure for taking x-ray images from many different angles and then assembling them into a cross-section of the body. This technique is generally used to visualize bone.

**corticosteroids:** A type of medicine used to reduce inflammation. Corticosteroid drugs mimic a substance produced naturally by the body. In asthma, corticosteroids are often taken through an inhaler for long-term control. They may also be taken orally or given intravenously for a short time if asthma symptoms get out of control.

**deep brain stimulation (DBS):** A neurosurgical treatment utilizing a neurostimulator placed in the brain to deliver electrical signals to specific parts of the brain to help control unwanted movements such as in Parkinson disease or regulate the firing of neurons in the brain to help control the symptoms of disorders such as epilepsy or depression.

**depression:** Lack of interest or pleasure in daily activities, sadness and feelings of worthlessness or excessive guilt that are severe enough to interfere with working, sleeping, studying, eating and enjoying life.

**diabetes:** A disease in which blood glucose (blood sugar) levels are above normal.

**disability insurance:** An insurance plan that pays some of a person's income when he or she is disabled from an illness or injury and cannot work. The two main types of disability insurance are short-term disability and long-term disability. Short-term disability may last for up to 2 years. Long-term disability usually begins after short-term disability ends and may last for a person's lifetime.

**dopamine:** A chemical messenger, deficient in the brains of people with Parkinson disease, that transmits impulses from one nerve cell to another.

**employment network (EN):** An employment network is a qualified public or private organization under contract to coordinate and deliver employment services, vocational rehabilitation services, or other support services to beneficiaries who are participating in the Ticket to Work program.

**exercise:** A type of physical activity that involves planned, structured, and repetitive bodily movement done to maintain or improve one or more components of physical fitness.

**hearing aid:** An electronic device that brings amplified sound to the ear; it usually consists of a microphone, amplifier, and receiver.

**human immunodeficiency virus (HIV):** Human immunodeficiency virus infects and destroys the body's immune cells and causes a disease called "acquired immunodeficiency syndrome" (AIDS).

**hypertension:** Also called "high blood pressure," it is having blood pressure greater than 140 over 90 mmHg (millimeters of mercury). Long-term high blood pressure can damage blood vessels and organs, including the heart, kidneys, eyes, and brain.

**immune system:** A complex network of specialized cells, tissues, and organs that defends the body against attacks by disease-causing microbes.

**learning disability:** A disorder in basic psychological processes involved in understanding or using language, spoken or written, that may manifest itself in an imperfect ability to listen, think, speak, read, write, spell or use mathematical calculations. The term includes conditions such as perceptual disability, brain injury, minimal brain dysfunction, dyslexia, and developmental aphasia.

**long-term care:** Services and supports necessary to meet health or personal care needs over an extended period of time.

**magnetic resonance imaging (MRI):** A noninvasive procedure that uses magnetic fields and radio waves to produce three-dimensional computerized images of areas inside the body.

**Medicaid:** Joint federal and state public assistance program for financing healthcare for low-income people. It pays for healthcare services for those with low incomes or very high medical bills relative to income and assets. It is the largest public payer of long-term care services.

**Medicare:** Federal program that provides hospital and medical expense benefits for people over age 65, or those meeting specific disability standards. Benefits for nursing home and home health services are limited.

**obesity:** Having too much body fat. Obesity is more extreme than being overweight, which means weighing too much.

**occupational therapy (OT):** Services given to help you return to usual activities (like bathing, preparing meals, and housekeeping) after illness either on an inpatient or outpatient basis.

**osteoporosis:** Literally means "porous bone." This disease is characterized by too little bone formation, excessive bone loss, or a combination of both, leading to bone fragility and an increased risk of fractures of the hip, spine, and wrist.

**over-the-counter (OTC):** Diseases, including ulcerative colitis (UC) and Crohn disease, that cause swelling in the intestine and/or digestive tract, which may result in diarrhea, abdominal pain, fever, and weight loss. People with inflammatory bowel disease (IBD) are at an increased risk for osteoporosis.

**physical therapy (PT):** Treatment of injury and disease by mechanical means, like heat, light, exercise, and massage.

**plan of care:** Written doctors orders for home health services and treatments based on the patient's condition. The plan of care is developed by the doctor, the home health team, and the patient. The home health team keeps the doctor up-to-date on the patient's condition and updates the plan of care as needed. It's the doctor, and not the home health team, that authorizes what services are needed and for how long.

**protein:** A molecule made up of amino acids. Proteins are needed for the body to function properly. They are the basis of body structures, such as skin and hair, and of other substances such as enzymes, cytokines, and antibodies.

**psychotherapy:** Treatment of mental illness by talking about problems rather than by using medication. Treatment for first episode psychosis is based on cognitive behavioral therapy principles and emphasizes resilience training, illness and wellness management, and coping skills.

**rehabilitation engineering:** The use of engineering science and principles to develop technological solutions and devices to assist individuals with disabilities, and aid the recovery of physical and cognitive functions lost because of disease or injury.

**rehabilitation services:** Special healthcare services that help a person regain physical, mental, and/or cognitive (thinking and learning) abilities that have been lost or impaired as a result of disease, injury, or treatment. Rehabilitation services help people return to daily life and live in a normal or near-normal way.

**rheumatoid arthritis (RA):** An inflammatory disease that causes pain, swelling, stiffness, and loss of function in the joints. It occurs when the immune system, which normally defends the body from invading organisms, attacks the membrane lining the joints. Studies have found an increased risk of bone loss and fracture in individuals with RA.

**Social Security Disability Insurance (SSDI):** Social Security Disability Insurance provides benefits to disabled or blind persons who are insured by workers' contributions to the Social Security trust fund. These contributions are based on your earnings (or those of your spouse or parents). Your dependents may also be eligible for benefits from your earnings record.

**speech therapy:** This is the study of communication problems. Speech therapists assist with problems involving speech, language, and swallowing. Communication problems can be present at birth or develop after an injury or illness, like a stroke.

**spina bifida:** Spina bifida is a condition that affects the spine and is usually apparent at birth. It is a type of neural tube defect (NTD).

**stroke:** Also known as a "cerebrovascular accident" (CVA); caused by a lack of blood to the brain, resulting in the sudden loss of speech, language, or the ability to move a body part, and, if severe enough, death.

**support groups:** Groups of people who share a common bond (e.g., caregivers) who come together on a regular basis to share problems and experiences. May be sponsored by social service agencies, senior centers, religious organizations, as well as organizations such as the Alzheimer's Association.

**vaccine:** A product made from very small amounts of weak or dead germs that can cause diseases—for example, viruses, bacteria, or toxins. It prepares your body to fight the disease faster and more effectively so you will not get sick. Vaccines are administered through needle injections, by mouth, and by aerosol.

**vertebrae:** The 33 bones that make up the spinal column, characterized by a round opening through which the spinal cord passes and three flat projections to which muscles of the back attach.

**vitamin D:** A nutrient that the body needs to absorb calcium.

**vocational rehabilitation (VR):** The VR program is a public program administered by a State VR agency in each State or U.S. territory to help people with physical or mental disabilities become gainfully employed.

**x-ray:** A type of radiation used in the diagnosis and treatment of cancer and other diseases. In low doses, x-rays are used to diagnose diseases by making pictures of the inside of the body.

**yoga:** An ancient system of practices used to balance the mind and body through exercise, meditation (focusing thoughts), and control of breathing and emotions. Yoga is being studied as a way to relieve stress and treat sleep problems in cancer patients.

# Chapter 60 | Directory of Organizations That Provide Information about Physical Rehabilitation

## GOVERNMENT AGENCIES

### Administration for Community Living (ACL)

330 C St., S.W.
Washington, DC 20201
Toll-Free: 800-677-1116
Phone: 202-401-4634
Website: www.acl.gov

### Agency for Healthcare Research and Quality (AHRQ)

Office of Communications
5600 Fishers Ln.
Seventh Fl.
Rockville, MD 20847
Phone: 301-427-1104
Website: www.ahrq.gov

### Assistant Secretary for Planning and Evaluation (ASPE)

U.S. Department of Health and Human Services (HHS)
200 Independence Ave., S.W.
Rm. 415F
Washington, DC 20201
Phone: 202-690-7858
Website: aspe.hhs.gov

### Center for Parent Information and Resources (CPIR)

c/o Statewide Parent Advocacy Network (SPAN), U.S. Department of Education (ED)
35 Halsey St.
Fourth Fl.
Newark, NJ 07102
Phone: 973-642-8100
Website: www.parentcenterhub.org

Resources in this chapter were compiled from several sources deemed reliable; all contact information was verified and updated in November 2019.

**Centers for Disease Control and Prevention (CDC)**
1600 Clifton Rd.
Atlanta, GA 30329-4027
Toll-Free: 800-CDC-INFO (800-232-4636)
Phone: 404-639-3311
Toll-Free TTY: 888-232-6348
Website: www.cdc.gov
E-mail: cdcinfo@cdc.gov

**Centers for Medicare & Medicaid Services (CMS)**
7500 Security Blvd.
Baltimore, MD 21244
Toll-Free: 877-267-2323
Phone: 410-786-3000
Toll-Free TTY: 866-226-1819
Website: www.cms.gov

***Eunice Kennedy Shriver* National Institute of Child Health and Human Development (NICHD)**
NICHD Information Resource Center (IRC)
P.O. Box 3006
Rockville, MD 20847
Toll-Free: 800-370-2943
Phone: 301-496-5133
Toll-Free Fax: 866-760-5947
Website: www.nichd.nih.gov
E-mail: NICHDInformationResourceCenter@mail.nih.gov

**Federal Trade Commission (FTC)**
600 Pennsylvania Ave., N.W.
Washington, DC 20580
Phone: 202-326-2222
Website: www.ftc.gov

**Health Resources and Services Administration (HRSA)**
Information Center
5600 Fishers Ln.
P.O. Box 2910
Rockville, MD 20857
Toll-Free: 888-275-4772
Toll-Free TTY: 877-489-4772
Fax: 703-821-2098
Website: www.hrsa.gov
E-mail: ask@hrsa.gov

**National Cancer Institute (NCI)**
9609 Medical Center Dr.
BG 9609, MSC 9760
Bethesda, MD 20892-9760
Toll-Free: 800-4-CANCER (800-422-6237)
Website: www.cancer.gov
E-mail: NCIinfo@nih.gov

**National Center for Complementary and Integrative Health (NCCIH)**
Clearinghouse
9000 Rockville Pike
Bethesda, MD 20892
Toll-Free: 888-644-6226
Toll-Free TTY: 866-464-3615
Website: nccih.nih.gov
E-mail: info@nccih.nih.gov

**National Council on Disability (NCD)**
1331 F St., N.W., Ste. 850
Washington, DC 20004
Phone: 202-272-2004
Fax: 202-272-2022
Website: www.ncd.gov
E-mail: ncd@ncd.gov

### National Heart, Lung, and Blood Institute (NHLBI)

31 Center Dr.
Bldg. 31
Bethesda, MD 20892
Website: www.nhlbi.nih.gov

### National Institute of Arthritis and Musculoskeletal and Skin Diseases (NIAMS)

Information Clearinghouse, National Institutes of Health (NIH)
One AMS Cir.
Bethesda, MD 20892-3675
Toll-Free: 877-22-NIAMS (877-226-4267)
Phone: 301-495-4484
TTY: 301-565-2966
Fax: 301-718-6366
Website: www.niams.nih.gov
E-mail: NIAMSinfo@mail.nih.gov

### National Institute of Diabetes and Digestive and Kidney Diseases (NIDDK)

Health Information Center
Toll-Free: 800-860-8747
Toll-Free TTY: 866-569-1162
Website: www.niddk.nih.gov
E-mail: healthinfo@niddk.nih.gov

### National Institute of Neurological Disorders and Stroke (NINDS)

NIH Neurological Institute
P.O. Box 5801
Bethesda, MD 20824
Toll-Free: 800-352-9424
Website: www.ninds.nih.gov

### National Institute of Standards and Technology (NIST)

U.S. Department of Commerce (DOC)
100 Bureau Dr.
Gaithersburg, MD 20899
Phone: 301-975-2000
Website: www.nist.gov

### National Institute on Aging (NIA)

31 Center Dr., MSC 2292
Bldg. 31, Rm. 5C27
Bethesda, MD 20892
Toll-Free: 800-222-2225
Toll-Free TTY: 800-222-4225
Website: www.nia.nih.gov
E-mail: niaic@nia.nih.gov

### National Institute on Deafness and Other Communication Disorders (NIDCD)

National Institutes of Health (NIH)
31 Center Dr., MSC 2320
Bethesda, MD 20892-2320
Phone: 301-827-8183
Website: www.nidcd.nih.gov
E-mail: nidcdinfo@nidcd.nih.gov

### National Institutes of Health (NIH)

9000 Rockville Pike
Bethesda, MD 20892
Phone: 301-496-4000
Website: www.nih.gov

### NIH Osteoporosis and Related Bone Diseases—National Resource Center (NIH ORBD—NRC)

Toll-Free: 800-624-BONE (800-624-2663)
Phone: 202-223-0344
Fax: 202-293-2356
Website: www.bones.nih.gov
E-mail: NIHBoneInfo@mail.nih.gov

**Occupational Safety and Health Administration (OSHA)**
U.S. Department of Labor (DOL)
200 Constitution Ave. N.W.
Rm. N3626
Washington, DC 20210
Toll-Free: 800-321-OSHA
(800-321-6742)
Website: www.osha.gov

**Office of Disability Employment Policy (ODEP)**
U.S. Department of Labor (DOL)
200 Constitution Ave., N.W.
Washington, DC 20210
Toll-Free: 866-ODEP-DOL
(866-633-7365)
Website: www.dol.gov/odep
E-mail: odep@dol.gov

**Office of Disease Prevention and Health Promotion (ODPHP)**
Office of the Assistant Secretary for Health (OASH), Office of the Secretary
1101 Wootton Pkwy
Ste. LL100
Rockville, MD 20852
Fax: 240-453-8281
Website: health.gov
E-mail: odphpinfo@hhs.gov

**Office of Special Education and Rehabilitative Services (OSERS)**
U.S. Department of Education (ED)
400 Maryland Ave., S.W.
Washington, DC 20202-7100
Toll-Free: 800-872-5327
Phone: 202-245-7468
Website: www2.ed.gov/about/offices/list/osers/contacts.html

**Office on Women's Health (OWH)**
U.S. Department of Health and Human Services (HHS)
200 Independence Ave., S.W.
Rm. 712E
Washington, DC 20201
Toll-Free: 800-994-9662
Phone: 202-690-7650
Fax: 202-205-2631
Website: www.womenshealth.gov

**U.S. AbilityOne Commission**
1401 S., Clark St.
Ste. 715
Arlington, VA 22202-3259
Toll-Free: 800-999-5963
Phone: 703-603-7740
Website: www.abilityone.gov
E-mail: info@abilityone.gov

**U.S. Access Board**
1331 F St., N.W.
Ste. 1000
Washington, DC 20004-1111
Toll-Free: 800-872-2253
Phone: 202-272-0080
TTY: 202-272-0082
Toll-Free TTY: 800-993-2822
Fax: 202-272-0081
Website: www.access-board.gov
E-mail: info@access-board.gov

**U.S. Bureau of Labor Statistics (BLS)**
2 Massachusetts Ave., N.E.
Postal Square Bldg.
Washington, DC 20212-0001
Phone: 202-691-5200
Toll-Free TDD: 800-877-8339
Website: www.bls.gov

**U.S. Department of Health and Human Services (HHS)**
200 Independence Ave., S.W.
Washington, DC 20201
Toll-Free: 877-696-6775
Website: www.hhs.gov

**U.S. Department of Transportation (DOT)**
1200 New Jersey Ave., S.E.
Washington, DC 20590
Toll-Free: 855-368-4200
Phone: 202-366-4000
Website: www.transportation.gov

**U.S. Department of Veterans Affairs (VA)**
Toll-Free: 844-698-2311
Website: www.va.gov

**U.S. Food and Drug Administration (FDA)**
10903 New Hampshire Ave.
Silver Spring, MD 20993-0002
Toll-Free: 888-INFO-FDA
(888-463-6332)
Website: www.fda.gov

**U.S. National Library of Medicine (NLM)**
8600 Rockville Pike
Bethesda, MD 20894
Toll-Free: 888-FIND-NLM
(888-346-3656)
Phone: 301-594-5983
Website: www.nlm.nih.gov
E-mail: custserv@nlm.nih.gov

**U.S. Social Security Administration (SSA)**
Office of Earnings & International Operations (OEIO)
P.O. Box 17769
Baltimore, MD 21235-7769
Toll-Free: 800-772-1213
Toll-Free TTY: 800-325-0778
Website: www.ssa.gov

## PRIVATE AGENCIES

**Academy of Neurologic Physical Therapy (ANPT)**
5841 Cedar Lake Rd., S.
Ste. 204
Minneapolis, MN 55416
Phone: 952-646-2038
Website: www.neuropt.org
E-mail: info@neuropt.org

**American Academy of Neurology (AAN)**
201 Chicago Ave.
Minneapolis, MN 55415
Toll-Free: 800-879-1960
Fax: 612-454-2746
Website: www.aan.com
E-mail: memberservices@aan.com

**American Academy of Ophthalmology (AAO)**
P.O. Box 7424
San Francisco, CA 94120-7424
Phone: 415-561-8500
Fax: 415-561-8533
Website: www.aao.org

**American Academy of Physical Medicine and Rehabilitation (AAPM&R)**
9700 W. Bryn Mawr Ave.
Ste. 200
Rosemont, IL 60018
Toll-Free: 877-227-6799
Phone: 847-737-6000
Website: www.aapmr.org
E-mail: info@aapmr.org

**American Association of Naturopathic Physicians (AANP)**
300 New Jersey Ave., N.W.
Ste. 900
Washington, DC 20001
Phone: 202-237-8150
Fax: 541-500-2256
Website: www.naturopathic.org

**American Association of Neurological Surgeons (AANS)**
5550 Meadowbrook Dr.
Rolling Meadows, IL 60008-3852
Toll-Free: 888-566-AANS (888-556-2267)
Phone: 847-378-0500
Fax: 847-378-0600
Website: www.aans.org
E-mail: info@aans.org

**American Counseling Association (ACA)**
6101 Stevenson Ave.
Ste. 600
Alexandria, VA 22304
Toll-Free: 800-347-6647
Phone: 703-823-9800
Fax: 703-823-0252
Toll-Free Fax: 800-473-2329
Website: www.counseling.org

**American Neurological Association (ANA)**
1120 Rt. 73
Ste. 200
Mt. Laurel, NJ 08054
Phone: 856-638-0423
Website: myana.org
E-mail: info@myana.org

**The American Occupational Therapy Association Inc. (AOTA)**
4720 Montgomery Ln.
Ste. 200
Bethesda, MD 20814
Toll-Free: 800-729-2682
Phone: 301-652-6611
Website: www.aota.org

**American Optometric Association (AOA)**
243 N. Lindbergh Blvd.
First fl.
St. Louis, MO 63141
Toll-Free: 800-365-2219
Website: www.aoa.org

**American Physical Therapy Association (APTA)**
1111 N. Fairfax St.
Alexandria, VA 22314-1488
Toll-Free: 800-999-APTA
(800-999-2782)
Phone: 703-684-APTA
(703-684-2782)
Fax: 703-684-7343
Website: www.apta.org

**American Speech-Language-Hearing Association (ASHA)**
2200 Research Blvd.
Rockville, MD 20850-3289
Toll-Free: 800-638-8255
Phone: 301-296-5700
Fax: 301-296-8580
Website: www.asha.org
E-mail: actioncenter@asha.org

**Arthritis Foundation® (AF)**
National Office
1355 Peachtree St. N.E.
Ste. 600
Atlanta, GA 30309
Toll-Free: 844-571-4357
Phone: 404-872-7100
Toll-Free TTY: 800-283-7800
Website: www.arthritis.org

**Bastyr Center for Natural Health (BCNH)**
3670 Stone Way N.
Seattle, WA 98103
Phone: 206-834-4100
Fax: 206-834-4131
Website: bastyrcenter.org

**Institute for Natural Medicine (INM)**
4500 Ninth Ave., N.E.
Ste. 300
Seattle, WA 98105
Phone: 206-486-3380
Website: naturemed.org

**International Association of Functional Neurology and Rehabilitation (IAFNR)**
3317 S., Higley Rd.
Ste. 114-288
Gilbert, AZ 85297
Phone: 480-926-1115
Website: iafnr.org
E-mail: info@iafnr.org

**The National Rehabilitation Association (NRA)**
P.O. Box 150235
Alexandria, VA 22315
Toll-Free: 888-258-4295
Phone: 703-836-0850
Website: www.nationalrehab.org
E-mail: Info@Nationalrehab.Org

**Neuro-Developmental Treatment Association (NDTA™)**
1540 S. Coast Hwy
Ste. 204
Laguna Beach, CA 92651
Toll-Free: 800-869-9295
Fax: 949-376-3456
Website: www.ndta.org

# INDEX

# INDEX

Page numbers followed by 'n' indicate a footnote. Page numbers in *italics* indicate a table or illustration.

## A

# Index

## B

# Index

# Index

## D

# Index



## E

## G



## H

## I

## M

## N

## Index

## O

# Index

## Q

## R

## S

## T

## U

## V

## W